Explanations of

Channels and Points

Vol. 2

Explanations of Channels and Points

經

穴

解

Jīng Xué Jiě
by Yuè Hánzhēn 岳含珍

Translated by Michael Brown
Edited by Allen Tsaur

purple cloud
press

Library of Congress Control Number: 2021910164

ISBN: 9798502881616

Front cover image and interior illustrations from the Lèijīng Túyì 類經圖翼 (the Illustrated Wings of the Classified Canon) and the Yīzōng Jīnjiàn 醫宗金鑒 (the Golden Mirror of Medical Ancestry)

Cover Design: Anne-Maree Taranto
(contact@rhapsodica.com)

Layout Design: Tanya Steklova-Lawson
(personalevolution@hotmail.co.uk)

Published by Purple Cloud Press
purplecouldinstitute.com

Purple Cloud Vision

Purple Cloud Press was founded on the principle that only by merging theoretical knowledge and practical experience is one able to gain true understanding and grasp the nuances of pertinent writings. Therefore, all publications by Purple Cloud Press are underpinned by this principle of scholar-physician and scholar-practitioner into the following threefold mission;

> to publish the works of the founders of the Purple Cloud Institute and other author's finished works in the field of Eastern medicine, Asian religions and martial arts,
>
> to translate original ancient Asian texts into the English language,
>
> to commission writings about masters' and teachers' lineage traditions.

Purple Cloud Press incentivizes authors and translators by guaranteeing them a large percentage of the royalties in order to encourage continued translation projects as well as by providing a platform to reach the largest possible readership. Purple Cloud Press strongly believes that this will help make accessible the profundity of treasures previously hidden from the English-speaking world.

purple cloud
press

Testimonials

Writing in the Latter years of the Ming Dynasty and the first few decades of the Qing Dynasty, Yue Hanzhen wrote a detailed analysis of the channels and their acupuncture points. Explanations of Channels and Points (*Jing Xue Jie*) drew heavily from previous historical works, notably the Classic of the Bright Hall (*Ming Tang Jing*) which was originally a third famous acupuncture text alongside the Simple Questions (*Su Wen*) and the Spiritual Pivot (*Ling Shu*). Although lost in its original form the Classic of the Bright Hall has been cited many times, from the passages quoted in the Systematic Classic of Acupuncture & Moxibustion (*Zhen Jiu Jia Yi Jing*) in around 282 AD, to Volumes 6 and 7 of the Great Compendium of Acupuncture - Moxibustion (*Zhen Jiu Da Cheng*) in 1601. Throughout the text, Yue frequently cites *Su Wen, Ling Shu, Zhen Jiu Da Cheng* and *Tong Ren [Shu Xue Zhen Jiu Tu Jing]* ([Illustrated Classic of the Acupuncture Points on the] Bronze Man) as well as many other sources.

However, Yue Hanzhen has added something which was fairly unique at the time – detailed explanations of the rationale for why certain points treated certain indications. The literature abounds with point indications in prose, as well as many famous odes and songs, but rarely is any explanation offered. For example, the use of KI 1 to treat dry tongue and swollen pharynx is explained thus: *Explanation: dry tongue and swollen pharynx is fire qì ascending, it is appropriate to drain this point.*

There are a few minor textual inconsistencies, such as different distances given for the Kidney channel from the midline for some points, and some citations of needle retention times not matching the original text quoted, however these are helpfully highlighted in the translator's footnotes. Incidentally, the retention times which are mentioned are very short – between 3 and 10 respirations, which is similar to what is found in the Systematic Classic of Acupuncture & Moxibustion.

In this second volume of this very important work, Michael Brown and Allen Tsaur have brought us another piece of the puzzle to understanding channels and points. The importance of point indications has, in some quarters, been undervalued in recent years. The creation of systematised "point functions" in the 1950s has led some to believe that point functions alone, without a thorough study of point indications, is a sufficient basis for point selection. However, the bulk of the last two millenia of our historical acupuncture literature is all about indications. Very few other branches of medicine in the world today have anything approaching this treasure trove of collected clinical expertise, each author drawing from a detailed study of previous works, then adding their own commentary and insights based on their own personal clinical experiences. This is how traditional medicines continue to grow and thrive without losing connection to their roots.

John McDonald, PhD.,

Author of *Acupuncture Point Dynamics*

The *Jīngxué Jiě* is an inspiration for those seeking to cultivate a clinical practice rooted in the syncretic philosophy and natural science of the *Nèijīng*, wherein the body is taken as the basic unit of orderly space and physiology a construct of water flowing over a landscape. Yuè Hánzhēn pulls extensively from the *Sùwèn* and *Língshū*, particularly the unified vessel theory of Língshū Chapter 10, and integrates commentary on this chapter by Mǎ Shì from the *Huángdì Nèijīng Língshū Zhùzhèng Fāwèi* with the phase dynamics of *Nánjīng* 49 and 50 to narrate a journey through the human interior comparable to that of Yu the Great traversing the mountains and waterways to tame the floods and order the legendary Chinese state of Xia.

Explanations of Channels and Points is especially useful in that it equips a numbered point system familiar in contemporary practice. More importantly Yuè Hánzhēn demystifies point names and explains their functions in terms of the interplay between physiological structure and flow at that location as well as their sequential arrangement and coordinated action as part of the larger totality. I further appreciate included details on the complimentary use of herbal and needle therapies as well as his tactful commentary on vessel theory and pathomechanics interfused throughout the text.

Next to the *Língshū* I regard Michael Brown's annotated translation of the *Jīngxué Jiě* among my most valued resources on needle therapy. No other clinical reference in the English language models the thought and clinical strategy of the *Nèijīng* as does the work of the distinguished military general, physician, and ardent student of Qí Bó and the Yellow Emperor, Yuè Hánzhēn.

Justin Penoyer, L.Ac. (Doctor of Acupuncture and Chinese Medicine),

Author of *Roots of Accordance: Political, Ecological, and*

Medical Holism in the Huangdi Neijing, forthcoming Spring 2022

Dedication

To my mother.

Sending you my love.

醫，仁術也。

Medicine is a benevolent skill.

Yīmén Fǎlù 醫門法律 (*Axioms of Medicine,* 1658 CE)

Contents

Foreword

By Henry McCann

Years ago when I was in first in school studying East Asian medicine I remember asking one of my Japanese acupuncture teachers about various protocols listed in one of our texts, which were laid out according to western biomedical diagnoses. My questions were simple: "Where did this come from? How were these points selected, and why did the author list them?" The answer I got was also simple – the points were "just empirical."

Even though I had very little clinical experience back then, that answer felt completely unsatisfactory and incomplete to me. How could it be implied that for any given condition, the physician simply experimented with all points on the body until they found the best treatment options? While I understand the role and importance of experience, it could not account for the sum total of what we do clinically. At its foundation, Chinese medicine is based on a deep understanding of Universal Principle (理) and its application to the body. If this were not the case then our classical foundational texts wouldn't spend so much time on this basic fact! The Su Wen would not give us such forceful statements as 'Yin and Yang are the Dao of Heaven and Earth.'

Today what we often see with acupuncture point rationale is reductionist in two ways. First, is that everything is reduced to the empirical, as that one instructor had told me. Second, we see acupuncture reduced to a simplistic reproduction of herbal medicine treatment principles applied with needles rather than medicinals. In the latter option, acupuncture points are described to have functions much like herbs do, and this approach, while seemingly good for the integration of medicines and needles, gives us an all too facile and simple an understanding of what acupuncture points are, how they work, and when they should be applied. Clearly this cannot be the sum total of the Dao of Acupuncture as practiced by those brilliant physicians of years past.

In my own practice I have tried to not only apply needles but also to understand the deeper mechanism behind that application. In my teaching I've also worked to convey this idea. An understanding of Yin-Yang, the dynamic interaction of the Five

Phases, the Three Burners, and how they are manifest on the body, in channels, in point categories, etc... allows an acupuncturist to effectively choose and combine needles in clinical practice. Thus, we can move beyond simple memorization of point functions, protocols and the limitations this imposes on our use of needles.

All of this is precisely why Explanations of the Channels and Points by Yue Hanzhen is my kind of book, and, more importantly, the kind of book that contemporary acupuncturists need. It thoroughly discounts what I was told so many years ago - that points are chosen simply through empiricism - as totally false and representing a shallow understanding of medicine. Throughout the Explanations Yue describes the mechanisms behind why a point works, and he does this through the lens of an acupuncturist, not an herbalist trying to apply needles using an herbal paradigm. In doing so, the reader is lead to an understanding of the deeper workings of points, channels, and treatment methods. Yue also sources his statements from earlier and more authoritative works such as the Yellow Emperor's Inner Classic (Huang Di Nei Jing) and the Great Compendium (Zhen Jiu Da Cheng), demonstrating his profound understanding of medical literature. His meticulous explanation of point indications and the meaning of point names is eye opening, even for those of us with decades of clinical experience.

One of the things that is particularly exciting about this second volume of Explanations is the inclusion of a section that discusses the Eight Extraordinary Vessels (奇經八脈). With a few exceptions, what I have seen in modern English language acupuncture texts is the same very basic retelling of Extraordinary Vessels diagnosis and point protocols, based mostly on the use of the eight confluent points (交會穴). And what we teach our students is this very basic approach.

The Eight Extraordinary Vessels is a topic that is important and often misunderstood. To make up for a real depth of understanding, many acupuncturists fill in the gap with material that would never have been found in classical or other pre-modern literature, including instead quite a bit of Orientalist fantasy. In Explanations Yue describes each of the vessels, diagnosis (including pulse) and clinical applications. Yue also goes through and actually analyzes each of the points on these Vessels, tying his analysis into classical literature such as the Neijing, and the clinical recommendations of other important texts and physicians. Reading through this section has already caused me to think again about the Extraordinary Vessels in a more thoughtful and more clinically relevant manner.

We all owe Michael Brown and Allen Tsaur a debt of gratitude for their translation and edit of this text. I am sure Yue Hanzhen would be pleased that his work continues to spread the Dao of Acupuncture to more clinicians. My sincere hope is that this work will help eliminate suffering and the cause of suffering for all who read it and use its wisdom to help people.

Dr. Henry McCann 馬爾博

Written during Qing Ming 清明 (Clear and Bright)

Xin Chou (辛丑) Year – 2021

Madison, New Jersey

Translator's Preface

By Michael Brown

Hello, thank you for taking the time to read this, and support our work. This has not been an easy road to complete this work, it has taken longer than I would have liked, but this is it, it is finally finished! When I finished my Chinese medicine studies in 2009, I never dreamed that I would have complete a translation of a book, yet alone a book of this this size. I feel incredibly lucky that I had the opportunity to work on this text with Allen and bright it to a new audience, and from the feedback we have received on Volume 1 I hope that it will also provide you with a particular and nuanced view of the medicine that isn't commonly read nor taught.

Every time we work and complete a book, there are always things we learn, or want to improve. So in Volume 2 there are some minor changes in terminology in this book which we detailed in the introduction. I hope you can forgive us for implementing these changes after Volume 1 as there were too important to wait, however, we will certainly update Volume 1 in the future to reflect the changes we have adopted for Volume 2.

Before I finished Volume 1, COVID-19 had not struck and the world was as we had always known. Since that time, many things have changed, especially how we live our lives. We have become quite isolated from each other, and it was always my hope to meet my Chinese medicine friends and colleagues from around the world sooner, but that has been delayed. Wherever you are, please make sure you are taking the time to check on your friends and family, to see that they are okay, and you also take time to reflect upon yourself and your health, both mental and physical. It is important that we support each other and help those in need. To quote one of my favourite lyrics from the artist Pain of Salvation, do not support "those who help make solidarity ideologically untrendy."

While I have this platform, I will continue to discuss issues which I see as crucial to Chinese medicine. Primarily, the lack of emphasis of studying on Chinese medical texts as opposed to Randomised Clinical Trails (RCTs). We must remember that Chinese medicine had stood on the back of the Neijing (Suwen and Lingshu), Shanghan Zabing Lun, Maijing and Zhenjiu Jiayi Jing. The knowledge in these texts can never substituted or replaced by reading RCTs. I beleive that Chinese medicine is a source-based medicine, in which we base our theories on our earliest sources, such as those texts mentioned above, and we are guided by later works and clinical experience of famous doctors of the last 2,000 years. To believe that one will gain same level of information from as RCT compared to the foundational texts is akin to drinking sea water when thirsty. More and more excellent works in Chinese medicine are becoming readily available, and I honestly foresee a better future for Chinese medicine if we are able to educate ourselves with these texts, rather than relying on RCTs to dictate our clinical decision making. However, we must also live up to the high standards that our medical ancestors bestowed upon us, we must study daily, review our formulae and acupuncture points, and discuss and critique difficult cases with our friends and colleagues, challenge ourselves amongst our peers so that we can elevate ourselves. Then, I believe that our medical ancestors will rest easy (except for Xú Dàchūn 徐大椿, that guy had no chill).

I will leave with my favourite passage from Mengzi 孟子, which I feel is even more true today than when it was written.[1]

孟子曰：「仁，人心也；義，人路也。

舍其路而弗由，放其心而不知求，哀哉！

人有雞犬放，則知求之；有放心，而不知求。

學問之道無他，求其放心而已矣。」

Mèngzǐ says, "benevolence, it is the heart-mind of humanity; righteousness, it is the path of humanity.

For those who have become lost on this path and failed to follow it, abandoned their heart-mind and are unaware how to locate it, this is truly lamentable!

When people's dogs or chickens are lost, they would know to search for them; yet when they lose their heart-mind, they do not know to how to find it.

In this great dào of learning, there is nothing else but to seek one's lost heart-mind."

---

[1] With assistance from Allen.

Acknowledgements

Once again, as I stated in the first book, I owe a thousand (and more) thanks to Allen. This book, in its current readable form, simply would not and could not be without his guidance at all times during the process. He helped me numerous times with extremely difficult parts that I would simply be incapable of doing on my own. This work is as much his as it is mine. I feel incredibly lucky to work with him, and bring our collaborative effort to the reader.

To Johan, I am not sure if people will ever know how much their encouragement and company pushed me to finish what seemed like an impossible task that I started all these years ago. Johan works behind the scenes, he's always there when you need him with kind words and advice.

To Will, thank for your diligence in checking this work. It took longer than we anticipated, but the notes that you left us were worth the wait. The feedback once again validates that a scholar, physician or translator needs to be in constant dialogue with those at the top of their field to facilitate nuanced discussion of difficult topics. You improved the work more than you will realise.

To Bhumi (Oana Budica), thank you for your helping in reading the manuscript. Like Will, you found many of our mistakes (those that remain, blame me) that we missed after having read the work many times. Having your eyes scour the book for errors was much needed, and hopefully, I haven't scared you off from working with us in the future.

To Henry, thank you for your amazing foreword. It is a privilege to have someone such as yourself help provide a platform for those preceding you. I hope one day, I can do the same for others.

To John, thank you not only for your endorsement but also for the communication we've had over the years, and during my formative years at school. Your scholarship and questioning of questionable material had a deep influence on me that I am forever grateful.

To Justin, thank you for the feedback you gave after the first book, and the endorsement for the second book. I hope the second volume will continue to give you valuable clinical reasoning for your patients.

To my wife, parents, grandparents and teachers. I would not be here without you. One last thanks to you for all you have done, and continue to do.

Editor's Preface

By Allen Tsaur

In March 2019, on a transpacific flight to Japan, within the confined space of my economy seat abroad a Boeing 787 Dreamliner, I read from the tilted screen of my Chromebook a preliminary translation draft, which was entitled *Explanations of Channels and Points*.

As I read through it, I scolded myself for my folly in having agreed to review this draft, a task that I found to be a delicate balancing act – I could neglect most issues and leave very little comments to appease the author, but to the detriment of the profession, it would not improve the accuracy or quality of the translation; alternatively, I could leave comments and edits on all the issues I noticed to improve the translation as much as possible, but it would not only diminish the author's input but also would certainly offend the author. As I knew very little about its author at the time, an internet acquaintance named Michael Brown whom I had never met in person, I was at a loss on how I should approach.

Perhaps, bothered by the discomfort of working in such a clustered space, along with countless silent curses while struggling with my unwieldy touchpad, I became increasingly irritated after leaving the first few courteous comments; in no time, all came loose and unfiltered. Inconsiderably, I simply wrote out whatever came to mind to improve the translation, with little to no regard for how Michael would receive it. Little did I know that my cavalier opinions that day would later drag me into a closer collaboration with Michael.

To this day, I still have no clue how Michael has managed to receive all my blunt comments and edits. Though I do try to incorporate humour and positive feedback as much and as often as I can, an edited document inevitably results in hundreds of corrections as well as numerous differences in interpretation, which can become heavy, overwhelming, or even personal. Being an author myself, I find it extremely challenging to detach my personal attachment to my work and often become defensive whenever I receive any feedback; however, Michael has such a genuine willingness to receive critiques and, perhaps, an obsession to better his translation, that he has not only been receptive to my suggestions but he also stood his ground whenever I made any mistakes; thus, we have been able to collaborate and learn from each other in this never-ending quest of faithfully reconstructing the voice of Yuè Hánzhēn. To be frank, I simply find myself lucky to be abroad this vessel, which is steered by its genial captain, Michael, and bounded for an arduous but rewarding journey.

From 2019 to 2021, the world has changed, so have we. As I now look over the translation that we published two years ago, I am filled with both astonishment and despair: I am greatly impressed that we were able to carry the work through with consistency and accuracy in translation that I still find acceptable; however, I also see vast room for improvement, from small nuances of terminology to grammar and readability. After gruesome lessons learned from Zhang Jingyue's work last year, Michael and I have grown much as translators, and hence my despair, that is, how should we approach this translation? Should we maintain the style we established in the first volume of this work, for the sake of consistency? Or should we bring everything up to the standard we now hold ourselves, for the sake of readability? This is an issue that has haunted me throughout the editing process of this translation. And, like before, with my usual indecision, while I have been mostly able to enforce consistency in terminology, I once again stumbled on grammar and style; irresponsibly, I kept most of Michael's translation style intact and applied sporadic changes for the sake of readability. The result is, once again, an inconsistent rendering[2] that certainly falls short of the gold standard of literal translation; for that, I apologize, but hopefully you will still find this work worthwhile even with this shortcoming.

As this years-long journey came to an end, I must once again express my deepest gratitude to Michael Brown and Johan Hausen for trusting my inputs and making me a part of this team in this worthy endeavour. My most indebted gratitude to my family, who have sacrificed much to make me who I am today and tolerated with every bit of my irrational impulses in life. Also, my most profound thanks to Bhikkhu Prof. Dhammadipa Sak, who has kept me sane and inspired to write for years. And thank you, dear reader, for your generous support to keep the textual tradition of Chinese medicine alive.

---

[2] Regarding the eternal debate on translation style and consistency, lately, I have found myself infinitely fascinated by the approach of the late Prof. Richard Gombrich from University of Oxford, a prominent scholar of Sanskrit, Pali, and Buddhism, whose mastery of the languages and understanding of the subject matters allowed him to reject the inflexibility of literal consistency and adopt instead a contextual-based translation with deliberate inconsistency.

Translation Style Changes from Vol. 1

In Volume 2 of *Explanations of Channels and Points* we have made some minor changes to the terminology we used. We have adopted more of the Wiseman TCM terminology, whereas in Volume 1 we used some alternate terms.

The biggest changes the reader will notice is three terms, which are

- *tonify* is now *supplement*
- *deficiency* is now *vacuity*
- *excess* is now *repletion*

There may be other minor changes, but we thought it important to highlight these three as they are the most common, and sometimes confusing for new readers of Wiseman TCM Terminology. We apologise for these changes, but felt they were necessary to enact.

The Foot Shàoyīn
Kidney Channel & Points

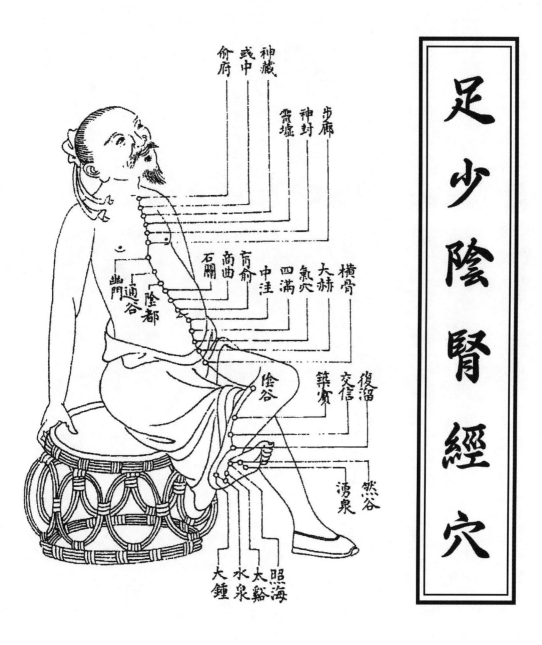

足少陰腎經穴

The Foot Shàoyīn Kidney Channel & Points
足少陰腎經

Overview of the Foot Shàoyīn Kidney Channel
足少陰腎經總論

思蓮子曰：腎經爲足少陰，氣多而血少，與膀胱爲表裏。

Master Sīlián says, the kidney channel is the foot shàoyīn, its qì is copious and blood is scant, it is an exterior-interior [pair] with the bladder.

其經起於足小指之下，斜趨足心之湧泉穴，轉出內踝前起大骨之下然谷穴，下循內踝後之太谿穴，別入足跟中之大鍾，又前行內踝下之照海，又斜行太谿下之水泉，乃折自大鍾之外，上循內踝，上行足厥陰、足太陰兩經之後，經本經復溜、交信二穴，過脾經之三陰交，上足之腨內，循築賓，出膕之內廉，抵陰谷，

This channel commences at the bottom of the little toe and converges obliquely towards Yǒng Quán (KI-1) at the centre of the foot. It turns and emerges at Rán Gǔ (KI-2) below the large bone that protrudes in front of the inner ankle [bone].

It descends to follow Tài Xī (KI-3) behind the inner ankle [bone] and Dà Zhōng[3] (KI-4) that diverges to enter the heel. It continues to travel to the front to Zhào Hǎi (KI-6) below the inner ankle [bone]. It continues to travel obliquely to Shuǐ Quán (KI-5) that is below Tài Xī (KI-3); thereupon, it returns to the outside of Dà Zhōng (KI-4), ascends following the inner ankle [bone], ascending behind the two channels of the foot juéyīn and foot tàiyīn, and passes through the two points of this channel, Fù Liū (KI-7) and Jiāo Xìn (KI-8). It traverses Sān Yīn Jiāo (SP-6) of the spleen channel, ascends the inside of the calf, following it to Zhú Bīn (KI-9). It emerges at the inner ridge at the back of the knee to arrive at Yīn Gǔ (KI-10).

上股內後廉，貫脊，會足太陽於督之長强，還出於前，上小腹，循本經之橫骨、大赫、氣穴、四滿、中注凡五穴，皆挾中行一寸而上行，同衝脈並上於腹，至臍

---

[3] This point is usually written as "Dà Zhōng 大鍾" instead of "Dà Zhōng 大鍾," the latter of which is consistently used throughout this work.

旁肓腧之所，臍之左右，僅挾臍五分，屬內腎，下臍過任脈之關元、中極，而絡膀胱焉；

It ascends the rear ridge of the inner thigh, pierces the spine, and meets with the tàiyáng [channel] at Cháng Qiáng (DU-1) of the dū [channel]. It returns to emerge at the front, ascends the lower abdomen, follows five points of this channel, Héng Gǔ (KI-11), Dà Hè (KI-12), Qì Xué (KI-13), Sì Mǎn (KI-14), and Zhōng Zhù (KI-15), ascending while clasping all of them at 1 cùn from the midline; together with the chōng vessel, it ascends the abdomen to arrive at the place of Huāng Shù (KI-16) beside the umbilicus, clasping the umbilicus at only 5 fēn to the left and right sides of the umbilicus; thereupon, it adjoins inwards to the kidneys, descends the umbilicus to traverse Guān Yuán (REN-4) and Zhōng Jí (REN-3) of the rèn [channel], and continues to network with the bladder.

其直行者，從肓腧屬腎處，復同衝脈挾中行僅五分而上行，循本經之商曲、石關、陰都、通谷貫肝，上循幽門上膈，歷步廊，挾中行各二寸，而上行入肺中，循神封、靈墟、神藏、或中、腧府，而上循喉嚨，並人迎，挾舌本而終；

For the vertical pathway, from Huāng Shù (KI-16), it adjoins to the place of the kidneys; it then returns to join together with the Chōng vessel, clasps the midline at only 5 fēn while ascending, follows Shāng Qū (KI-17), Shí Guān (KI-18), Yīn Dū (KI-19), and Tōng Gǔ (KI-20) of this channel, and pierces the liver. It ascends to follow Yōu Mén (KI-21) and further ascend the diaphragm, where it passes through Bù Láng (KI-22) while clasping the midline at 2 cùn on each side. It continues to ascend and enter into the lung, following Shén Fēng (KI-23), Líng Xū (KI-24), Shén Cáng (KI-25), Yù Zhōng (KI-26), and Shù Fǔ (KI-27). It continues to ascend following the throat, [traverses] besides Rén Yíng (ST-9), clasps at the root of the tongue, and terminates there.

其支者，自神藏別出繞心，注胸之膻中，以交於手厥陰心包絡經也。

From Shén Cáng (KI-25), a branch diverges to encircle the heart, pours into Dàn Zhōng (REN-17),[4] [where] it intersects with the hand juéyīn pericardiac network channel.

衝脈之上行者，既自橫骨穴，同足少陰經出於頏顙，滲諸陽，灌諸經，而又有一歧下行，自橫骨注於少陰之大絡大鍾穴，起於腎下，出於氣街，循陰股內廉，斜入委中，伏行骭骨內廉，並少陰之經入足下；

From Héng Gǔ (KI-11), the ascending pathway of the chōng vessel emerges at the nasopharynx together with the foot shàoyīn channel, and permeates all the yáng and irrigates all the channels.

---

[4] Dàn Zhōng is also the name of the anatomical place, the chest centre.

In addition, there is one forking pathway [of the chōng vessel] that descends; from Héng Gǔ (KI-11), it pours into the great network-vessel of shàoyīn [channel], [which connects to] the point Dà Zhōng (KI-4).[5] [The great network-vessel] commences from below the kidneys, emerges at Qì Jiē (ST-30),[6] follows the inside ridge of the yīn of the thigh, travels obliquely to enter Wěi Zhōng (BL-40), becomes concealed as it travels along the inner ridge of the shin bone, and joins with the shàoyīn channel to enter the bottom of the foot .

其支者，並於少陰，滲三陰，斜入踝，伏行出屬跗屬，下循跗上，入大指之間，滲諸絡而溫足脛肌肉，故其脈常動，別絡結則跗上不動，不動則厥，厥則寒矣。

A branch joins with the shàoyīn [channel] to permeate into the three yīn. It obliquely enters the ankle [bone], becomes concealed as it travels [along the ankle bone] and emerges to adjoin to the instep, descends following the surface of the instep to enter the space between the big toe [and second toe], where it permeates into all the network-vessels in order to warm the muscles and flesh of the feet and lower leg; thus, its vessel there is constantly pulsating. When the divergent network-vessel is bound, the instep [vessel] will cease to pulsate; when [the vessel] fails to pulsate, there will be reversal; when there is reversal, there will be cold.

又衝脈爲十二經之海，其腧上出在於大杼，下出與巨虛之上下廉。又衝爲血海，有餘，常想其身大，怫然不知其所病，不足，亦常想其身小，狹然不知其所病。

Moreover, the chōng vessel is the sea of the twelve channels, its transport point emerges above at Dà Zhù (BL-11), and it emerges below at Jù Xū Shàng Lián (ST-37) and Jù Xū Xià Lián (ST-39). In addition, the chōng [vessel] is also the sea of blood; when there is superabundance [in the sea of blood], one often feels oneself to have a large physical stature of the body, with an indignant attitude and an inability to recognise where the disease is located; when there is insufficiency, one often feels oneself to have a small physical stature of the body, with a reserved attitude and an inability to recognise where the disease is located.

---

[5] This point name, "Dà Zhōng (KI-4)," seems to be an inline annotation added to this original passage from *Língshū* Chapters 38 and 62. In the original passage, once the great network-vessel is mentioned, it immediately follows up to explain its trajectory, as the next sentence demonstrated. Nevertheless, the addition of this point proves problematic, as now we have to explain the relationship between this point and the network-vessel, hence the previous text in bracket; in addition, as it interrupts the original passage, we also have to bring back the subject in the next sentence, hence another set of text in brackets.

[6] Qì Jiē is an alternate name for ST-30, it is commonly translated as qì thoroughfare or qì street.

Diseases of the Shàoyīn Kidney Channel
足少陰腎經病

是動病則爲饑而不欲食，蓋虛火盛也，饑不欲食者，脾氣弱也。面黑如炭色，則
腎之色黑形於外也。咳唾則有血，以脈入肺中，則爲咳而唾中有血，則腎主有損
矣。

**When there are changes, it will result in hunger with no desire to eat;
undoubtedly, this is exuberance of vacuity fire; regarding no desire to eat
despite hunger, this is weakness of the spleen qì. Regarding black facial
complexion like the colour of charcoal, it is the manifestation of the black
colour of the kidneys on the exterior. For coughing and spitting with blood, as
the [kidney] vessel enters into the lung, if there is cough with blood in the
spittle, it is indicative of detriment to the kidneys.[7]**

喝喝而喘者，脈入肺中，循喉嚨，挾舌本，火盛則水虧之症也。坐而欲起，陰虛
不能安靜也。目䀮䀮無所見，水虧腎弱也。心懸若饑，脈之支者，從肺出絡心
也。

**Regarding severe thirst and panting, as the [kidney] vessel enters into the
lung and follows the throat to clasp the root of the tongue, this is a sign of
water depletion caused by exuberant fire. For sitting with desire to stand up,[8]
this is one's inability to remain calm [due to] yīn vacuity. For blurred vision
with inability to see, this is water depletion and weakness of the kidneys.
When the heart feels suspended as if one is starving, this is because a branch
of the [kidney] vessel emerges from the lung to network with the heart.**

氣不足則善恐，心惕惕然如人將捕之者，腎在志爲恐，恐傷腎也。此皆腎主骨，
骨之氣逆而厥，是爲骨厥。

**When there is insufficiency of qì, there will be susceptibility to fear, and the
heart will be alarmed as if one is about to be seized by another person; as fear
is the emotion of the kidneys, fear damages the kidneys. Here, because the
kidneys govern the bones, when there is counterflow qì of the bones, there
will be reversal; thus, there is bone reversal.**

所生病爲口熱，爲舌乾，爲咽腫，爲上氣，爲咽乾及痛，蓋以脈循喉嚨，挾舌
本，而生是病也。又爲煩心，爲心痛，以脈從肺絡心也。又爲黃疸，乃爲女勞疸
也。又爲腸澼者，以腎之脈至臍下，緊挾臍，乃大腸之所也。爲脊後內廉痛，脈
所經處也。爲痿，乃骨痿也。爲厥，乃氣弱不至足也。爲嗜臥，骨痿則嗜臥也。
爲足下熱而痛，脈起足心湧泉穴也。以上諸病，邪氣盛則泄，正氣虛則補。熱盛

---

[7] Lit. detriment to that which the kidneys govern.
[8] I.e., agitation or inability to sit still.

則疾去鍼以泄之，寒則久留鍼以溫之。脈陷下者灸之，若不盛不虛，則止取本
經，不必求取於太陽膀胱經也。

For disease itself engenders, there is heat in the mouth, dry tongue, swollen pharynx, qì ascent, and dry pharynx with pain; undoubtedly, because the vessel follows the throat and clasps the root of the tongue, thus these diseases are engendered.

In addition, for heat vexation and heart pain, this is because the vessel networks with the heart from the lung. Also, for jaundice, this is surely jaundice caused by sexual taxation. Regarding intestinal aggregations, this is because the kidney vessel reaches below the umbilicus, where it tightly clasps the umbilicus, this is surely the place of the large intestine. For pain on the inner ridge of the back spine, this is the place where the vessel travels.

For wilting, this is surely bone wilting. For reversal, this is due to weakness of the qì that fails to reach the feet. For somnolence, when there is bone wilting, it will cause somnolence. For heat below the feet with pain, this is because the vessel commences at Yǒng Quán (KI-1) at the centre of the foot. For the various diseases [mentioned] above, when there is an exuberance of evil qì, it is to be drained; when there is a vacuity of the upright qì, it is to be supplemented.

When there is an exuberance of heat, quickly remove the needle in order to drain it; when there is cold, retain the needle in order to warm it. When the vessel is sunken, moxa it. When there is neither an exuberance nor vacuity, then only choose this channel, as there is no need to use the foot tàiyáng bladder channel.

如寸口較人迎之脈大者二倍，則少陰腎經爲實當泄，太陽膀胱爲虛當補。如寸口
較人迎之脈小者二倍，則腎經爲虛當補，膀胱爲實當泄。

When the cùnkǒu pulse in comparison to the rényíng pulse is two times larger, the shàoyīn kidney channel is replete, which ought to be drained; the tàiyáng bladder is vacuous, which ought to be supplemented. When the cùnkǒu pulse in comparison to the rényíng pulse is two times smaller, the kidney channel is vacuous, one ought to supplement it; the bladder is replete, one ought to drain it.

衝脈與腎脈，分上下而同行，故衝脈之爲病，並應責之少陰焉。衝脈爲病，氣逆
裏急，刺膚中陷者與胸下動脈。腹痛，刺臍左右動脈，按之立已，不已刺氣街，
按之立已。

The chōng vessel and the kidney vessel travel together in both areas above and below, thus when the chōng vessel is diseased, one should seek the shàoyīn [channel]. When the chōng vessel is diseased, there will be counterflow qì with internal urgency; pierce the depressions on the bosom as well as the pulsating vessels below the chest.[9] For abdominal pain, pierce the pulsating vessel on the left and right side of the umbilicus and then put pressure on it, [the pain] will immediately cease; if it does not cease, pierce Qì Jiē (ST-30) and then put pressure on it, [the pain] will immediately cease.[10]

爲厥逆，其症氣上衝咽不得息，而喘息有音不得臥。又爲痿厥，痿者，四肢痿軟也；厥者，四肢如火或如冰也。若濕熱成痿，乃不足中之有餘也，宜泄；若精血枯涸成痿，乃不足中之不足也，宜補。

When there is reverse flow, there will be signs such as qì upthrust into the pharynx and inability to catch the breath, leading to audible panting and inability to lie down.[11] In addition, there is also wilting reversal; regarding wilting, there is atony[12] and weakness in the four limbs; regarding reversal, the four limbs may feel like fire or ice.[13] If the wilting is developed from damp-heat, this is superabundance within insufficiency, it is appropriate to drain; if the wilting is developed from desiccation of the essence and blood, this is insufficiency within insufficiency, it is appropriate to supplement.[14]

The Foot Shàoyīn Sinew Channel
足少陰經筋

足少陰之筋，起小指之下，並足太陰之經，斜走內踝之下，結於踵，與太陽之筋合而上結於內輔之下，並太陰之筋，上循陰股，結於陰器，循脊內挾膂，上至項，結於枕骨，與足太陽之筋合。其爲病轉筋，及所過而結者皆痛。又疾在外者不能俯，在內者不能仰。

The sinew [channel] of the foot shàoyīn commences from below the little toe and joins together with the channel of the foot tàiyīn. It travels obliquely to below the inner ankle [bone], knots at the heel, unites together with the sinew [channel] of the foot tàiyáng, and ascends to knot below the inner assisting [bone]. Together with the sinew [channel] of the tàiyīn, it ascends following

---

[9] From *Língshū* Chapter 26.

[10] From *Língshū* Chapter 26.

[11] From *the Lánshì Mìcáng* 蘭室秘藏 (*Secret Treasure of the Orchid Chamber*, 1276 CE) by Lǐ Dōngyuán and his student, chief disciple, Luó Tiānyì.

[12] While this is the same character as "痿 wilting," it means "atony" in this textual context.

[13] From *the Qíjīng Bāmài Kǎo* 奇經八脈考 (*An Investigation of the Eight Extraordinary Channels*, 1578 CE), where Lǐ Shízhēn attributes to Lǐ Dōngyuán; however, this line cannot be found in any extant work of the latter.

[14] Paraphrasing from Lǐ Shízhēn's comment within *the Qíjīng Bāmài Kǎo* 奇經八脈考 (*An Investigation of the Eight Extraordinary Channels*, 1578 CE).

the yīn of the thigh, knotting at the yīn organs.[15] It continues to follow the internal paravertebral sinews that clasp the spine, ascends to reach the nape, and knots at the occipital bone, where it unites together with the sinew [channel] of the foot tàiyáng.

When [the sinew channel] becomes diseased, there is cramping, as well as pain in the places where it traverses and knots. Also, when the disease is located on the exterior, there is inability to bend forward; when it is located on the interior, there is inability to bend backward.

First Point of the Kidney Channel
Yǒng Quán – Gushing Spring (KI-1)
腎經第一穴湧泉

一名地衝
Alternate name: Earth Surge

穴在足心陷中，屈足捲指宛宛中，白肉際，跪取之，非在足中心也。足少陰腎脈所出爲井木。實則泄之。《銅人》：鍼五分，無令出血，灸三壯。《素》注：鍼三分，留十呼。

This point is located in the depression in the centre[16] of the foot, in the depression when the foot and toes are curled. It is on the border of the white flesh that is located by kneeling, which is in fact not at the centre of the foot. The foot shàoyīn kidney vessel emerges here, as the well and wood point. When it is replete, drain it. *The Tóngrén* states, "Needle 5 fēn, do not allow it to bleed, and moxa 3 cones." *The Sùzhù* states, "Needle 3 fēn, and retain for 10 respirations."[17]

注：穴名湧泉者，此穴受太陽、少陰之交，而趨足心，又將上行，腎爲水也，故爲泉，自足下上行，有湧之象也，故曰湧泉。又少陰之井爲木，木性有上行之意，乃一身最下之處，而爲人之根本。

Explanation: this point is named Yǒng Quán (Gushing Spring); as this point is the intersection that transfers from the tàiyáng [channel] to the shàoyīn [channel], it then converges at the centre of the foot. In addition, [the channel] is about to ascend

---

[15] I.e., the external genitals.

[16] Lit. the heart/core.

[17] *The Sùzhù* and *Zhēnjiǔ Dàchéng* actually state "3 respirations" instead of "10 respirations" listed above.

[from there], as the kidneys are classified as water, thus it is a Quán (Spring). As [the channel] ascends from the bottom of the foot, it has the image of Yǒng (Gushing), thus it is called Yǒng Quán (Gushing Spring).

In addition, the shàoyīn well point is wood, and the nature of wood carries the meaning of upward movement; as this is the lowest location in the entire body, it is the root and foundation of a human being.

凡氣之上行而逆者，此穴一泄可下，故曰實則泄之，無令出血，不宜太深也，取氣而不取血之義。《素》注：鍼三分，酌乎中矣。

For all upward movement of qì that turns into counterflow, once this point is drained, then [the qì] will descend; thus, it is said, "When there is repletion, drain it;" however, do not allow it to bleed, and it is not appropriate to needle too deeply, this is the meaning of "seek the qì but do not seek the blood." *The Sùzhù* states, "Needle 3 fēn." This is to have discretion of moderation [in treatment].

腎之本病：足下熱，五指盡痛，足脛寒而逆，足下冷至膝，股內廉痛，屍厥，面黑如炭色，頭痛癲癲然。

Principal diseases of the kidneys: heat on the bottom of the feet, pain in all five toes, cold in the feet and lower leg with counterflow, cold from the bottom of the feet that reaches the knees, pain in the inner ridge of the thigh, deathlike reversal, black facial complexion like the colour of charcoal, and headache that resembles epilepsy.[18]

注：足下熱者，水少火偏勝也，刺此穴立愈。五指盡痛者，清濕之氣中此穴也，宜泄之。足脛寒而逆，中寒邪而逆也，宜鍼以去寒，更灸以溫之。足下冷至膝者，中清濕之氣也，宜泄以去其清濕。股內廉痛，乃腎經上行之氣有鬱也，宜泄此穴。

Explanation: heat on the bottom of the feet is due to scantness of water and prevalence of fire; pierce this point and there will be immediate recovery. Pain in all

---

[18] Note: The term, diān 癲, is a problematic one. From ancient usage, it seems to describe a disease that is equivalent to epilepsy; however, later on, it seems to describe a person with confusion and mania, which is commonly translated as "withdrawal" today (sincere gratitude to Will Ceurvels for pointing out this issue that we are unaware of). As there are two drastically different but possibly equally valid interpretations of the term, we will select the interpretation according to the context; however, the reader should be aware that there is a chance that our selection may result in misinterpretation. Another term, jiān 癇, is also translated to epilepsy, as the term is largely identical to what diān 癲 represents; the minor difference is that diān 癲 tends to describe acute epilepsy, whereas jiān 癇 tends to mean episodic epilepsy.

five toes is due to strike of cool damp[19] qì at this point, it is appropriate to drain this [point]. Cold in the feet and lower legs with counterflow is strike by cold evil leading to counterflow, it is appropriate to needle in order to eliminate cold and further moxa in order to warm this [point].

Cold from below the feet that reaches the knees is strike by cool damp qì, it is appropriate to drain in order to eliminate the cool-dampness. Pain in the inner aspect of the thigh is depression of the ascending qì of the kidney channel, it is appropriate to drain this point.

屍厥、面黑如炭色，乃腎氣全鬱於下，並太陰之氣亦鬱，遂屍厥不知人事矣，故取此穴方活。頭痛癲癲者，乃少陰頭痛也，病在上，泄下以治之。

Deathlike reversal and black facial complexion like the colour of charcoal are because the kidney qì is entirely depressed in the lower; at the same time, the qì of tàiyīn is also depressed; as a result, there will be deathlike reversal with loss of consciousness, thus choose this point and the life will be saved. Headache that resembles epilepsy is a shàoyīn headache; as the disease is in the above, drain the below in order to treat it.

腎之舌咽病：舌乾咽腫，上氣咽乾，喉閉舌急失音，咽中痛不可納食，瘖不能言，頭痛，身項痛而寒且痠。

Tongue and pharynx diseases of the kidneys: dry tongue and swollen pharynx, qì ascent with dry pharynx, throat block with tension of the tongue and loss of voice, pain in the pharynx with inability to swallow food, loss of voice with inability to speak, headache, and pain in the body and nape with both chills and aches.

注：舌乾咽腫，火氣上昇也，宜泄此穴。上氣咽乾，火氣有餘而上行也，宜泄此穴。喉閉舌急至於失音，氣鬱之極也，宜泄之。咽中痛不可納食，乃氣逆而熱極所致，宜泄。

Explanation: dry tongue and swollen pharynx is fire qì ascending, it is appropriate to drain this point. Qì ascent with dry pharynx is upward movement of fire qì due to superabundance, it is appropriate to drain this point. Throat block with tension of the tongue causing loss of voice is extreme depression of qì, it is appropriate to drain this [point]. Pain in the pharynx with inability to swallow food is a result of qì counterflow leading to extreme heat, it is appropriate to drain.

---

[19] Cool damp is a disease in category of cold damp evils, to which, the 中医大辞典 *Great Dictionary of Chinese Medicine* states, "因寒湿之气下坠，致病时可见下肢痠麻痹痛，浮肿，屈伸不利，膝肿痛或腹痛水泻等症 it is caused by the down bearing of cold damp qì, it will present with signs such as aching, numbness, impediment, and pain in the lower limbs, puffy swelling, pain and swelling of the knee, abdominal pain, and watery diarrhoea."

瘖不能言，乃腎氣不足，不能上通於舌，鍼泄其火，更宜用補腎之藥。頭痛乃腎氣有餘也，宜泄此穴。身項痛而寒且痠者，亦腎氣之滯也，泄之以舒其氣。

Loss of voice with inability to speak is a result of the inability of kidney qì to ascend to communicate with the tongue due to its insufficiency, needle [this point] to drain the fire; furthermore, it is even more appropriate to utilise herbs that supplement the kidneys. Headache is a result of kidney qì superabundance, it is appropriate to drain this point. Pain in the body and nape with both chills and aches is also stagnation of kidney qì, drain it in order to soothe the qì.

腎之肺病：咳吐有血，鼻衄不止，渴而喘，喘而脊脇相引，悲欠，咳嗽身熱，風疹，胸脇滿悶，少氣寒厥，痿厥嗜臥，舌乾引飲。

Lung diseases of the kidneys: coughing and spitting of blood, incessant nosebleed, thirst with panting, panting with pulling between the lumbus and rib-side, sorrow and yawning, cough with generalised heat, wind papules, fullness and oppression in the chest and rib-side, scantness of qì with cold reversal, wilting reversal with somnolence, and dry tongue [with desire] to drink fluids.

注：咳吐有血，水虧火有餘也，鍼泄其火，更用藥以補腎水。鼻衄不止，乃肺氣上逆也，宜泄。渴而喘、喘而脊脇相引，水不足，氣有餘也，宜泄。悲欠，悲者，肺症也，子有病及其母也；欠者，精不足也，故取此穴。

Explanation: coughing and spitting of blood is depletion of water with superabundance of fire, needle [this point] to drain the fire; moreover, use herbs in order to supplement kidney water. For incessant nosebleed, this is a result of counterflow ascent of lung qì, it is appropriate to drain [this point]. For thirst with panting and panting with pulling between the lumbus and rib-side, this is insufficiency of water and superabundance of qì, it is appropriate to drain. For sorrow and yawning, sorrow is a lung sign, this is the child's disease affecting the mother. For yawning, it is the insufficiency of essence, thus choose this point.

咳嗽身熱，水不足，火有餘也，宜泄。風疹乃肺中風邪，及於皮毛也，母有餘則泄其子。胸脇滿悶，腎氣上入肺者，逆而急也，宜泄。少氣寒厥，乃清濕之氣重也，取此穴以泄清濕之氣。

Cough with generalised heat is insufficiency of water and superabundance of fire, it is appropriate to drain [this point]. Wind papules is a result of the lung struck by wind evil, which has implicated the skin and body hair; when the mother has abundance, drain the child. Fullness and oppression of the chest and rib-side is the kidney qì ascending to enter the lung; as this counterflow [of the kidney qì] is causing the tension [in the lung], it is appropriate to drain [this point]. Scantness of qì with cold reversal is a result of considerable cool-damp qì, choose this point in order to drain the cool-damp qì.

痿厥嗜臥，陽明症也，泄腎之火，即所以泄衝脈之火，而解陽明之熱也。舌乾引飲，水不足而火上逆也，宜泄。

Wilting reversal with somnolence is a yángmíng sign; by draining the fire of the kidneys, it will drain the fire of the chōng vessel; as a result, the heat of yángmíng will be resolved. Dry tongue [with desire] to drink fluids is insufficiency of water leading to counterflow ascent of fire, it is appropriate to drain [this point].

腎之肝病：坐欲起，目䀮䀮無所見，善恐，如人將捕之，風癇。

Liver diseases of the kidneys: a desire to stand up while sitting, blurry vision with inability to see, susceptibility to fear with feeling as if about to be seized by another person, and wind epilepsy.

注：坐欲起，魂不定也，邪入腎，則瞳人為邪所蔽，而目無所見，宜泄之。善恐、如人將捕之，膽怯也，膽繫於肝，宜資腎以養肝，腎不足，則肝病及膽，而有是症也。風癇，痰火積於命門，而及於肝也，宜泄此穴。

Explanation: desire to stand up while sitting is due to an unstable ethereal soul. When the evil enters the kidneys, the pupil will be covered by the evil, leading to an inability to see, it is appropriate to drain [this point]. Susceptibility to fear with feeling as if about to be seized by another person is timidity of the gallbladder, as the gallbladder attaches to the liver, it is appropriate to support the kidney in order to nourish the liver; when the kidney is insufficient, the liver disease will affect the gallbladder, causing these signs. Wind epilepsy is phlegm fire accumulation in the mìngmén, which has subsequently affected the liver, it is appropriate to drain this point.

腎之心病：煩心心痛，心中結熱，卒心痛，癲病挾臍痛，忽忽喜忘。

Heart diseases of the kidneys: vexation of the heart with heart pain, heat bind in the heart, sudden heart pain, epileptic disease and pain that clasps the umbilicus, carelessness and forgetfulness.

注：煩心者，腎氣有餘，上逆於心也，宜泄。心痛，亦腎氣上逆於心也，宜泄。心中結熱，氣火有餘也，取此穴以泄之，心中之火自消。

Explanation: vexation of the heart is superabundance of kidney qì that counterflows upwards into the heart, it is appropriate to drain [this point]. Heart pain is also kidney qì that counterflows upwards into the heart, it is appropriate to drain [this point]. Heat bind in the heart is superabundance of qì and fire, choose this point in order to drain [the qì and fire], so that the fire in the heart will naturally disperse.

卒心痛，素無心痛，而忽有是症，非同於胃脘痛也，此屬急症，宜急取此穴以泄之。

For sudden heart pain, if [the person] does not typically have heart pain but suddenly has this sign, this is not the same as stomach duct pain, this is an urgent sign, it is appropriate to urgently choose this point in order to drain it.

癲病，陰病也，挾臍痛，乃腎脈所行之地也，故亦泄此穴。忽忽喜忘，志不足也，腎水不足，乃有此症，雖當泄，還宜用藥以補之。

Epileptic disease is a yīn disease; pain that clasps the umbilicus is because it is the place where the kidney vessel travels, thus drain this point. For carelessness and forgetfulness, this is insufficiency of the will; as the kidney water is insufficient, there are these signs; although one should drain [this point], it is furthermore appropriate to use herbs in order to supplement [the kidneys].

腎之腎病：轉胞不得溺，腰痛大便難，小腹急痛，泄而下重，男子如蠱，女子如娠，婦人無子，腸癖，腎積奔豚，風入腸中，小腹痛，腰痛，腹脹不欲食。

Kidney diseases of the kidneys: shifted bladder with inability to urinate, lumbar pain with difficult defecation, tense pain[20] in the lower abdomen, diarrhoea with lower body heaviness, resemblance of gǔ in males, resemblance of pregnancy in females, infertility in women, intestinal aggregation, kidney accumulation with running piglet, wind entering the intestines, pain in the lower abdomen, and abdominal distension with no desire to eat.

注：腎司二便，轉胞不得溺、腰痛大便難，急取此穴，以調其氣。小腹急痛、泄而下重，腎氣鬱也，亦取此穴。

Explanation: as the kidney controls the urine and stool, when there is shifted bladder with inability to urinate and lumbar pain with difficult defecation, urgently choose this point in order to regulate the qì. Tense pain in the lower abdomen and diarrhoea with lower body heaviness are due to kidney qì depression, also choose this point.

氣積於臍下，而有脹滿之形，如蠱如娠焉，宜泄此穴，再取足跗上血絡盛處，皆出血。婦人無子，腎脈鬱而滯也，取此穴以通其氣。腸癖而亦責腎者，以腸在臍下腎之部分，取此穴，氣流通則無積矣。

When there is qì accumulation below the umbilicus, it will lead to the formation of distension and fullness, which resemble gǔ or pregnancy, it is appropriate to drain this point; further choose locations of exuberant blood vessels on the dorsal aspect of the foot and let blood on all these [vessels]. Infertility in women is due to depression of the kidney vessel leading to stagnation, choose this point in order to free the qì. For intestinal aggregation, the kidneys can also be

---

20 "急痛 Tense pain" could also be translated as urgent pain.

responsible, as the intestines are located below the umbilicus in the area of the kidneys, choose this point; [once] the qì flows freely, there will be no more accumulations.

腎積奔豚者，氣積也，宜泄腎之逆氣。風入腸中、小腹痛，亦腎氣之有餘也，泄此穴。腰痛、腹脹不欲食，清濕之氣入於腹也，泄此穴。

Kidney accumulation with running piglet is qì accumulation, it is appropriate to drain the counterflow qì of the kidneys. Wind entering the intestines and lower abdominal pain are [both] superabundance of kidney qì, drain this point. Lumbar pain and abdominal distension with no desire to eat are due to the qì of cool-dampness entering the abdomen, drain this point.

腎之脾病：黃疸，霍亂轉筋。

Spleen diseases of the kidneys: jaundice, and sudden turmoil with cramps.

注：黃疸者，多因醉飽行房所得，飲食在腹，脾不能運化，遂成濕熱，發黃在面。黃者，土色也，尅腎之色也，急調腎之本源，使腎氣上行，小便下降，以去濕熱，此藥中治黃必用茵陳利小便之義。

Explanation: jaundice is predominantly caused by having sexual intercourse after intoxication and excessive food and drink; as food and drink are in the abdomen, which the spleen fails to transport and transform, they become damp heat, resulting in yellowing of the face. Yellow is the colour of earth, it is [also] the colour that restrains the kidneys; thus, urgently regulate the root and source of the kidneys to make the kidney qì move upwards and make the urine descend, so that damp heat can be eliminated. This is the reason why in the treatment of yellowing by herbs, one must utilise Yīn Chén[21] to disinhibit urination.

霍亂，氣亂也，轉筋，則筋之在後者，勢欲在前，股之筋在後者，腎之所主也，故取此穴，以降其邪而順其氣。

When there is sudden turmoil, the qì is in turmoil; for cramping, the sinews located in the rear are pulled towards the front; as the sinews of the thigh that are located in the rear are governed by the kidneys, thus choose this point in order to descend the evil and smooth the qì.

---

[21] I.e., Yīn Chén 茵陳 (Artemisiae Scopariae Herba), which is commonly called virgate wormwood.

15

Second Point of the Kidney Channel
Rán Gǔ – Blazing Valley (KI-2)
腎經第二穴然谷

一名龍淵
Alternate name: Dragon in the Abyss

穴在內踝前起大骨下陷中，一云內踝下在前一寸，別於足太陰之郄，腎脈所溜爲
滎火。《銅人》：鍼三分，灸三壯，留五呼。不宜見血，令人立饑欲食。如誤刺足
下布絡中脈，血不出爲腫。

This point is located in the depression below the large bone that protrudes in front of inner ankle [bone]. One source states, "It is 1 cùn in front of the bottom of the inner ankle [bone]." It diverges to the cleft of the foot tàiyīn. The kidney vessel gushes here, as the brook and fire point. *The Tóngrén* states, "Needle 3 fēn, moxa 3 cones, and retain for 5 respirations. It is not appropriate to bleed; [if it is bled], then it will immediately cause the person to become hungry. When one by mistake pierces directly on the vessels of spreading network-vessel on the lower [aspect] of the foot, if there is no discharge of blood, it will become swollen."

　　注：穴名然谷者，火之始灼曰然，此穴接湧泉之脈上行，湧泉爲木，然谷
爲火，水之所溜爲谷，故曰然谷。一名龍淵，亦象淵中有龍上騰之象。僅在內踝前
大骨下，若誤刺布絡，則出血，血將不止，不出血，則爲腫矣。

Explanation: this point is named Rán Gǔ (Blazing Valley), because when fire begins to scorch, it is said to Rán (Blaze). This point succeeds the ascent of vessel from Yǒng Quán (KI-1); as Yǒng Quán (KI-1) is wood, Rán Gǔ (Blazing Valley) is fire. The place where water gushes is a Gǔ (Valley), thus it is called Rán Gǔ (Blazing Valley).

An alternate name is Lóng Yuān (Dragon in the Abyss), because it also has the image of a Lóng (Dragon) rising from an Yuān (Abyss).[22] As [this point] is located near and below the large bone in front of the inner ankle [bone], if one mistakenly pierces the spreading network-vessel, there will be bleeding, and the bleeding will be incessant; however, if there is no bleeding, it will become swollen.

腎之本病：足跗腫不得履地，淋瀝白濁，婦人無子，痿厥，胻痠不能久立，足一
寒一熱，男子泄精，陰挺出，月事不調，陰癢，小腹脹，上搶胸。

---

[22] This alludes to the fourth line of hexagram qián (hexagram 1) in *the Yìjīng*, "九四：或躍在
淵，无咎。On the fourth nine (yáng), [the dragon] may leap from the abyss. There will be
no mistake."

Principal diseases of the kidneys: swelling of the instep and foot with inability to step on the ground, dribbling urination and white turbid [urine], infertility in women, wilting reversal, inability to stand for long periods due to aching calves, one foot is cold while the other is hot, seminal discharge in men, vaginal protrusion, irregular menstruation, pudendal itch, distension in the lower abdomen, and surging [sensation] into the chest.

注：足跗腫不得履地，腫者，濕也，濕勝者，火不足也，宜鍼此穴，以除其濕，更灸以溫之。淋瀝者，腎氣不足，白濁者，腎中濕熱，宜取腎之火穴，而除濕熱，以調腎中之氣。婦人無子，腎虛也，補腎中之火穴以滋腎。

Explanation: for swelling of the instep and foot with inability to step on the ground, this swelling is indicative of dampness; when dampness is prevalent, there is an insufficiency of fire, it is appropriate to needle this point in order to eliminate the dampness; in addition, moxa it in order to warm it. Dribbling urination is due to kidney qì insufficiency; white turbid [urine] is due to damp-heat within the kidneys, it is appropriate to choose the fire point of the kidneys in order to eliminate damp heat, so that the qì of the kidneys can be regulated. Infertility in women is because of kidney vacuity, supplement the fire point of the kidneys in order to enrich the kidneys.

痿厥者，氣不至足也，取腎火穴，以引腎中之氣。胻痠不能久立、足一寒一熱者，腎有二，一水一火，火少則寒，水少則熱，然多左寒右熱，故取此穴，以補泄其水火。

Wilting reversal is a failure of the qì to reach the feet, choose the kidney fire point in order to guide the qì within the kidneys. For inability to stand for long periods due to aching calves, as well as one foot is cold while the other is hot, these are because there are two kidneys; one [kidney] is water while the other is fire; when fire is scant, there will be cold; when water is scant, there will be heat. Nevertheless, in general, the left [foot] is cold while the right [foot] is hot, thus choose this point in order to drain the water and fire.

男子泄精，非腎之寒而滑，即腎之熱而溢，寒則補，熱則泄。陰挺出，肝病也，以腎氣之有餘，故泄腎之火穴。陰癢，亦腎火之熾也，故泄腎火。小腹脹、上搶胸者，腎脈同衝脈上至胸，乃腎氣、衝氣之逆也，宜泄此穴。

For seminal discharge in men, if it is not efflux caused by cold of the kidneys, it will be spillage caused by heat of the kidneys; when there is cold, supplement it; when there is heat, drain it. Vaginal protrusion is a liver disease due to a superabundance of the kidney qì, thus drain the fire point of the kidneys. Pudendal itch is also due to the blazing of kidney fire, thus drain the kidney fire [point]. For distension in the lower abdomen and surging [sensation] into the chest, as the kidney vessel ascends together with the chōng vessel to reach the chest, this is counterflow of the kidney qì and chōng qì, it is appropriate to drain this point.

腎之肝病：心恐懼，如人將捕之，寒疝，小兒臍風口噤。

Liver diseases of the kidneys: dread and fear in the heart, feeling as if about to be seized by another person, cold mounting, and infantile umbilical wind with clenched jaw.

注：心恐懼、如人將捕之，膽怯也，肝衰也，腎敗也，宜補腎之火穴。寒疝，肝病也，然必腎寒，而後有此症，宜補此穴。小兒臍風口噤，先受寒，次受熱之症也，急泄腎火。

Explanation: for dread and fear in the heart along with feeling as if about to be seized by another person, these are caused by gallbladder timidity, liver debilitation, or kidney vanquishment, it is appropriate to supplement the fire point of the kidneys. Cold mounting is a liver disease; yet, this sign can only appear if the kidneys are cold; thus, it is appropriate to supplement this point. Regarding infantile umbilical wind with clenched jaw, this is a pattern that initially contracts cold and subsequently contracts heat, urgently drain the kidney fire [point].

腎之脾病：消渴。

Spleen disease of the kidneys: dispersion-thirst.

注：消渴者，火有餘也，泄腎之火，再用補腎水之藥。

Explanation: dispersion-thirst is the superabundance of fire, drain the fire [point] of the kidneys, further utilise herbs that supplement the kidney water.

腎之心病：舌縱煩滿，心痛如刺，暴脹，胸脇支滿，無積。

Heart diseases of the kidneys: protracted tongue with vexation and fullness, heart pain that resembles being stabbed, sudden distension, and propping fullness in the chest and rib-sides but the absence of any accumulations.

注：舌者，心之竅，為火，然谷亦腎之火穴，脈上注舌，氣逆則舌長，宜泄。心痛如刺、暴脹、胸脇支滿、無積者，邪客於足少陰之絡所致，乃腎心痛之急症也，刺此穴出血立已。

Explanation: the tongue is the orifice of the heart, it is fire; as Rán Gǔ (KI-2) is also the fire point of the kidneys and the [kidney] vessel ascends to pour into the tongue, when there is counterflow qì, the tongue will be extended, it is appropriate to drain. For heart pain that resembles being stabbed, sudden distension, and propping fullness in the chest and rib-side yet without any accumulations, these are caused by evils lodging in the network-vessel of the foot shàoyīn; surely, this is an urgent sign of heart pain caused by the kidneys; pierce this point, [the pain] will immediately cease once bleeding occurs.

腎之肺病：咽內腫，不能納唾，不能出唾，涎出喘呼少氣，咳唾血，喉痹，自汗盜汗。

Lung diseases of the kidneys: swelling inside the pharynx, inability to swallow spittle, inability to expectorate drool, expectorating of drool with distressing panting[23] and scantness of qì, coughing of spittle and blood, throat impediment, spontaneous sweating and night sweats.

注：腎脈循喉嚨，挾舌本，火有餘，遂咽腫不能出唾焉，宜泄。左取右，右取左。涎出者，腎液上溢也，喘呼少氣，乃氣逆在肺也，泄此穴，以下上逆之氣。

Explanation: the kidney vessel follows the throat to clasp the root of the tongue; when there is superabundance of fire, the pharynx will be swollen with the inability to expectorate spittle, it is appropriate to drain; for [swelling on] the left, choose the right [point]; for the right, choose left. Expectoration of spittle is the upward spillage of kidney humour; distressing panting and scantness of qì are caused by counterflow qì in the lung; drain this point in order to descend the upward counterflow qì.

咳唾血，腎火盛而上尅肺金也，宜泄。喉痹，亦腎脈上挾喉嚨之所致，自汗盜汗，乃腎火上逆也，泄此穴，使火不上逆，則汗不作矣。

Coughing of spittle and blood is exuberance of kidney fire that ascends to restrain lung metal, it is appropriate to drain. Throat impediment is because the kidney vessel ascends to clasp the throat; for spontaneous sweating and night sweats, they are a result of counterflow ascent of kidney fire, drain this point, so that the fire will no longer counterflow and ascend; as a result, the [abnormal] sweating will no longer occur.

Third Point of the Kidney Channel
Tài Xī – Great Ravine (KI-3)
腎經第三穴太谿

一名呂細
Alternate name: Thin Spine[24]

---

[23] "喘呼少氣 distressing panting with scantness of qì" is originally "呼吸少氣 scantness of qì in respiration" in the primary manuscript. The editors of this manuscript, Zhāng and Zhà, have amended it according to the secondary manuscript and the *Zhēnjiǔ Dàchéng.*

[24] *Grasping the Wind* names it "Small Lǚ." We are interpreting Lǚ 呂 as the spine according to the *Shuōwén Jiězì* 説文解字 (*Explaining Graphs and Analysing Characters*, 2nd century CE).

穴在內踝後五分，跟骨上動脈陷中，屈足五指乃得穴。男、婦病，有此脈則生，無則死，足少陰所注爲腧土。《素》注：鍼二分，留七呼，灸三壯。

This point is located 5 fēn behind the inner ankle [bone], in the depression above the heel bone, on the pulsating vessel; by contracting the five toes, the point will be located. For the diseases of men and women, if this pulse is present, there will be life; if absent, there will be death. The foot shàoyīn pours here, as the stream and earth point. *The Sùzhù* states, "Needle 2 fēn,[25] retain for 7 respirations, and moxa 3 cones."

注：穴名太谿者，腎爲人身之水，自湧泉發源，尚未見動之形，溜於然谷，亦未見動之形，至此而有動脈可見。谿乃水流之處，有動脈則水之形見，故曰太谿。谿者，水之見也；太者，言其淵不測也。

Explanation: this point is named Tài Xī (Great Ravine), as the kidneys are the water of the human body: at the commencing source at Yǒng Quán (KI-1), there is yet an observable appearance of the pulse; as it gushes into Rán Gǔ (KI-2), again, there is yet an observable appearance of the pulse; yet, once arriving here,[26] the pulsating vessel becomes observable.

Xī (Ravine) is the place where water flows; where a pulsating vessel is present, the form of water can be observed [there], thus it is called Tài Xī (KI-3). Whereas Xī (Ravine) is the water that can be observed, Tài (Great) is depicting its immeasurable abyss.

腎之本病：熱病汗不出，默默嗜臥，溺黃，傷寒手足厥冷，大便難，消癉。

Principal diseases of the kidneys: febrile disease with absence of sweating, taciturnity with somnolence, yellow urine, cold damage with reversal cold of the hands and feet, difficult defecation, and pure-heat dispersion [thirst].

注：熱病汗不出，默默嗜臥，乃寒邪直中少陰，真少陰症也，宜補之。溺黃者，膀胱熱也，腎與膀胱爲表裏，泄此穴以去其熱。

Explanation: for febrile disease with absence of sweating and taciturnity with somnolence, these are due to the direct strike of cold evil at the shàoyīn; these are true shàoyīn signs, it is appropriate to supplement this [point]. Regarding yellow urine, because the kidneys and the urinary bladder are an exterior-interior [pair], drain this point in order to eliminate the heat.

---

[25] For "3 fēn" *the Zhēnjiǔ Dàchéng* actually has "2 fēn."
[26] I.e., KI-3.

傷寒手足厥冷，寒甚矣，泄之以去其寒。大便難者，腎司二便，氣化則出，泄此穴則氣調，而大便出矣。消癉者，下消也，乃房事不滿欲之症，腎之邪氣盛，而正氣將絕，急刺此穴，以復正去邪。

When there is cold damage with reversal cold of the hands and feet, this is severe cold, drain this [point] in order to eliminate the cold. Regarding difficult defecation, as the kidneys control both the urine and stool, which will be discharged when qì transformation takes place,[27] by draining this point, the qì will be regulated and the stool will be discharged.

Pure-heat dispersion is dispersion [thirst] in the lower [jiāo], this sign is due to an insatiable desire for sexual intercourse; as evil qì is exuberant in the kidneys and the upright qì is on the verge of expiration, urgently pierce this point in order to restore the upright [qì] and eliminate the evil.

腎之肝病：寒疝，胸脇痛，瘦瘠，寒熱，久瘧咳逆。

Liver diseases of the kidneys: cold mounting, pain of the chest and rib-side, emaciation and frailty, chills and fever, enduring malaria with cough and counterflow.

注：寒疝，肝病也，不宜責腎之穴。胸脇痛、瘦瘠者，胸雖爲腎經、衝脈所行之部分，而胸乃肝經所行之地，取此穴以降其上行之逆。

Explanation: cold mounting is a liver disease, it is not appropriate to seek this point of the kidney [channel]. For pain of the chest and rib-side, emaciation and frailty, although the chest is an area where the kidney channel and chōng vessel travel, yet the chest is also the place where the liver channel travels, choose this point in order to descend the counterflow ascent.

寒熱乃少陽膽經之病也，水不生木，故有此病，此穴爲水所見行之處，取此穴以補水。久瘧咳逆者，取此穴以扶脾土，而降肝上逆之氣。

Chills and fever are the disease of the shàoyáng gallbladder channel; when water fails to engender wood, this disease manifests; as this point is the place where the flow of water becomes observable, choose this point in order to supplement water. For enduring malaria with cough and counterflow, choose this point in order to support spleen earth, so that the counterflow ascent of liver qì can be descended.

---

[27] "When qì transformation takes place" is a quote from *Sùwèn* Chapter 8, which the majority view attributes it only to the function of bladder; yet, here Yuè Hánzhēn appears to hold the view that this phrase refers to every organ listed in the chapter, not only the bladder. See the footnote in "Overview of the Hand Shàoyáng Sānjiāo" for further discussion.

腎之脾病：嘔吐痰實，口中如膠，善噫，痿，牙齒痛，痃癖。

Spleen diseases of the kidneys: vomiting and spitting of replete phlegm, gluey sensation in the mouth, frequent belching, wilting, toothache, strings and aggregations.[28]

注：嘔吐痰實如膠，胃熱極矣，泄此水中之土穴，以去胃之濕熱。善噫者，脾氣鬱也，取此穴以去胃中之鬱。

Explanation: for vomiting and spitting of replete phlegm that is gluey, this is due to extreme stomach heat, drain the earth point of water in order to eliminate the damp-heat of the stomach. Frequent belching is due to depression of the spleen qì, choose this point in order to eliminate depression within the stomach.

痿者，宜導濕熱，引胃氣出行，不令濕土尅腎水，其穴在太谿。牙齒痛者，其症宜責腎、責胃，故牙齒痛堪治。痃癖者，冷積腎水，邪氣太勝，土不能治也，故取此穴，以治積之根。

For wilting, it is appropriate to abduct[29] damp-heat, guide stomach qì to move outwards as to prohibit damp-heat from restraining kidney water; [to accomplish] this, use the point that is located at Tài Xī (KI-3). For the sign of toothache, it is appropriate to seek both the kidneys and stomach, thus [this point] is also able to treat toothache.

Strings and aggregations are cold accumulations of kidney water, which is a great prevalence of the evil qì that the earth is unable to govern, thus choose this point in order to treat the root of the accumulations.

腎之心病：心痛如錐刺，心脈沉，手足寒至節，喘息者死，唾血。

Heart diseases of the kidneys: heart pain that resembles being stabbed by an awl, deep heart pulse, and cold sensation from the hands and feet to the joints;[30] those who pant will die, and there will be spiting of blood.

注：心痛如錐刺，真心痛也，乃腎水上尅心火之象，急泄此穴。嗽血責肺，唾血則責腎矣，泄此穴以降上逆之氣。

---

[28] According to *the Practical Dictionary*, "Strings are elongated masses located at the side of the umbilicus; aggregations are masses located in the rib-side that occur intermittently with pain and at other times are not detectable by palpation. The two conditions belong to the category of concretions, conglomerations, accumulations, and gatherings, and are usually referred to together."

[29] According to *the Practical Dictionary* "導 abduct" means "to carry away, specifically to carry stagnant food down the digestive tract."

[30] We speculate these joints to be knees and elbows.

Explanation: pain that resembles being stabbed by an awl is true heart pain, this is the manifestation of kidney water ascending to restrain heart fire, urgently drain this point. When there is coughing of blood, the lung is responsible; when there is spitting of blood, the kidneys are responsible, drain this point in order to descend the counterflow ascent of qì.

腎之肺病：咳嗽不嗜食，咽腫。

Lung diseases of the kidneys: cough with no pleasure in eating, and swollen pharynx.

注：咳嗽不嗜食，子病及母也，泄此土穴，以去土之濕熱，則能食矣。咽腫，心脈上至咽喉，故泄此穴，以降上逆之火。

Explanation: cough with no pleasure in eating is the child affecting the mother, drain the earth point in order to eliminate the damp-heat of the earth, then one will be able to eat. Regarding swollen pharynx, the heart vessel ascends to arrive at the pharynx and throat, thus drain this point in order to descend the upward counterflow fire.

Fourth Point of the Kidney Channel
Dà Zhōng – Large Goblet (KI-4)
腎經第四穴大鍾

穴在足跟後踵中，大骨上兩筋間。《素》注：在內踝後，動脈應手。足少陰絡，別走太陽。《銅人》：鍼二分，灸三壯，留七呼。

This point is located behind the heel, above the great bone, between the two sinews. *The Sùzhù* states, "It is located behind the inner ankle [bone], where the pulsating vessel resonates with the hand. It is the foot shàoyīn network point that diverges towards the foot tàiyáng." *The Tóngrén* states, "Needle 2 fēn, moxa 3 cones, and retain for 7 respirations."

注：穴名大鍾者，言其部分之形也，其穴在內踝後，有細動脈應手，在太谿之上，其形空懸如鍾，所以吸腎脈之上行者，故曰大鍾。乃少陰之別絡，而走足太陽，正少陰交太陽之路也。

Explanation: this point is named Dà Zhōng (Large Goblet), because it depicts the shape of this area. This point is located behind the inner ankle [bone], where a fine pulsating vessel resonates with the hand. The shape above Tài Xī (KI-3) is hollow and suspended like a Zhōng (Goblet), which is what siphons the kidney vessel to travel upwards; therefore, it is called Dà Zhōng (Large Goblet). [This point] is also the shàoyīn network point, which diverges to go to the foot tàiyáng; this is exactly the route where the shàoyīn intersects with the tàiyáng.

即有別出之脈，並本經脈氣之行，以上，走於手厥陰心包絡之經，其下者，外則貫於腰脊間也。

Here, a diverging vessel emerges and travels together with the vessel qì of this channel; in the above, it goes to the channel of the hand juéyīn pericardiac network; in the below, it moves externally and pierces the middle of the lumbar spine.

其別之脈逆，則爲煩心，邪氣有餘而實，則爲閉癃，以腎通於二便也，正氣不足而虛，則爲腰痛，皆取此別脈大鍾之穴以治之。

When there is counterflow in the diverging vessel, there will be vexation of the heart; when there is repletion due to the superabundance of evil qì, there will be dribbling urinary block, as the kidney [controls] the flow of urination and defecation; when there is an insufficiency of the upright qì leading to vacuity, there will be lumbar pain; in all cases, choose the diverging vessel point Dà Zhōng (Large Goblet) in order to treat these [signs].

腎之本病：腰脊痛，淋瀝，腹脊強，善驚恐不樂，口中熱，多寒，欲閉户而處，閉癃。

Principal diseases of the kidneys: pain in the lumbar spine, dribbling urination, stiffness of the abdomen and spine, frequent fright and fear with unhappiness, heat in the mouth, excessive chills, desire to close the door [of the house] and remain inside, and dribbling urinary block.

注：腰脊痛，責此穴者，以腰爲腎之府也，腎虛則腰痛，補此穴。淋瀝，責此穴者，腎氣不足也，補此穴。腹脊強，腹在前，脊在後，腎氣不順則強，泄此穴。善驚恐不樂，腎之志爲恐，補此穴以定腎志。

Explanation: for pain in the lumbar spine, seek this point, because the lumbus is the residence of the kidneys; when the kidney is vacuous, there will be lumbar pain, supplement this point. For dribbling urination, this point is sought because the kidney qì is insufficient, supplement this point. Regarding stiffness of the abdomen and spine, while the abdomen is in the front, the spine is in the rear, when kidney qì is not smooth, there will be stiffness, drain this point. For frequent fright and fear with unhappiness, as the emotion of the kidneys is fear, supplement this point in order to stabilize the emotion of the kidneys.

口中熱，熱在內也，多寒，寒在外也，腎中之火上昇，故口熱，在下皆陰氣，故多寒，欲閉户而處，則陰氣太甚矣，泄之以去其陰氣。閉癃者，腎氣實也，宜泄此穴。

Whereas heat in the mouth is due to heat located in the interior, excessive chills is due to cold located in the exterior, this is the ascension of fire from within the kidney, thus there will be heat in the mouth; yet, all the yīn qì will be located in the below, thus there will be excessive chills. Regarding the desire to close the door [of the house] and remain inside, the yīn qì is at its utmost extreme, drain this [point] in order to eliminate the yīn qì. Dribbling urinary block is repletion of the kidney qì, it is appropriate to drain this point.

腎之脾病：嘔吐，腹滿便難，嗜臥。

Spleen diseases of the kidneys: retching and vomiting, abdominal fullness with difficult defecation, and somnolence.

注：嘔吐者，腎氣上逆也，泄之，使氣不上逆。腹滿便難，腎氣不動則腹滿，腎氣不順則便難，泄之以調腎氣。嗜臥雖爲脾倦之症，然精不足，則亦嗜臥，補之以養腎之精。

Explanation: retching and vomiting are due to counterflow ascent of kidney qì, drain this [point] in order to cease the counterflow ascent of qì. Regarding abdominal pain with difficult defecation, when the kidney qì fails to move, there will be abdominal fullness; when kidney qì is not smooth, there will be difficult defecation; drain this [point] in order to regulate the kidney qì. Although somnolence is a sign of spleen lassitude, yet, when the essence is insufficient, there can also be somnolence, supplement this [point] in order to nourish the essence of the kidneys.

腎之心病：舌乾。

Heart disease of the kidneys: dry tongue.

注：舌乾者，心之竅雖通於舌，而舌之下有廉泉穴，乃腎水上昇之源也，腎水竭，則舌爲之乾，取此穴以泄腎之火，而補腎之水。

Explanation: regarding [the disease of] dry tongue, even though the orifice of the heart communicates with the tongue, Lián Quán (REN-23) [is located] underneath the tongue, which is the source [of saliva] from the ascending kidney water; when the kidney water is exhausted, the tongue will become dry, choose this point in order to drain the fire of the kidneys, as well as supplement the water of kidneys.

腎之肺病：肺脹喘息，少氣不足，洒淅，咽中食噎不得下，喉中鳴，咳唾氣逆，煩悶。

Lung diseases of the kidneys: lung distension with panting, scantness of breath with insufficiency, [sensation] as though after a soaking, choking of

food in the throat that is unable to descend, rales from within the throat, coughing of spittle with qì counterflow, and vexation with oppression.

注：胸脹喘急，腎脈直行者入腹，支者從肺出絡心注胸，腎氣逆，則有此症，宜泄以降腎氣。少氣不足者，肺統一身之氣，腎爲肺子，子衰則母亦病，補此穴。

Explanation: regarding chest distention and rapid panting, as the vertical pathway of the kidney vessel enters the abdomen, a branch emerges from the lung to network with the heart and pour into the chest; when there is counterflow of the kidney qì, there will be this sign, it is appropriate to drain [this point] in order to descend the kidney qì. For scantness of breath with insufficiency, as the lung controls the qì of the whole body and the kidney is the child of the lung, when the child is debilitated, the mother will also become ill, supplement this point.

洒淅者，肺寒也，肺寒者，子衰也，急補此穴。咽中食噎不得下者，腎脈挾喉嚨，挾舌本，腎有火，故有此症，宜泄。咳而唾、氣逆煩悶，腎爲痰之本，氣逆於肺，則煩悶，急泄此穴。

[Sensation] as though after a soaking is due to lung cold; lung cold is indicative of a debilitated child,[31] urgently supplement this point. Regarding choking of food in the throat that is unable to descend, as the kidney vessel clasps the throat and clasps the root of the tongue, when there is a presence of fire in the kidneys, there will be this sign, it is appropriate to drain [this point]. For coughing with spittle, counterflow of qì, and vexation with oppression, the kidneys are the root of phlegm; in addition, when there is counterflow qì in the lung, there will be vexation and oppression, urgently drain this point.

Fifth Point of the Kidney Channel
Shuǐ Quán – Water Spring (KI-5)
腎經第五穴水泉

穴在太谿下一寸，內踝下，少陰郄。《銅人》：鍼四分，灸五壯。

This point is located 1 cùn below Tài Xī (KI-3), below the inner ankle [bone]. It is the shàoyīn cleft point. *The Tóngrén* states, "Needle 4 fēn, and moxa 5 cones."

注：腎之脈爲大鍾既吸之而上，又折而下行爲水泉，爲少陰郄者，以此穴受大鍾下降之水，腎之脈至此而大見，故爲郄也。

---

[31] I.e., the kidneys.

Explanation: precisely at Dà Zhōng (KI-4), the kidney vessel is syphoned to travel upwards; thereupon, it turns and descends to Shuǐ Quán (Water Spring). Regarding its designation as the shàoyīn cleft point, as this point (KI-5) receives the water that descends from Dà Zhōng (KI-4), once the vessel of the kidneys arrives at this place, it becomes readily visible; therefore, it is the cleft point.

腎之本病：小便淋瀝。

Principal disease of the kidneys: dribbling urination.

注：上症乃腎氣之不足也，補此穴以助腎氣。

Explanation: the above sign is due to insufficiency of the kidney qì, supplement this point in order to assist the kidney qì.

腎之肝病：目眈眈不能視遠，月事不來，陰挺出。

Liver diseases of the kidneys: blurred vision with inability to see distant [objects], absence of menstruation, and vaginal protrusion.

注：目之所以視者，腎之水也，不能遠視，腎水虛也，補之以益腎水。月事不來，肝血虛也，而實腎水之不足，補之以益肝血。陰挺出雖為肝病，取此穴以扶腎水，而不益肝木之邪。

Explanation: what enables the eyes to see is the water of the kidneys; thus, when there is an inability to see distant objects, this is vacuity of the kidney water, supplement this [point] in order to benefit the kidney water. Absence of menstruation is [often attributed to] liver blood vacuity; yet, in this case, it is actually insufficiency of the kidney water, supplement this [point] in order to benefit liver blood. Although vaginal protrusion is a liver disease, choose this point in order to support the kidney water without [mistakenly] increasing the evil of liver wood.[32]

腎之脾病：腹中痛。

Spleen disease of the kidneys: pain in the abdomen.

注：腹者，乃腎脈所行之部分，痛者，腎有邪也，泄此穴以去腎邪。

Explanation: regarding the abdomen, it is indeed the area where the kidney vessel travels; regarding pain [in the abdomen], this is because of the presence of evil in the kidneys, drain this point in order to eliminate the kidney evil.

---

[32] This appears to be an indirect treatment to support liver wood without directly agitating it with liver channel point, where one treats the child by treating the mother.

Sixth Point of the Kidney Channel
Zhào Hǎi – Shining Sea (KI-6)
腎經第六穴照海

穴在內踝下四分，前後有筋，上有踝骨，下有軟骨，其穴居中，陰蹻脈所生。
《素》注：鍼四分，留六呼，灸三壯。《銅人》：鍼三分，灸七莊。《明堂》：
灸三壯。

**This point is located 4 fēn below the inner ankle [bone], with sinews in front
and behind, the ankle bone above, and soft bone[33] below, this point resides in
the middle. It is where the yīnqiāo vessel is engendered.** *The Sùzhù states,*
"**Needle 4 fēn, retain for 6 respirations, and moxa 3 cones.**" *The Tóngrén states,*
"**Needle 3 fēn, and moxa 7 cones.**"[34] *The Míngtáng states,* "**Moxa 3 cones.**"

注：穴名照海者，以此穴又折而上，俯視湧泉、水泉，有海之象焉，而穴
居其上，有以上照下之義，故名曰照海。乃陰蹻脈所生之源，女子以此爲蹻脈，蓋
男子數其陽，女子數其陰，正此穴也。

Explanation: this point is named Zhào Hǎi (Shining Sea), because [the
pathway] turns around at this point, and ascends to look down at Yǒng Quán (KI-1)
and Shuǐ Quán (KI-5); as such, [this point] has an image of the Hǎi (Sea); moreover,
as this point resides above [them], it [also] bears the meaning of Zhào (Shining)
down from the above; therefore, it is called Zhào Hǎi (Shining Sea). Indeed, it is the
source where the yīnqiāo vessel is engendered, which is the qiāo vessel in women;
thus, "in men, the yáng [vessel] is counted, in women, the yīn [vessel] is counted;"[35]
it is precisely referring to this point.

---

[33] I.e., cartilage.

[34] For "7 cones," *the Tóngrén* actually states "3 cones."

[35] From *Língshū* Chapter 17. Note: the "counted" likely refers to a dilemma encountered in
Língshū Chapters 15-17, where its author worked to accommodate for a theoretical
framework of 28 vessels in the body, as stated in *Língshū* Chapter 15, "人經脈上下左右前
後二十八脈，周身十六丈二尺，以應二十八宿。In the above, below, left, right, front, and
rear, the twenty-eight channel-vessels of the human are in total 16 zhàng and 2 chǐ in
length throughout the body, so that they correspond to the twenty-eight constellations of
stars." As the beginning paragraph of *Língshū* Chapter 17 accounts for 26 out of 28 vessels
already (double-counting the 12 vessels as they occur on left and right sides, in addition to
the rèn and dū vessels), leaving only 2 slots for the yīnqiāo and yángqiāo vessels, which
would end up with 30 vessels in total if they are both counted (since both sides have to be
counted). So, to resolve this dilemma, in men, the yángqiāo vessels are counted among the
28 vessels while the yīnqiāo vessels are demoted to network-vessels; in females, the
yīnqiāo vessels are counted among the 28 vessels while the yángqiāo vessels are demoted
to network-vessels. This may be what "counted" means in this paragraph, as well as what
it means by "the qiāo vessel in women" – because according to *Língshū* Chapter 17,
yīnqiāo is the qiāo vessel in women while yángqiāo is the qiāo network-vessel in women.

凡癇之夜發者，則取此穴以灸之。陰蹻脈起於跟中、足少陰然谷之後，同足少陰循內踝下照海穴，上內踝上之二寸，以交信穴爲郄，直上入陰股，循胸裏入缺盆，上出人迎之前，至喉嚨，交貫衝脈，入頄內廉，上行屬目內眥，與手足太陽、足陽明、陽蹻五脈，會於睛明穴而上行，寸口脈後左右彈者，陰蹻脈也。

In general, for epilepsy that occurs at night, choose this point and moxa it. The yīnqiāo vessel commences from within the heel and behind Rán Gǔ (KI-2) of the foot shàoyīn [channel]; together with the foot shàoyīn [channel], it follows Zhào Hǎi (Shining Sea) below the inner ankle [bone], ascends to 2 cùn above the inner ankle [bone], with Jiāo Xìn (KI-8) serving as the cleft [point of the yīnqiāo vessel]. [It continues and] ascends vertically to enter the yīn of the thigh, follows the interior of the chest to enter Quē Pén (ST-12), ascends and emerges in front of Rén Yíng (ST-9), arrives at the throat, intersects and pierces the chōng vessel, enters the inner ridge of the cheekbone, and ascends to adjoin to the inner canthus, where it meets with the five vessels, the hand and foot tàiyáng, foot yángmíng, [yīnqiāo],[36] and yángqiāo [vessels], at Jīng Míng (BL-1); thereupon, it continues to ascend. When the pulse flicking behind the cùnkǒu [position] on both the left and right, this is the yīnqiāo pulse.[37]

張氏曰：蹻者，捷疾也，二脈起於足，使人蹻捷也。陰蹻在肌肉之下，陰脈所行，通貫五脈，主持諸裏，故名爲陰蹻之絡焉。

Mister Zhāng[38] says, "Regarding 'qiāo', it means swift movement; as the two [qiāo] vessels commence from the foot, they allow people to be agile on foot. The yīnqiāo [vessel] is located underneath the flesh, which is where the yīn vessels travel, so that it communicates and pierces the five vessels,[39] as well as takes charge of the interior; thus, it is named as the yīnqiāo network-vessel."[40]

腎之本病：小腹痛，小腹偏痛，淋。

Principal diseases of the kidneys: pain in the lower abdomen, unilateral pain in the lower abdomen, and strangury.

---

[36] Note: The other vessels only add up to four vessels. Yīnqiāo vessel is the fifth and the missing one here, based on the information presented in BL-1.

[37] From *Màijīng* Vol. 10.

[38] The *Qíjīng Bāmài Kǎo* 奇經八脈考 (*An Investigation of the Eight Extraordinary Channels*, 1578 CE) attributes this quote to Zhāng Jiégǔ 張潔古 (commonly known by his given name Zhāng Yuánsù 張元素). Nevertheless, we cannot find this quote in any surviving work by Zhāng Jiégǔ 張潔古.

[39] For "it communicates and pierces the five vessels," the *Qíjīng Bāmài Kǎo* 奇經八脈考 (*An Investigation of the Eight Extraordinary Channels*, 1578 CE) has "it communicates and pierces the five zàng-viscera" instead.

[40] From the *Qíjīng Bāmài Kǎo* 奇經八脈考 (*An Investigation of the Eight Extraordinary Channels*, 1578 CE).

注：腎脈由少腹上行，小腹痛及小腹偏痛，皆腎氣之逆也，宜泄此穴，淋者，膀胱熱也，腎與膀既為表裏，此穴爲腎脈上行之始，宜泄其熱。

Explanation: as the kidney vessel ascends on the lower abdomen, when there is lower abdominal pain as well as unilateral lower abdominal pain, these are both counterflow of kidney qì, it is appropriate to drain this point. Strangury is because of bladder heat; as the kidney and bladder are an exterior-interior [pair], in addition, this point is the beginning of the kidney vessel's ascent, it is appropriate to drain the heat.

腎之肝病：卒疝，不寐，大風默默不知所痛，視如見星，婦女經逆，月水不調，四肢淫濼，四肢怠惰，陰暴跳起或癢，漉清汁，陰挺出，目赤痛自目內眥始。

Liver diseases of the kidneys: sudden mounting,[41] sleeplessness, great wind[42] with taciturnity and lack of awareness to pain, vision as if seeing stars, menstrual counterflow, irregular menstruation, pain and weakness of the four limbs, fatigue of the four limbs, sudden erection and possibly genital itchiness, dripping of clear [vaginal discharge], vaginal protrusion, pain and redness of the eyes that originate from the inner canthus.

注：疝者，肝病也，然未有腎不虛而有此症者，肝腎之部位相近，必兩求之始當。不寐者，腎有邪也，宜泄此穴，大風默默不知所痛，乃風邪中肝之其也，腎者，作強之官，陰蹻脈閉，則一身之動機全息，故默默矣，視如見星者，二蹻之脈，上屬於目，視如見星，陰蹻之脈寒也，故取此穴，以去陰蹻之滯。

Explanation: mounting is a liver disease; however, it is unprecedented to have this sign without kidney vacuity, as the liver and kidney are very close to each other in their [respective] locations; thus, [for this disease], it is only proper to seek both of these. Sleeplessness is due to evil in the kidneys, it is appropriate to drain this point. For great wind, taciturnity, and lack of awareness to pain, these are due to wind evil striking the liver; since the kidneys are the official of action and strength,[43] when yīnqiāo vessel is blocked, the mechanism of movement in the whole body completely ceases, thus there is taciturnity; regarding vision as if seeing stars, as the two qiāo vessels ascend to adjoin with the eyes, when the vision is as if seeing stars, this is cold in the yīnqiāo [vessel], choose this point in order to eliminate the stagnation in the yīnqiāo [vessel].

---

[41] *The Practical Dictionary* defines mounting as, "any of various diseases characterized by pain or swelling of the abdomen, groin, or scrotum."

[42] I.e., leprosy. For which, *Sùwèn* Chapter 55 states, "骨節重，鬚眉墮，名曰大風。 In the presence of heaviness in bones and joints, loss of one's hair and eyebrows, this is called the great wind."

[43] This is referring to *Sùwèn* Chapter 8.

婦人以陰蹻之脈爲主，所以司其經脈之流通也，如經逆、月水不調，皆陰蹻之脈上逆、及衝脈之所爲也，故宜取此穴。四肢淫濼者，火勝水枯也，補此穴以濟水之枯。四肢怠惰，蹻脈有傷，而舉動艱難也，宜取此穴。

Women are governed by the vessel of the yīnqiāo, which is what controls the circulation and flow of the channels; if there is menstrual counterflow or irregular menstruation, both of these are [caused by] ascending counterflow of the yīnqiāo vessel and the action of the chōng vessel,[44] thus it is appropriate to choose this point. Pain and weakness of the four limbs is the prevalence of fire with the exhaustion of water, supplement this point in order to relieve the exhaustion of water. Fatigue of the four limbs is due damage to the qiāo vessels;[45] as a result, there is difficult movement, it is appropriate to choose this point.

陰暴跳起、或癢、漉清汁、陰挺出，皆陰蹻有傷也，宜泄此穴。目赤痛自內眥始，內眥者，睛明穴也，腎與膀胱爲表裏，補腎之陰，即所以退太陽之陽也。

For sudden erection and possibly genital itchiness, dripping of clear [vaginal discharge], and vaginal protrusion, these are all due to damage to the yīnqiāo [vessel], it is appropriate to drain this point. For pain and redness of the eyes that originate from the inner canthus, the inner canthus is [the location of] Jīng Míng (BL-1); as the kidney and bladder are an exterior-interior [pair], supplementing the yīn of the kidneys is precisely what allows one to abate the yáng of tàiyáng.

腎之脾病：嘔吐嗜臥，唏。

Spleen diseases of the kidneys: retching and vomiting, somnolence, and gasping.

注：嘔吐不止者，腎氣上逆也，嗜臥，則蹻脈有傷，而懶於動矣，但取此穴，以降上逆之氣，而調舉動之機。

Explanation: incessant retching and vomiting is counterflow ascent of the kidney qì; as for somnolence, as there is damage to the qiāo vessels, the person becomes too lazy to move, choose only this point in order to descend the counterflow ascent of qì, so that the mechanism of lifting and moving can be regulated.

唏者，陰氣盛而陽氣虛，陰氣疾而陽氣徐，陰氣勝陽氣絶所致也，當泄此穴，補申脈穴。

---

[44] Alternatively, since 及 can be read as "and" as well as "reach," this line can be read as, "both of these are caused by the ascending counterflow of the yīnqiāo vessel, which has affected the chōng vessel."

[45] This could be read as vessel (i.e., only the yīnqiāo vessel) or vessels (i.e., both the yīnqiāo vessel and yángqiāo vessels), as the nouns in Chinese are not designated as singular or plural.

For gasping, the yīn qì is exuberant while the yáng qì is vacuous; since the yīn qì manifests with racing [qì] while the yáng qì manifest with steady [qì], [gasping] is caused by the prevalence of yīn qì and the expiration of yáng qì, one should drain this point and supplement Shēn Mài (BL-62).[46]

腎之肺病：咽乾，心悲不樂。

Lung diseases of the kidneys: dry pharynx, sorrow and unhappiness in the heart.

注：咽乾者，以腎之經上循咽喉，腎火上逆則咽乾，泄之。心悲不樂，乃肺之燥也，肺爲腎母，母病及子，乃蹻脈不上昇，心腎不交，而肺有此症，補此穴以交心腎。

Explanation: dry pharynx is because the kidney channel ascends to follow the pharynx and throat; thus, when there is counterflow ascent of kidney fire, there will be dry pharynx, drain this [point]. Sorrow and unhappiness in the heart is dryness of the lung, as the lung is the mother of the kidneys, this is the mother's disease affecting the child; because the qiāo vessel fails to ascend, the heart and kidney are unable to interact, hence this sign occurs in the lung, supplement this point in order to [promote] interaction between the heart and kidney.

Seventh Point of the Kidney Channel
Fù Liū – Recover Flow (KI-7)
腎經第七穴復溜

一名伏白
Alternate name: Deep-Lying White

一名昌陽
Alternate name: Glorious Yáng

穴在內踝上二寸，筋骨陷中，前傍骨，是復溜，後傍筋，是交信，二穴只隔一條筋，足少陰腎脈所行爲經金，腎虛補之。《素》注：鍼三分，留七呼，灸五壯。《明堂》：灸七壯。

This point is located 2 cùn above the inner ankle [bone], in the depression [between] the sinew and bone; whereas Fù Liū (KI-7) is in front and beside this bone, Jiāo Xìn (KI-8) is behind and beside the sinew, these two points are only separated by the sinew.[47] The foot shàoyīn kidney vessel flows here, as

---

[46] I.e., the yángqiāo vessel.
[47] Lit. separated by one strip of sinew.

the river and metal point. When the kidney is vacuous, supplement this [point]. *The Sùzhù* states, "Needle 3 fēn, retain for 7 respirations,[48] and moxa 5 cones." *The Míngtáng* states, "Moxa 7 cones."

注：此穴承照海之脈而上行，流而不居，故曰復溜。又脈絶者，取此穴則脈生，亦有復溜之義。與交信穴共居一處，止隔一條筋，亦有復溜之義，乃腎經離踝上行之第一穴也，其脈動而不休，故爲經。

Explanation: the vessel ascends from Zhào Hǎi (KI-6) and continues to this point, as it Liū (Flows) and does not remain idle, thus it is called Fù Liū (Recover Flow). Also, when the pulse is expired, by choosing this point, the pulse can be restored, that is also the meaning of Fù Liū (Recover Flow). Together with Jiāo Xìn (KI-8), they both reside in the same place, only separated by one strip of sinew, this is also the meaning of Fù Liū (Recover Flow), because this is the first point of the ascending kidney channel as it departs from the [inner] ankle [bone]. As this vessel pulsates ceaselessly, thus it is the river[49] [point].

腎之本病：腰脊引痛，不得俯仰起坐，足痿不收履，胻寒不自溫，五淋血淋，小便如散火，骨寒熱，脈微細或時無脈。

Principal diseases of the kidneys: pain that radiates between the lumbus and spine, inability to bend forward and backward or stand and sit, wilting of the legs with inability to contract one's feet, coldness of the lower leg that fails to become warm by itself, five stranguries and blood strangury, urination that feels as though it is scattered fire, heat and cold of the bones, faint and fine pulse or the periodic absence of the pulse.

注：腰脊引痛，不得俯仰起坐，乃腎氣上逆，腰脊既爲腎府，而又爲膀胱、腎經表裏之所，故泄之，以降腎經之逆，若遇春時無見血，若見血，則腎氣不能復，以春木旺則水衰也，足痿不收履，胻寒不自溫，皆腎氣之滯而不行也，取此穴以通腎氣。

Explanation: for pain that radiates between the lumbus and spine, as well as inability to bend forwards and backwards or stand and sit, this is due to counterflow ascent of kidney qì; the lumbus and spine are not only the residence of the kidneys, but also the location for the exterior-interior [pair] of the bladder and kidney channels, thus drain this [point] in order to descend the counterflow of the kidney channel. When one [utilises this point] in spring, one must not cause bleeding; if bleeding occurs, one will not be able to recover[50] the kidney qì; this is because in

---

[48] For "7 respirations," *the Sùzhù* actually states "3 respirations."

[49] In early literature, the character jīng 經 (channel/river point) can also be defined as "great rivers" or "regular" as something that is constantly present. Here, Yuè Hánzhēn likely refers to the early definition.

[50] "Recovered" likely refers to the point name Fù 復.

spring, wood is effulgent, thus water is debilitated. For wilting of the legs and inability to contract one's feet, coldness of the lower leg that fails to become warm by itself, both of these are due to the lack of kidney qì movement because of stagnation, choose this point in order to free the kidney qì.

五淋血淋，小便如散火，腎之火熱所致也，泄之以去其腎熱。寒熱至於骨，則病入裏，非取腎之穴，不足以致之。取復溜者何也？以此穴爲腎脈上行之始，有生脈之力，故取此穴，以定其寒熱。脈雖屬心，而所以生脈之根，乃腎爲之主，此穴乃腎脈上行之始，其力甚銳，故有生脈之力，故脈微細無見，或時無脈者，則補此穴以生脈焉。

For five stranguries and blood strangury, urination that feels as though it is burning hot, these are a result of the fire and heat in the kidneys, drain this point in order to eliminate the kidney heat. Regarding cold and heat that has reached the bones, the disease has entered the interior; as such, without choosing the kidney points, it will not be enough to produce an effect. Why should one choose Fù Liū (KI-7)? Because this point is where the kidney vessel begins to ascend, it has the power to revive the pulse, thus choose this point in order to stabilize heat and cold. Although the vessels belong to the heart, however, the kidneys govern the root of that which revives the pulse; as this point is where the kidney vessel begins to ascend, its force is extremely vigorous, thus it has the power to revive the pulse; therefore, when the pulse is faint and thin or absent in observation, or when the pulse is periodically absent, supplement this point in order to revive the pulse.

腎之肝病：目視眈眈，善怒。

Liver diseases of the kidneys: blurred vision and frequent anger.

注：目視眈眈眛者，腎水不足也，補此穴以益腎水。善怒者，肝有餘也，子有餘則泄其母。

Explanation: blurred vision is due to insufficiency of kidney water, supplement this point in order to boost kidney water. Frequent anger is due to superabundance of the liver, when the child is superabundant, drain the mother.

腎之脾病：胃熱，蟲動涎出，腹中雷鳴，腹脹如鼓，四肢腫，五種水病，青、黃、赤、白、黑，青取井，赤取滎，黃取腧，白取經，黑取合。如白水，則取此經之經穴，泄後腫，齒齲。

Spleen diseases of the kidneys: stomach heat, stirring of worms and drooling of spittle, thunderous rumbling in the abdomen, drum-like abdominal distention, and swelling of the four limbs. For the five types of water disease: green-blue, yellow, red, white, or black, when it is green-blue, choose the well point; when it is red, choose the spring point; when it is yellow, choose the stream point; when it is white, choose the river point; when it is black, choose

the uniting point. If there is white water [disease], then choose the river point of this channel.[51] [It also treats] swelling after diarrhoea, and tooth decay.

注：胃熱者，腎脈挾胃氣上行，氣有餘所致，宜泄。蟲動涎出者，涎爲腎之液，腎氣上行，則鼓涎上溢，而胃中之蟲，亦隨氣而動，故涎出焉，宜泄之以降腎氣。

Explanation: regarding stomach heat, as the kidney vessel clasps the stomach, when there is an ascent of qì, [stomach heat] will occur due to the superabundance of qì, which is caused by the qì ascent of the kidney vessel that clasps the stomach, it is appropriate to drain [this point]. Regarding stirring of worms and drooling of spittle, as drool is the fluid of the kidneys,[52] when kidney qì ascends, it stirs the drool to spill upwards; in addition, worms in the stomach will also move by following the qì; thus, drool will be ejected, it is appropriate to drain this [point] in order to descend kidney qì.

腹中雷鳴、腹脹如鼓，皆腎之逆氣也，泄之以降腎氣。腎爲水之本，白取經者，以經爲金，其色白，故取經穴以泄水。泄後腫者，水氣有餘也，泄之。齒齲，乃陽明經症，而取此穴者，以齒爲腎骨之餘，泄之以降腎火。

For thunderous rumbling in the abdomen and drum-like abdominal distension, these are both due to counterflow qì of the kidneys, drain this [point] in order to descend qì. As the kidneys are the root of water, for one to choose the river point in the presence of white [water disease], this is because the river point is metal, which is white in colour, thus choose the river point in order to drain water [diseases]. Swelling after diarrhoea is due to superabundance of water qì, drain this [point]. As tooth decay is a yángmíng channel sign, for one to choose this point, this is because "the teeth are the abundance of the bones,"[53] [which are governed by] the kidneys, drain this [point] in order to descend kidney fire.

腎之心病：舌乾多言。

Heart disease of the kidneys: dry tongue and being overly talkative.

注：腎脈挾舌本，火有餘則舌乾，泄之以降腎火，多言者，水不足而心火勝也，補之以助腎水。

---

[51] This long sentence regarding the five types of water disease seems to be an inline annotation inserted into this passage, which can possibly explain the reason why it seems out of place along with other indications.

[52] This statement may be an error as according to *Sùwèn* Chapter 23, 涎 drool belongs to the spleen, while 唾 spittle belongs to the kidneys; however, *Nànjīng* Difficulty 44 does state the kidneys govern the body fluids.

[53] This seems to be a paraphrase of *Sùwèn* Chapter 1 commentary by Wáng Bīng, where he noted, "齒爲骨之餘也 the teeth, they are the abundance of the bones."

Explanation: as the kidney vessel clasps the root of the tongue, when there is superabundance of fire, the tongue will be dry, drain this [point] in order to descend kidney fire. When one is overly talkative, this is prevalence of heart fire due to insufficiency of water, supplement this [point] in order to assist kidney water.

腎之肺病：盜汗不止，腸澼，血痔。

Lung diseases of the kidneys: incessant night sweats, intestinal aggregation, and bleeding haemorrhoids

注：盜汗不止，陰氣虛也，腎虛火動而衛熱，故有此症，泄之以降腎火。腸澼，下焦之氣不能運也，下焦之氣主腎肝，取此穴以運腎氣，而動腸中之積，使流轉而不停滯。血痔雖大腸病，而實下焦之火妄動所致，宜泄此穴，以降下焦之火。

Explanation: incessant night sweats is vacuity of yīn qì, when the kidneys are vacuous with fire stirring, it will lead to heat in the wèi-defence [aspect]; as such, there will be this sign, drain this [point] in order to descend kidney fire. Intestinal aggregation is because the qì of the lower jiāo fails to be transported; as the qì of the lower jiāo is governed by the kidneys and liver, choose this point in order to transport the kidney qì, so that it will move the accumulations in the intestines and circulate [the kidney qì] to prohibit lodging and stagnation. Although bleeding haemorrhoids is a large intestine disease, this is actually a result of frenetic stirring of fire in the lower jiāo, it is appropriate to drain this point in order to descend the fire of the lower jiāo.

Eighth Point of the Kidney Channel
Jiāo Xìn – Intersection Fidelity[54] (KI-8)
腎經第八穴交信

穴亦在足內踝上二寸，少陰前，太陰後廉，筋骨間，陰蹻脈之郄。《銅人》：鍼四分，留十呼，灸三壯。

This point is also located 2 cùn above the inner ankle [bone], in front of the shàoyīn [channel], on the ridge behind the tàiyīn [channel], and between the sinew and bone; it is the cleft point of the yīnqiāo vessel. *The Tóngrén* states, "Needle 4 fēn, retain for 10 respirations,[55] and moxa 3 cones."

---

[54] *Grasping the Wind* names it "Intersection Reach." Note: for Xìn 信, we are translating it as fidelity in accordance with the explanation below.

[55] *The Tóngrén* actually states "5 respirations" instead of "10 respirations" listed above.

注：穴名交信者，按各經之穴，皆未有一經之穴，兩穴並立一處者，此穴
與復溜，俱在內踝上二寸，僅隔一條筋，一在筋裏，一在筋外，有交之義焉。脈之
細微不見，取復溜，女人之月事不來，取交信，有信之義焉，故曰交信。

Explanation: this point is named Jiāo Xìn (Intersection Fidelity), because from my observation, for the points on every channel, it is unprecedented that two points for a single channel would be located side by side at the same place. This point and Fù Liū (KI-7) are both located 2 cùn above the inner ankle [bone], only separated by one strip of sinew – one of them is located in front of the sinew, while the other one is located behind the sinew – thus, there is the meaning of Jiāo (Intersection). For a pulse that is fine or faint, or cannot be observed, choose Fù Liū (KI-7); for absence of menses in females, choose Jiāo Xìn (Intersection Fidelity), as it carries the meaning of Xìn (Fidelity),[56] thus it is called Jiāo Xìn (Intersection Fidelity).

又爲陰蹻之郄。陰蹻之脈，始見於照海，上內踝上二寸，而再會於此穴，
直上循陰股，入陰股，上循胸裏，入缺盆，上出人迎之前，至喉嚨，交貫衝脈，入
頄內廉，上行屬目內眥，與手、足太陽、足陽明、陽蹻五脈，會於睛明穴而上行
焉。

Furthermore, it is the cleft point of the yīnqiāo. The vessel of the yīnqiāo is first observed at Zhào Hǎi (KI-6), it continues to ascend to 2 cùn above the inner ankle [bone], and meets at this point;[57] [it continues and] ascends vertically following the yīn of the thigh, enters the yīn of the thigh, follows the interior of the chest to enter Quē Pén (ST-12), ascends and emerges in front of Rén Yíng (ST-9), arrives at the throat, intersects and pierces the chōng vessel, enters the inner ridge of the cheekbone, and ascends to adjoin to the inner canthus, where it meets with the five vessels, the hand and foot tàiyáng, foot yángmíng channels, [yīnqiāo],[58] and yángqiāo [vessels], at Jīng Míng (BL-1); thereupon, it continues to ascend.

腎之本病：氣淋，氣熱癃，股內樞痛，大小便難，女子漏血不止，月事不來，小
腹偏痛。

Principal diseases of the kidneys: qì strangury, qì heat with dribbling urination, pain at the joint of the inner thigh, difficult urination and defecation, incessant spotting of blood in women, absence of menstruation, and unilateral pain in the lower abdomen.

---

[56] Based on the context, this "信 fidelity" here likely refers to "月信 monthly fidelity" (i.e., menses), which means "按月而至，如潮有信。 that which arrives monthly, just as tides occur with fidelity."

[57] I.e., KI-8.

[58] Note: The other vessels only add up to four vessels. Yīnqiāo vessel is the fifth and the missing one here, based on the information presented in BL-1.

注：氣淋及諸淋，皆腎之熱也，取此穴以泄腎火而去熱。氣熱則癃，亦腎熱也，亦宜泄此穴。股內樞，腎之部分也，被寒則痛，泄此穴以去腎之寒邪。

Explanation: regarding qì strangury and other types of stranguries, they are all due to heat of the kidneys, choose this point in order to drain kidney fire and eliminate the heat. With heat in the qì [aspect], there is dribbling urination, which is also kidney heat, it is also appropriate to drain this point. Regarding the joint of the inner thigh, this is the area of the kidneys; when it contracts cold, there will be pain, drain this point in order to eliminate the cold evil in the kidney [channel].

三焦司二便，爲決瀆之官，右腎將之，二便難，乃腎氣不調也，取此穴以調腎氣。

The sānjiāo controls urination and defecation, it is the official of dredging the sluices, which is commanded by the right kidney; when one has difficulty in urinating and defecating, this is due to discord of the kidney qì, choose this point in order to regulate kidney qì.

女子漏下不止，宜補此穴，以止其滑脫。月事不來，腹偏痛，乃血之凝也，又宜泄此穴，以通其滯，此穴專主女子月事者，以腎主下焦之血也。

For incessant spotting of blood in women, it is appropriate to supplement this point in order to stop efflux desertion. Regarding absence of menstruation and unilateral abdominal pain, these are due to congealed blood; for both [diseases], it is appropriate to drain this point in order to free the stagnation; this point specialises in governing women's menstruation [diseases], because the kidney governs the blood of the lower jiāo.

腎之肝病：癩疝，陰急，婦人陰挺出。

Liver diseases of the kidneys: slumping mounting,[59] genital tension, and vaginal protrusion.

注：三症皆肝病也，而取此穴者，以腎爲水母，母之邪盛，則泄母即所以泄子也。

Explanation: these three signs are all liver diseases, hence choose this point because the kidney is the water and mother [of the liver]; when the evil of the mother is exuberant, drain the mother so as to drain the child.

腎之脾病：四肢淫濼。

Spleen disease of the kidneys: pain and weakness in the four limbs.

注：上症乃水不足，而火有餘也，補此穴，使水上行以救火。

---

[59] According to *the Practical Dictionary*, "癩疝 slumping mounting" is a "condition of the yīn sac (scrotum) characterized by swelling, ulceration, and flowing forth of pus and blood."

Explanation: the above sign is superabundance of fire due to insufficiency of water, supplement this point to ascend water in order to stem fire.

腎之肺病：泄利赤白，盜汗。

Lung diseases of the kidneys: red and white diarrhoea, and night sweats.

注：赤白利，乃大腸瘀熱也，大腸雖與肺爲表裏，而腎實司二便，下焦之熱，亦熱火有餘也，泄此穴以清下焦之火。盜汗者，榮血虛，而衛氣不周也，必寐中之火動，而始致之，取此穴以清陰血之火。

Explanation: red and white diarrhoea is because of stasis and heat in the large intestine; although the large intestine and the lung are an exterior-interior [pair], yet, it is the kidneys that actually control urination and defecation; as heat of the lower jiāo is also a superabundance of heat and fire, drain this point in order to clear the fire of the lower jiāo. Night sweats is failure of the wèi-defensive qì to circulate due to vacuity of the yíng-nutritive blood;[60] thus, this certainly occur after fire is stirred during sleep, choose this point in order to clear the fire in the yīn and blood.

Nineth Point of the Kidney Channel
Zhú Bīn – Guest House (KI-9)
腎經第九穴築賓

穴在內踝上腨分中，陰維之郄。《銅人》：鍼三分，留五呼，灸五壯。《素》注：鍼三分，灸五壯。

This point is located above the inner ankle [bone] on the calf aspect, it is the cleft point of the yīnwéi [vessel]. *The Tóngrén* **states, "Needle 3 fēn, retain for 5 respirations,[61] and moxa 5 cones."** *The Sùzhù* **states, "Needle 3 fēn, and moxa 5 cones."**

注：足少陰腎之經，而陰維始於此，有賓之象焉。維者，所以維內防出也，有牆之象，有築之義，故曰築賓。又陰維由踝而上循陰分，而上脇至咽，行於榮分諸陰之交，其所會之經，則足太陰脾也，足厥陰肝也，本出之經，足少陰腎也，足陽明胃也，而俱會於脾經之府舍穴焉。

---

[60] The text actually states "榮 róng-nutritive," however, as yíng and róng are often used interchangeably to represent the nutritive aspect, so we have followed the modern convention and rendered it as yíng instead.

[61] "Retain for 5 five respirations" is absent in *the Tóngrén*.

Explanation: this is the channel of the foot shàoyīn kidneys, yet, the yīnwéi [vessel] begins at this [point]; thus, it has the image of a Bīn (Guest). The wéi[62] [vessel] is that which links the interior together to prevent it from emerging outwards, which has the image of walls and carries the meaning of Zhú (House); therefore, it is called Zhú Bīn (Guest House). Also, from the ankle [bone], the yīnwéi ascends following the yīn aspects [of the body], it continues to ascend the rib-sides to arrive at the pharynx. It travels in the yíng-nutritive aspect where it intersects with all of the yīn [channels]; for the channels it meets, there is the foot tàiyīn spleen and foot juéyīn liver; for the channels that it emerges from, there is the foot shàoyīn kidney and foot yángmíng stomach, both of which meet [with the yīnwéi vessel] at Fǔ Shè (SP-13) of the spleen channel.

府舍穴在脾經腹結穴下二寸，去中行四寸半，又上行，會足太陰於大橫、腹哀。大橫穴在腹哀下三寸五分，腹哀在日月下一寸五分，二穴俱去中行各四寸半。日月乃膽經穴，在期門下五分。又循脅肋，會足厥陰肝經之期門，在乳下二肋端，不容旁一寸五分，肝之募也，乃足厥陰、太陰、陰維之會。

Fǔ Shè (SP-13) is located 2 cùn below Fù Jié (SP-14) of the spleen channel, at 4 and a half cùn from the midline; [after the yīnwéi vessel re-emerges at Fǔ Shè (SP-13)], it continues to ascend, meeting with Dà Héng (SP-15) and Fù Āi (SP-16) of the foot tàiyīn [channel]. Dà Héng (SP-15) is located 3 cùn 5 fēn below Fù Āi (SP-16) on the abdomen; Fù Āi (SP-16) is located 1 cùn 5 fēn below Rì Yuè (GB-24); these two points are both 4 and a half cùn from the midline. Rì Yuè (GB 24) is a gallbladder channel point, it is located 5 fēn below Qí Mén (LR-14); [after these points], it follows the rib-sides, meets with Qī Mén (LR-14) of the foot juéyīn liver channel, which is located at the tip of the two [floating] ribs below the breast, at 1 cùn 5 fēn to the side of Bù Róng (ST-19), which is the gathering point of the liver and the meeting of foot juéyīn, tàiyīn [channels], and yīnwéi [vessel].

又上行胸膈挾咽，與任脈會於天突、廉泉，至項前而終。觀陰維之行，始於足少陰築賓之穴，而上會足三陰，並足陽明胃經，而上行於小腹、脅肋、胸膈，與任脈會於天突、廉泉，皆維於諸陰之脈，主乎榮，而司乎裏者也。

[The yīnwéi vessel] continues and ascends through the chest and diaphragm, clasping the pharynx while meeting with Tiān Tū (REN-22) and Lián Quán (REN-23) of the rèn vessel, and arrives at the front of the nape and terminates. Consider the pathway of the yīnwéi [vessel], it commences at the point Zhú Bīn (Guest House) of the foot shàoyīn [channel] and ascends to meet with the three foot yīn [channels] as well as the foot yángmíng stomach channel. It continues and ascends through the lower abdomen, rib-sides, diaphragm, and chest, thereupon meeting with Tiān Tū (REN-22) and Lián Quán (REN-23) of the rèn vessel. As such, [the yīnwéi vessel]

---

[62] Note: This character, "wéi 維," have been translated as link/linking when it is not used in conjunction with the vessel.

links all of the yīn vessels together, governs the yíng-nutritive, and controls the interior.

故陰維爲病苦心痛，所以然者，陰維之脈，雖交三陰，而實與任脈同歸，故心痛多屬少陰、厥陰、任脈之經，上衝而然。按之少止者爲虛，不可近者爲實。又陰維不能維於陰，則悵然失志。

Thus, when the yīnwéi [vessel] is diseased, one will suffer from heart pain; the reason why it occurs is that although the vessel of the yīnwéi communicates with the three yīn [vessels], it actually converges with the rèn vessel; therefore, heart pain is commonly caused by an upsurge in the channels of shàoyīn and juéyīn as well as the rèn vessel. If [the heart pain] is alleviated upon placing pressure [to the chest], that is vacuity; if [the chest] cannot be touched, that is repletion. Moreover, when the yīnwéi [vessel] is unable to link the yīn [channels] together, there will be disappointment and frustration with loss of will.

陰維之脈，從少陰斜至厥陰，是陰維脈也，診得陰維脈，沉大而實者，苦胸中痛，脇下支滿。其脈如貫珠者，男子兩脇下實，腰中痛，女子陰中痛，如有瘡狀。

As for the pulse of the yīnwéi, it stretches obliquely from the shàoyīn to the juéyīn,[63] this is the yīnwéi pulse. When one is diagnosed with a yīnwéi pulse that is deep and large with repletion, [that person] will suffer from pain in the chest and propping fullness below the rib-sides. When the pulse resembles a string of pearls, in men there will be repletion below both of the rib-sides and pain of the lumbus; in women there will be pain in the genitals as if there were sores.

《內經》云：飛揚之脈，令人腰痛，怫怫然，甚則悲以恐。王氏注云：此陰維脈也，在內踝上五寸腨分中，並足少陰經而上也，乃築賓穴也。

The Nèijīng states, "When the vessel of Fēi Yáng (BL-58) appears,[64] the person will have lumbar pain, depression and dejection; when it is severe, there will be sorrow that leads to fear."[65] To this, Mister Wáng [Bīng] commentates, "This is the yīnwéi vessel; located 5 cùn above the inner ankle [bone] on the calf,[66] it ascends with the foot shàoyīn channel." Of which, he refers to Zhú Bīn (Guest House).

---

[63] I.e., from the guān (bar) to the chǐ (cubit) pulse positions on left arm.

[64] Note: based on the context of this chapter of Sùwèn, this is a blood vessel, varicosity, or abnormity in pulsation, skin colour, temperature, or texture that will appear around the location of BL-58 in the presence of a disease.

[65] From Sùwèn Chapter 41.

[66] "內踝上五寸腨分中 5 cùn above the inner ankle [bone] on the calf" is originally "內踝上五分腨肉中 5 fēn above the inner ankle [bone] within the flesh of calf" in the primary manuscript. The editors of this manuscript, Zhāng and Zhà, have amended it according to the secondary manuscript and the Sùzhù.

由中行而數之，任之外，爲足少陰，則衝脈上行之分也，而陰蹻之直行者，亦在乎此，而少陰之外，則爲足陽明下行之胃經，胃經外乃足太陰上行之脾經，而陰維自腎之築賓上行入腹者，乃同脾經而上行也，至脾之府舍與肝經會，又上行而與肝之期門會，乃遠而入裏，與任之天突、廉泉會而終焉，此陰維自下而上行之部分也。

To count it from the midline, outside of the rèn [vessel], it is the foot shàoyīn, which is the area where the chōng vessel ascends; in addition, the vertical pathway of the yīnqiāo [vessel] is also located here. Moreover, on the outside of the shàoyīn [channel], it is the descending pathway of the foot yángmíng stomach channel; on the outside of the stomach channel, it is the ascending pathway of the foot tàiyīn spleen channel. For the ascending pathway of the yīnwéi [vessel] that commences from Zhú Bīn (Guest House) to enter the abdomen, it ascends together with the spleen channel; upon arriving at Fǔ Shè (SP-13) of the spleen [channel], it meets with the liver channel; it continues to ascend to meet with Qī Mén (LR-14) of the liver [channel]. Thereupon, it winds around and enters the interior, meeting with Tiān Tū (REN-22) and Lián Quán (REN-23) of the rèn [vessel], where it terminates. These are the areas where the yīnwéi [vessel pathway] ascends and travels through from the below.

腎之本病：足腨痛。

Principal disease of the kidneys: foot and calf pain.

注：足腨乃本經穴部分，陰維、腎經，受清濕則痛，泄之以去其清濕。

Explanation: the foot and calf are the areas where this channel [travels] and [moreover] where this point [is located]; when the yīnwéi [vessel] and kidney channel contract cool damp, there will be pain; drain it in order to eliminate the cool damp.

腎之肝病：癲疝，小兒胎疝痛，不得乳，癲疾狂易，妄言怒罵。

Liver diseases of the kidneys: downfall mounting, infantile foetal mounting and pain, inability to breastfeed, epileptic disease and mania, raving and angry shouting.

注：凡疝病，皆不宜責腎，以腎脈由少腹上行，與厥陰肝經會，故取此穴，以泄肝木之母也。癲疾屬陰，陰維所主在裏，故取此穴。

Explanation: for all mounting diseases, it is never appropriate to blame the kidneys; however, from the lower abdomen, the kidney vessel ascends to meet with the juéyīn liver channel, thus choose this point in order to drain the mother of liver wood. Epileptic disease and mania belong to yīn, as the yīnwéi [vessel] governs the interior, thus choose this point.

腎之脾病：嘔吐涎沫。

Spleen disease of the kidneys: vomiting with spitting of drool and foam.

注：陰經會脾脈於府舍，陰維有邪及於脾，故取此穴，以泄脾中之濕。

Explanation: as the yīn channels meet with the spleen vessel at Fǔ Shè (SP-13), when there is a presence of evil in the yīnwéi [vessel] it will affect the spleen, thus choose this point in order to drain the dampness within the spleen.

腎之心病：吐舌。

Heart disease of the liver: protrusion of the tongue.

注：陰維會任之天突、廉泉，有邪及於任則吐舌，故取此穴，以泄陰維之逆。

Explanation: the yīnwéi [vessel] meets with Tiān Tū (REN-22) and Lián Quán (REN-23) of the rèn [vessel]; therefore, when the evil affects the rèn [vessel], there will be protrusion of the tongue, thus choose this point in order to drain the counterflow of the yīnwéi [vessel].

Tenth Point of the Kidney Channel
Yīn Gǔ – Yīn Valley (KI-10)
腎經第十穴陰谷

穴在膝內輔骨後，大筋下，小筋上，動脈應手，屈膝乃得之，足少陰脈所入爲合水。《銅人》：鍼四分，留七呼，灸三壯。

This point is located behind the assisting bone on the inside of the knee,[67] below the large sinew, above the small sinew, where the pulsating vessel resonates with the hand; bend the knee to locate it. The foot shàoyīn vessel enters here, as the uniting and water point. *The Tóngrén* states, "Needle 4 fēn, retain for 7 respirations, and moxa 3 cones."

注：此穴爲少陰經所入，衝脈由上而下行者，亦由於此。陰維脈由下而上行者，亦由於此，並本經之上行者，俱入於此穴。谷，言其深也；陰，言衆陰之所聚也，故曰陰谷。又少陰爲一身水之本，水之所入而合者，非谷而何。

Explanation: this point is the place where the shàoyīn channel enters; in addition, the descending pathway of the chōng vessel also passes through here from above; moreover, the ascending pathway of the yīnwéi vessel also passes through

---

[67] Note: The assisting bone is namely the fibula.

here, where it joins with the ascending pathway of this channel;[68] all of them enter this point. Gǔ (Valley) is speaking of its depth, while Yīn (Yīn) is referring to the gathering of the multitude of yīn [vessels], thus it is called Yīn Gǔ (Yīn Valley). In addition, the shàoyīn is the foundation of the entire body's water; for the place where water enters and unites, how can it be anything else but a Gǔ (Valley)?

腎之本病：膝痛如錐刺，不得屈伸，小便難，急引陰痛，陰痿，股內廉痛，婦人漏下不止，腹脹滿不得息，小便黃，男子如蠱，女子如娠。

Principal diseases of the kidneys: knee pain that resembles being stabbed by an awl, inability to bend and stretch [the knee], difficult urination, tension and pain that radiate to the genitals, genital wilting, pain in the inner aspect of the thigh, incessant spotting, abdominal distension and fullness with inability to breathe, yellow urine, resemblance of gǔ in males,[69] and resemblance of pregnancy in females.

注：膝痛如錐刺，不得屈伸，本穴部分受邪也，宜取此穴，以去其邪。小便難而急引陰痛，皆腎氣不調，泄此穴以通其氣。陰痿，腎氣不足也，補此穴以助腎氣。股內廉痛，亦部分之氣逆也，泄之。婦人漏下不止，則腎氣脫，宜補此穴。腹脹、如蠱如娠，俱腎經及陰維之氣上逆，而皆聚於小腹，宜泄以舒其氣。

Explanation: for knee pain that resembles being stabbed by an awl, and inability to bend and stretch [the knee], the area of this point has contracted the evil, it is thus appropriate to choose this point in order to eliminate the evil. For difficult urination that leads to tension and pain that radiates to the genitals, in all cases, this is discord of the kidney qì, drain this point in order to free the qì. Genital wilting is because of kidney qì insufficiency, supplement this point in order to assist kidney qì. Pain in the inner aspect of the thigh is also due to qì counterflow of this area, drain this [point]. When there is incessant spotting in women, there will be kidney qì desertion, it is appropriate to supplement this point. For abdominal distension that resembles gǔ [in males] or pregnancy [in females], both are due to gathering in the lower abdomen caused by counterflow qì ascent of the kidney channel and yīnwéi [vessel], it is appropriate to drain this point in order to soothe the qì.

---

[68] I.e., the kidney channel.

[69] Gǔ 蠱 is Yìjīng's hexagram 18 (correcting), which is depicted with the mountain trigram above and the wind trigram below. The mountain is yáng on the above and in the exterior but is yīn and hollow inside. This is an imagery of a type of fullness that is hollow inside, like a drum. For the lower trigram, the movement of wind is being obstructed by the mountain above, this is obstruction of qì. As such, we speculate this to be a drum-like distension and fullness with qì stagnation and an unknown origin.

Eleventh Point of the Kidney Channel
Héng Gǔ – Transverse Bone[70] (KI-11)
腎經第十一穴橫骨

一名下極

Alternate name: Lower Extreme

穴在大赫下一寸，陰上橫骨中，宛曲如仰月中央，去腹中行各一寸。《銅人》：
灸三壯，禁鍼。

This point is located 1 cùn below Dà Hè (KI-12), on the transverse bone above the genitals, in the middle of where it winds like an upturned moon, 1 cùn on each side of the abdominal midline. *The Tóngrén* **states, "Moxa 3 cones, and needling is contraindicated."[71]**

注：腎經由股後廉直上，行至此穴，則橫入裏行，故曰橫骨。始接衝脈之由胞向外，浮而上行者會。蓋衝脈自胞中發源分三歧，一由脊裏上行，一由胞中浮而外出，起於足陽明氣衝穴，在小腹毛中兩旁各二寸，橫骨兩端，動脈宛宛中，歷大赫、四滿、中注、肓腧、商曲、石關、陰都、通谷、幽門，至胸中而散，又會於咽喉，別而繞唇口。

Explanation: from the outer ridge of the thigh, the kidney channel ascends vertically to arrive at this point; thereupon, [it travels] Héng (Transversely) to the interior, thus it is called Héng Gǔ (Transverse Bone). It is the first [point] that meets with the ascending pathway of the chōng vessel, which moves outwards from the womb and floats to the surface. Undoubtedly, from within the womb, the chōng vessel emerges to split into three pathways: One ascends along the interior of the spine. Another one floats outwards and emerges from within the womb, it commences at Qì Chōng (ST-30) of the foot yángmíng, which is located at 2 cùn on each side of the lower abdomen [midline] at the [pubic] hair, at the tips of the pubic bone, in the depression of the pulsating vessel. It then passes through Dà Hè (KI-12), Sì Mǎn (KI-14), Zhōng Zhù (KI-15), Huāng Shù (KI-16), Shāng Qū (KI-17), Shí Guān (KI-18), Yīn Dū (KI-19), Tōng Gǔ (KI-20), and Yōu Mén (KI-21), arrives at the chest and dissipates. It further meets at the pharynx and throat, then diverges to encircle the lips.

岐伯曰：衝脈者，五臟六腑之海也。其上者出於頏顙，滲諸陽，灌諸經；其下者，著於少陰之大絡，起於腎下，出於氣衝，循陰股內廉，斜入膕中，伏行骭骨內廉，並少陰之經，入內踝之後，入足下，其別者，並於少陰，滲三陰，斜入

---

[70] *Grasping the Wind* names it "Pubic Bone."
[71] "Needling is contraindicated" is actually absent in *the Tóngrén*.

踝，伏行出屬跗，下循跗，入大指間，滲諸脈而溫足脛肌肉，故其脈常動。別絡結
於跗上，脈不動，不動則厥，厥則寒矣。

Qíbó states, "Regarding the chōng vessel, it is the sea of the five zàng-viscera and six fǔ-bowels...[72] The ascending [pathway] emerges at the nasopharynx [region], where it permeates all yáng [vessels] and irrigates all channels.[73] The descending [pathway] attaches itself to the great network of shàoyīn[74] and commences from below the kidneys; it then emerges at Qì Chōng (ST-30),[75] follows the inner ridge of the yīn of the thigh,[76] obliquely enters the back of the knee; thereupon, while concealed, it travels along the inner ridge of the shin bone, together with the channel of the shàoyīn, it enters behind the inner ankle and continues to enter the bottom of the foot. Its divergent [pathway] joins with the shàoyīn to permeate the three yīn[77] [channels], it obliquely enters the ankle, becomes concealed as it travels [along the ankle bone] and emerge to adjoin to the instep, descends along the instep, and enters the space [next to] the big toe, where it permeates all the vessels in order to warm the flesh and muscles of the feet and lower legs, thus the vessel is constantly pulsating.[78] When its divergent network-vessel is bound on the instep, the vessel will cease to pulsate; when [the vessel] fails to pulsate, there will be reversal; when there is reversal, there will be cold."[79]

又云：衝脈爲十二經之海，其輸上在於大杼，下出於巨虛之上下廉。衝脈
又爲血海，血海有餘，則常想其身大，怫然不知其所病。血海不足，則常想其身
小，狹然不知其所病。

It also states, "The chōng vessel is the sea of the twelve channels, its transport point emerges above at Dà Zhù (BL-11), and it emerges[80] below at Jù Xū

---

[72] From the original passage in *Língshū* Chapter 38, the quote continued with "五藏六府皆稟爲 five zàng-viscera and six fǔ-bowel are all endowed by it" which is absent in this text.

[73] For "灌諸經 irrigates all channels," it is actually "灌諸精 irrigates all essence" in *Língshū* Chapter 38.

[74] For "著於少陰之大絡 attaches to the great network of the shàoyīn," it is actually "注於少陰之大絡 pours into the great network of shàoyīn" in *Língshū* Chapter 38.

[75] "Emerges at Qì Chōng 氣衝 (ST-30)" is actually "emerges at Qì Jiē 氣街 (qì thoroughfare)" in *Língshū* Chapter 38. Note: Qì Jiē is listed as an alternate name for ST-30.

[76] The yīn of the thigh is synonymous with the inner thigh.

[77] While we speculate the "three yīn" to be the "three yīn channels," it is ambiguous what this "three yīn" is; alternatively, it could be the point SP-6.

[78] This line, "thus the vessel is constantly pulsating," seems to be an addition found in Mǎ Shì's annotation, as it is not found in the original passage in the *Língshū*.

[79] From *Língshū* Chapter 38.

[80] For "出 emerge," it is originally "在 located" in the primary manuscript. The editors of this manuscript, Zhāng and Zhà, have amended it according to the secondary manuscript and *Língshū* Chapter 33.

Shàng Lián (ST-37) and Jù Xū Xià Lián (ST-39)."[81] Furthermore, the chōng vessel is the sea of blood, "When the sea of blood has superabundance, one often feels oneself to have a large physical stature of the body, with an indignant attitude and an inability to recognize where the disease is located. When the sea of blood is insufficient, one often feels oneself to have a small physical stature of the body, with a reserved attitude and also an inability to recognize where the disease is located."[82]

又云：脈來中央堅實，徑至關者，衝脈也，動則苦小腹痛，上搶心。又為疝瘕遺溺，支脇煩滿，女子絕孕。又云：尺寸俱牢，直上直下，此為衝脈，胸中有寒氣也。

In addition, it states, "When a pulse that is hard and replete in the centre arrives directly on the guān [position], this is the chōng [vessel] pulse; when it is stirred, one will suffer from pain in the lower abdomen, which ascends to prod the heart. Also, there will be mounting-conglomeration with enuresis, propping of the rib-sides with vexation and fullness, and infertility in women."[83]

It also states, "When the entire [pulse] from chǐ to cùn [positions] is firm, in which the entire pulse [in three positions] go up and down together, this is the chōng pulse, and there will be cold qì in the chest."[84]

腎之本病：五淋小便不通，陰器下縱，小腹滿，五臟虛竭，失精。

Principal diseases of the kidneys: five stranguries with urinary stoppage, protraction of the genitals, fullness in the lower abdomen, vacuity and exhaustion of the five zàng-viscera, and seminal emission.

注：五淋小便不通，氣滯而熱也，灸之以調腎氣。陰器下縱，肝腎有邪也，灸之以泄其邪。小腹，腎之部分。滿者，氣滯也。灸之，腹中氣响，則氣散而滿消矣。五臟虛竭、失精者，寒也，急灸此穴以補腎寒。

Explanation: the five stranguries with urinary stoppage are due to qì stagnation leading to heat, moxa it in order to regulate the kidney qì.[85] Protraction of

---

[81] From *Língshū* Chapter 33. Note: Some commentators, such as Unschuld, only list ST-37 as the lower transport point of the chōng vessel, we have opted for both ST-37 and ST-39.

[82] Also from *Língshū* Chapter 33.

[83] From Vol 2, "平奇經八脈病第四 Chapter 4, the General Diseases of the Eight Extraordinary Vessels" in the *Màijīng*.

[84] Also from the aforementioned source in the *Màijīng*. Note: "胸中有寒氣 there will be cold qì in the chest" was originally "胸中有寒疝 there will be cold-mounting in the chest" in the primary manuscript. The editors of this manuscript, Zhāng and Zhà, have amended it according to the secondary manuscript.

[85] Note: This is likely a co-acting treatment also known as paradoxical treatment, see BL-16 from the first volume for discussion.

the genitals is due to the presence of evil in the liver and kidneys, moxa it in order to drain the evil. The lower abdomen is the area of the kidneys; [the sign of] fullness is due to qì stagnation, moxa it and the qì within the abdomen will make a sound; subsequently, the qì will be dissipated and the fullness will be dispersed. Vacuity and exhaustion of the five zàng-viscera and seminal emissions are due to cold, urgently moxa this point in order to supplement the kidney [to eliminate] the cold.

腎之肝病：目赤痛，自內眥始。

Liver disease of the kidneys: reddening of the eyes with pain that begins at the inner canthus.

注：按足少陰經穴，自橫骨上行，歷大赫、氣穴、四滿、中注、肓腧、商曲、石關、陰都、通谷、幽門，凡十一穴，臍上六穴，臍下五穴，無不治目赤痛、自內眥始何也？蓋腎經挾任脈而上行，又同衝脈上行，目內眥部分，亦緊挾中脈之旁，故皆有治此脈之功。

Explanation: by examining the foot shàoyīn channel points, from Héng Gǔ (KI-11), [the pathway] ascends to pass through Dà Hè (KI-12), Qì Xué (KI-13), Sì Mǎn (KI-14), Zhōng Zhù (KI-15), Huāng Shù (KI-16), Shāng Qū (KI-17), Shí Guān (KI-18), Yīn Dū (KI-19), Tōng Gǔ (KI-20), and Yōu Mén (KI-21), in total there are eleven points, with six points above the umbilicus and five points below the umbilicus; without exception, all of them treat reddening of the eyes with pain that begins at the inner canthus, why is this? Undoubtedly, it is because the kidney channel clasps the rèn vessel and accompanies with the chōng vessel as it ascends to the area of the inner canthus,[86] which is located besides these vessels that clasp the midline, thus all [of these points] have the capability to treat these vessels [that reach the inner canthus].

---

[86] Note: Yuè Hánzhēn seems to argue that since these three vessels are located on the midline or closely clasp the midline, they should be able to reach the inner canthus, as it is close to the midline; however, none of the three vessels actually reach the inner canthus. The yīnqiāo vessel might be a better candidate as it intersects with both the chōng vessel and the kidney channel and reaches the inner canthus; furthermore, it is specifically mentioned to be able to treat this sign, as Língshū Chapter 23 states, "目中赤痛，從內眥始，取之陰蹻。For reddening of the eyes with pain that begins at the inner canthus, choose the yīnqiāo" Nevertheless, Yuè Hánzhēn may have intentionally disregarded the yīnqiāo vessel as it is unclear where it is on the abdomen, while it is clear that the kidney channel shares an intimate relationship with the chōng vessel and is located near the rèn vessel. On a side note, this association of the treatment of inner canthus with abdominal points of the kidney channel was not found in earlier text such as the reconstructed Míngtáng Jīng, Sūn Sīmiǎo's works, or even the authoritative compendium of Tóngrén; as it first appeared in the Zhēnjiǔ Jùyīng 針灸聚英 (Gathered Blooms of Acupuncture and Moxibustion, 1529 CE), a highly influential compilation that is infamously marred with countless errors, it is highly possible that this was a mistake or perhaps a new discovery made in this text. As the Dàchéng copied extensively from the Zhēnjiǔ Jùyīng, it appears in our text here.

Twelfth Point of the Kidney Channel
Dà Hè – Great Eminence[87] (KI-12)
腎經第十二穴大赫

一名陰維

Alternate name: Yīn Link

一名陰關

Alternate name: Yīn Pass[88]

穴在氣穴下一寸，去中行各一寸，橫與中行膀胱之募中極對，腎、肝、脾至此，
會於任之中極，足少陰、衝脈之會。《銅人》：灸五壯，鍼三分。《素》注：鍼
一寸，灸三壯。

**This point is located 1 cùn below Qì Xué (KI-13), at 1 cùn from the midline on
each side; horizontally, it is a counterpart to Zhōng Jí (REN-3) on the midline,
which is the collecting point of the bladder; furthermore, the kidney, liver, and
spleen arrive there to meet with Zhōng Jí (REN-3) of the rèn vessel. [Dà Hè
(KI-12)] is the meeting of the foot shàoyīn and chōng vessels. *The Tóngrén*
states, "Moxa 5 cones, and needle 3 fēn." *The Sùzhù* states, "Needle 1 cùn, and
moxa 3 cones."**

注：穴名大赫者，前名橫骨之穴，部分猶在骨際，至此穴，初入腹中，內
之所藏，深廣不測，故曰大赫。又名陰關，以足少陰之脈，離骨入腹，有關之象
焉。

Explanation: regarding the point name Dà Hè (Great Eminence), it is behind
the point that is named Héng Gǔ (KI-11), which is still located in the area that
borders the [transverse] bone; yet, upon arriving at this point, [the kidney channel]
begins to enter the abdomen; what is stored inside [the abdomen] is deep and broad
beyond measure, thus it is called Dà Hè (Great Eminence). It is also named Yīn Guān
(Yīn Pass), because as the vessel of the foot shàoyīn departs the [transverse] bone to
enter the abdomen, [this point] has the image of a Guān (Pass).

又曰陰維者，以陰維之脈入腹，而特此名以示人，恐人隻知少陰與衝脈在
此穴，而遺陰維之脈亦在此穴也。過此穴而陰維之脈，則會足太陰、足厥陰、足陽
明、足少陰於府舍，又會足太陰於大橫、腹哀，循脅肋而會足厥陰於期門，不與足
少陰腎脈同行矣，故於此特示人以別之。

---

[87] *Grasping the Wind* names it "Great Manifestation."
[88] *Grasping the Wind* names it "Yīn Gate."

It is also called Yīn Wéi (Yīn Link)[89] because the vessel of the yīnwéi enters the abdomen [here], so it is specifically named as such in order to express this to people, due to the fear that people may only be aware of the presence of shàoyīn and chōng vessel at this point but are unaware that the yīnwéi vessel is also present at this point. Traversing from this point, the vessel of the yīnwéi meets with the foot tàiyīn, foot juéyīn, foot yángmíng, and foot shàoyīn [channels] at Fǔ Shè (SP-13); it further meets the foot tàiyīn [channel] at Dà Héng (SP-15) and Fù Āi (SP-16); thereupon, it follows the rib-sides and meets with the foot juéyīn at Qī Mén (LR-14); as such, [the yīnwéi vessel] does not travel together with the shàoyīn kidney vessel, thus, here, [its name] specifically demonstrates this [concept] so that people can scrutinize it.

腎之本病：虛勞失精，男子陰器結縮，莖中痛，婦人赤帶。

Principal diseases of the kidneys: vacuity taxation with seminal emission, bound up and retracted genitals as well as pain in the penis in men, and red vaginal discharge in women.

注：虛勞失精，補此穴以治下脱。陰器結縮，乃肝腎過勞，而後總筋鬱滯所致，泄此穴以通其滯，而莖中痛亦愈矣。婦人赤帶，乃小腸之熱下滲膀胱，此穴緊在陰器之旁，宜泄以去其熱。

Explanation: for vacuity taxation with seminal emission, supplement this point in order to treat desertion in the lower [jiāo]. Retraction of the genitals is due to excessive taxation of the liver and kidneys, which subsequently results in depression and stagnation in the ancestral sinews,[90] drain this point in order to free the stagnation, so that the pain in the penis will be relieved. Red vaginal discharge in women is due to heat of the small intestine descending and permeating into the bladder, as this point is closely nearby the genitals, it is appropriate to drain [this point] in order to eliminate the heat.

腎之肝病：目赤痛，自内眥始。

Liver diseases of the kidneys: reddening of the eyes with pain that begins at the inner canthus.

注：見橫骨穴。

Explanation: see Héng Gǔ (KI-11).

---

[89] It should be noted that Yīn Wéi is both the name of the point and the vessel discussed here; when the point instead of the vessel is discussed, its name will follow in parenthesis.

[90] "Zōngjīn 宗筋 (ancestral sinew)" is actually "zǒngjīn 總筋 (chief sinew)" in the manuscript, which is likely a scribal error, as zōng 宗 and zǒng 總 are homophones.

Thirteenth Point of the Kidney Channel
Qì Xué – Qì Point[91] (KI-13)
腎經第十三穴氣穴

一名胞門
Alternate name: Uterine Gate

一名子戶
Alternate name: Infant's Door

穴在四滿下一寸，去腹中行一寸，橫與中行小腸之募關元對，而腎經之脈至此處，與肝經、脾經會於下紀，下紀者，關元也，足少陰、衝脈之會。

《銅人》：鍼三分，灸三壯。《素》注：鍼一寸，灸五壯。

This point is located 1 cùn below Sì Mǎn (KI-14), 1 cùn from the abdominal midline; horizontally, it is a counterpart to Guān Yuán (REN-4) on the midline, which is the collecting point of the small intestine. Upon arriving at this place, the vessel of the kidney channel further meets with the liver channel and spleen channel at Xià Jì;[92] as for Xià Jì, it is referring to Guān Yuán (REN-4). Moreover, [Qì Xué (KI-13)] is the meeting of the foot shàoyīn and chōng vessels. *The Tóngrén* states, "Needle 3 fēn, and moxa 3 cones."[93] *The Sùzhù* states, "Needle 1 cùn, and moxa 5 cones."

注：穴名氣穴者，以衝脈上行，而此穴其始。曰氣者，指衝脈而言也。曰胞門者，以衝脈自胞而出三歧，一由脊而上，一由股而下，一浮而出腹上行，至胸而散，而此其見端也。曰子戶者，婦人之孕娠，以胞爲主，而此穴乃其戶也。

Explanation: this point is named Qì Xué (Qì Point) because when the chōng vessel ascends, this Xué (Point) is where it begins. Regarding Qì (Qì), this is specifically referring to the chōng vessel. Regarding Bāo Mén (Uterine Gate), this is because the chōng vessel splits into three paths from the womb: one ascends along the spine; one descends along the thigh; and one moves outwards and floats to the surface at the abdomen, ascends to arrive at the chest and dissipates. Here, this [name] elucidates the beginning [of the chōng vessel]. It is also called Zi Hù (Infant's Door) because pregnancy in women is governed by the womb, and this point is precisely its door.

---

[91] *Grasping the Wind* names it "Qì Hole."
[92] This is named Lower Regulator, which is an alternate name for REN-4.
[93] "Moxa 3 cones" is actually "moxa 5 cones" in *the Tóngrén*.

腎之本病：奔豚氣上下行，引腰脊痛，泄利不止，月事不調。

Principal diseases of the kidneys: running piglet with qì moving up and down, pain that radiates into the lumbar spine, incessant diarrhoea, and irregular menstruation.

注：奔豚者，腎積也，衝脈內逆不行，積久遂生是病，其病無定處，而根在於小腹，泄之以降逆氣。泄利不止，氣下脫也，補之以收其氣。月事不調，衝之病也，宜取此穴。

Explanation: running piglets is due to kidney accumulation;[94] owing to the internal counterflow and failure of the chōng vessel to move, after accumulating over an extended period of time, such a disease will be engendered; this disease has no fixed location, moreover, its root is located in the lower abdomen, so drain this [point] in order to descend the counterflow qì. Incessant diarrhoea is because of desertion and sunken qì, supplement this [point] in order to contract the qì. Irregular menstruation is a disease of the chōng [vessel], it is appropriate to choose this point.

腎之肝病：目赤痛，自內眥始。

Liver diseases of the kidneys: reddening of the eyes with pain that begins at the inner canthus.

注：見橫骨穴。

Explanation: see Héng Gǔ (KI-11).

Fourteenth Point of the Kidney Channel
Sì Mǎn – Fourfold Fullness (KI-14)
腎經第十四穴四滿

一名髓府
Alternate name: Marrow Mansion

穴在中注下一寸，去腹中行各一寸，橫與石門對，足少陰、衝脈之會。《銅人》：鍼三分，灸三壯。

This point is located 1 cùn below Zhōng Zhù (KI-15), 1 cùn on each side of the abdominal midline; horizontally, it is a counterpart to Shí Mén (REN-7). It is

---

94 Note: There are five types of accumulation in total, as each zàng-viscus is designated an accumulation as per *Nànjīng* Difficulty 56.

the meeting of the foot shàoyīn and chōng vessels. *The Tóngrén* states, "Needle 3 fēn, and moxa 3 cones."

注：穴名四滿者，蓋足少陰之經，自橫骨入腹，至此穴爲四，而適當小腹飽滿之處，乃大腸迴疊層積之所，故曰滿也。又小腸、大腸、膀胱、廣腸，皆在其內，其數亦爲四，故曰四滿。

Explanation: this point is named Sì Mǎn (Fourfold Fullness); undoubtedly, from Héng Gǔ (KI-11), the channel of the foot shàoyīn enters the abdomen, and this is the Sì (Fourth) point. As this [point] is located precisely at a place where the lower abdomen becomes Mǎn (Full), which is where the large intestine curves and overlaps to amass layer upon layer, thus it is called Mǎn (Fullness). Moreover, the small intestine, large intestine, bladder, and rectum are all located on the interior of this [point], these also total to Sì (Four), thus it is called Sì Mǎn (Fourfold Fullness).

腎之本病：奔豚上下，月水不調，惡血疞痛，積聚疝瘕，腸癖，大腸有水，臍下切痛，振寒。

Principal diseases of the kidneys: running piglet that moves up and down, irregular menstruation, malign blood with tense pain, gatherings and accumulations with mounting-conglomeration, intestinal aggregations, water in the large intestine, stabbing pain below the umbilicus, and shivering with cold.

注：此穴在臍旁之下僅二寸，而在毛際橫骨之上已四寸，正大腸迴疊之處，故治積聚及大小腸有水、臍下切痛、腸癖、月水不調、奔豚上下諸症，皆用此穴，以散其滯氣，而破其積血也。振寒亦用此穴者何也？水積於下，則寒生焉，取此穴以散寒水，而寒自已也。

Explanation: this point is beside the umbilicus and only 2 cùn below it; as such, it is at the border of the pubic hair region and has already ascended 4 cùn past Héng Gǔ (KI-11), it is exactly at the place where the large intestine curves and overlaps; thus, to treat these various signs such as gatherings and accumulations with water in the large and small intestines, stabbing pain below the umbilicus, intestinal aggregations, irregular menstruation, and running piglet that moves up and down, in all cases, utilise this point in order to disperse the stagnant qì, so that the accumulated blood can be broken. Why does one utilise this point for those shivering with cold? Because when water accumulates in the below, cold will be engendered, choose this point in order to disperse the cold water, so that [the amassed] cold will cease naturally.

腎之肝病：目內眥赤痛。

Liver disease of the kidneys: reddening of the inner canthus with pain.

注：見橫骨穴。

Explanation: see Héng Gǔ (KI-11).

Fifteenth Point of the Kidney Channel
Zhōng Zhù – Central Pour[95] (KI-15)
腎經第十五穴中注

穴在肓腧下一寸，去腹中行各一寸，橫與中行之陰交穴對，足少陰、衝脈之會。
《銅人》：鍼一寸，灸五壯。

This point is located 1 cùn below Huāng Shù (KI-16), 1 cùn on each side of the abdominal midline; horizontally, it is counterpart to Yīn Jiāo (REN-7). It is the meeting of the foot shàoyīn and chōng vessels. *The Tóngrén* states, "Needle 1 cùn, and moxa 5 cones."

注：穴名中注者，乃人腹之上下，以臍爲中，肓腧僅挾臍旁一寸，而此穴乃肓腧之下，爲肓腧之所注，故曰中注。中注，自上而下之名，腎經自下而上，何亦以注名也？經無有不昇降，昇者其氣，降者其血，故亦曰注也。

Explanation: this point is named Zhōng Zhù (Central Pour), because from the upper to the lower abdomen of a person, the umbilicus is regarded as the Zhōng (Centre). Huāng Shù (KI-16) clasps the umbilicus closely at 1 cùn beside it; as this point is below Huāng Shù (KI-16), it is what Huāng Shù (KI-16) Zhù (Pours) into, thus it is called Zhōng Zhù (Central Pour). Regarding Zhōng Zhù (Central Pour), the name [infers] that it descends from above. As the kidney channel ascends from below, why does it include Zhù (Pour) in the name? Without exception, all channels ascend and descend; what is ascending, it is the qì; what is descending, it is the blood, thus it is also called Zhù (Pour).

腎之本病：小腸有熱，大便堅燥不利，泄氣上下引腰脊痛，月事不調。

Principal diseases of the kidneys: small intestine heat, hard dry stool that is inhibitive [to pass], discharge of qì[96] with pain radiating up and down the lumbar spine, and irregular menstruation.

注：小腸有熱，乃小腸之熱不傳入膀胱，而傳入大腸也，取此穴以泄大腸之氣，氣泄則熱除，而乾燥病愈矣。泄氣上下引腰脊痛，乃氣滯於臍之後，正內腎之對，泄此穴而氣散，則腰脊之痛除矣。月事乃衝脈之所司，不調者，寒熱不均也，泄此穴以調其寒熱。

---

[95] *Grasping the Wind* names it "Central Flow."
[96] Possibly flatulence.

Explanation: small intestine heat is due to the small intestine failing to transmit the heat into the bladder, but transmitting it into the large intestine instead, choose this point in order to drain the qì of the large intestine; when the qì is drained, heat will be eliminated, leading to recovery from the dryness disease. Discharge of qì with pain radiating up and down the lumbar spine is because of qì stagnation behind the umbilicus, which is exactly the counterpart to the kidneys inside, drain this point and the qì will disperse, and the pain of the lumbar spine will [also] be eliminated. Menstruation is what the chōng vessel controls, when it is unregulated, it is due to an uneven distribution of cold and heat, drain this point in order to regulate the cold and heat.

Sixteenth Point of the Kidney Channel
Huāng Shù – Huāng Transport Point (KI-16)
腎經第十六穴肓腧

穴在商曲下一寸，去腹中行各一寸，橫與中行之神闕對，足少陰、衝脈之會。
《銅人》：鍼一寸，灸五壯。

This point is located 1 cùn below Shāng Qū (KI-17), 1 cùn on each side of the abdominal midline; horizontally, it is a counterpart to Shén Què (REN-8). It is the meeting of the foot shàoyīn and chōng vessels. *The Tóngrén* states, "Needle 1 cùn, and moxa 5 cones."

注：此穴僅挾臍旁，肓者，膈也，膈所以遮上下、分清濁也。膈之上爲心肺清虛之所，膈之下爲水穀承化之所，而至臍以下，則又爲糟粕運出之所。膈在上，而此其司也，乃運輸生穀之精，以上行而潤膈之前者，至足太陽背後所載之膈腧，又所以司膈之後，一在督之旁，一在任之旁，督主一身之氣，任主一身之血。膈，前齊鳩尾，後附十一椎，有此一穴，而膈之氣血始備，故曰肓腧，所以別背後之膈腧也。

Explanation: [the location of] this point intimately clasps the sides of the umbilicus. Huāng (Huāng) is the diaphragm; the diaphragm is what separates above and below, divides the clear and turbid. Above the diaphragm is the clear and empty place of the heart and lung; below the diaphragm is the place where the undertaking of transformation of water and grain occurs; as for below the umbilicus, it is the place where filth and dregs are transported and expelled. As the diaphragm is located above [this point], what this [point] controls is that it moves and transports the essence engendered from grain, so that it can ascend and moisten the front of the diaphragm; furthermore, it also arrives at Gé Shù (BL-17, Diaphragm Transport Point), which the foot tàiyáng [channel] carries on the upper back; for that reason, it also controls the back of the diaphragm. One [point] is located beside the dū [vessel],[97] while the other one is located beside the rèn [vessel];[98] the dū [vessel] governs the qì of the whole body, while the rèn [vessel] governs the blood of the whole body. The diaphragm is level with Jiū Wěi (REN-15) on the front, and it is attached to the eleventh vertebra on the back. It is only with the existence of this one point that the qì and blood of the diaphragm are fully provided for, thus it is called Huāng Shù (Huāng Transport), as a way to distinguish it from Gé Shù (BL-17) on the upper back.

自下而上，屬於帶脈之橫者，而過之上行。凡經之自下而上，自上而下，無不過於帶脈者，此穴乃腎經過帶脈之處。

[The channel] ascends from the below to adjoin to the horizontal [pathway] of the dài vessel, traversing it as it ascends. For all the channels that ascend from below or those that descend from above, without exception, they all traverse the dài vessel; and this point is precisely at the location where the kidney channel traverses the dài vessel.

腎之本病：寒疝，大便燥。

Principal diseases of the kidneys: cold mounting and dry stool.

注：疝，肝病也，腎虛而後肝易中寒邪，未有腎不虛，而有疝症者，故肝腎之穴，疝病皆責之也。此穴以寒由臍入，腹前之寒，皆自臍入，而此穴在臍之旁，故取之。腎司二便，此穴正在小腸、大腸之際，闌門之下，故大便之症，亦責此穴，而調其氣。

Explanation: mounting is a liver disease, yet, when there is kidney vacuity, the liver will subsequently become susceptible to the strike by cold evil; for those with the sign of mounting, without exception, all of them have kidney vacuity; thus, for the mounting diseases, seek the points of both the liver and kidney [channels]. This point is for cold that enters the umbilicus; for all cold [evils] at the front of the abdomen, they always enter from the umbilicus, since this point is located to the sides of the umbilicus, thus choose it. The kidneys control urination and defecation; as this point is located exactly in the region of the small and large intestines and below the screen gate,[99] thus for signs relating to defecation, also seek this point in order to regulate the qì.

腎之脾病：腹切痛，腹滿響響然不便，心下有寒。

Spleen diseases of the kidneys: stabbing pain in the abdomen, abdominal fullness with echoing sounds and inability to defecate, and coldness below the heart.

---

[97] I.e., BL-17.

[98] I.e., KI-16.

[99] I.e., the ileocecal valve, which is one of the seven gates between the mouth and the anus as outlined in *Nànjīng* Difficulty 44.

注：腹切痛，衝氣之逆也，取此穴以降衝之逆氣。腹滿響響然不便者，氣滯也，泄之以降其氣。心下有寒，乃胃中有寒邪也，取此穴以降寒邪。

Explanation: stabbing pain in the abdomen is due to counterflow of the chōng [vessel] qì, choose this point in order to descend the counterflow qì of the chōng [vessel]. Abdominal fullness with echoing sounds and inability to defecate is caused by qì stagnation, drain this [point] in order to descend the qì. Coldness below the heart is due to the presence of cold evil in the stomach, choose this point in order to descend the cold evil.

腎之肝病：目赤痛，自內眥始。

Liver diseases of the kidneys: reddening of the eyes with pain that begins at the inner canthus.

注：見橫骨穴。

Explanation: see Héng Gǔ (KI-11).

Seventeenth Point of the Kidney Channel
Shāng Qū – Shāng Bend (KI-17)
腎經第十七穴商曲

穴在石關下一寸，去腹中行各一寸五分，足少陰、衝脈之會。《銅人》：鍼一寸，灸五壯。

This point is located 1 cùn below Shí Guān (KI-18), 1 cùn 5 fēn on each side of the abdominal midline. It is the meeting of the foot shàoyīn and chōng vessels. *The Tóngrén* states, "Needle 1 cùn, and moxa 5 cones."

注：此穴在臍上第一穴，挾中行任脈水分穴一寸五分，正大、小腸會處，自此際滲入膀胱，而爲溺便，穀之渣穢，則自闌門而傳送於大腸，肺屬金，大腸亦屬金，金爲商，故曰商曲。

Explanation: this point is the first point [of the kidney channel] located above the umbilicus, it clasps Shuǐ Fēn (REN-9) of the rèn vessel at 1 cùn 5 fēn from the midline. It is exactly the place where the large and small intestines join together. From this place, [digested food and drink] permeate into the bladder, where it is excreted as urine; as for the dregs and filth of the grain, they are conveyed to the large intestine through the screen gate.[100] As the lung belongs to metal, the large intestine also belongs to metal; the metal [tone] is Shāng (Shāng), thus it is called Shāng Qū (Shāng Bend).

---

100 See previous footnote.

腎之脾病：腹痛，腹中積聚時切痛，腹中痛不嗜食。

Spleen diseases of the kidneys: abdominal pain, accumulations and gatherings in the abdomen with periodic stabbing pain, and pain in the abdomen with no pleasure in eating.

注：腹痛者，臍之上下皆痛也，腎經同衝脈過臍之上下，其在內，皆與胃、大、小腸相關，故腹痛取此穴，以降其逆氣。腹內積聚，胃中有積也，非腹中之積，時切痛，乃氣逆而不行也，取此穴以通腹之逆氣。腹中痛不嗜食，乃闌門氣逆，食物不下所致，取此穴以通闌門之氣。

Explanation: regarding [this type of] abdominal pain, one feels pain in both [areas] above and below the umbilicus; as the kidney channel traverses together with the chōng vessel above and below the umbilicus, they are associated with the stomach, large and small intestines inside, thus for abdominal pain, choose this point in order to descend the counterflow qì. For accumulations and gatherings in the abdomen, the accumulations are present in the stomach, they are not accumulations within the abdomen; for periodic stabbing pain, this is due to counterflow qì that is not moving, choose this point in order to unblock the counterflow qì in the abdomen. Abdominal pain with no pleasure in eating is because of counterflow qì at the screen gate, as a result, there will be no pleasure in eating, choose this point in order to free the qì at the screen gate.

腎之肝病：目赤痛，自內眥始。

Liver diseases of the kidneys: reddening of the eyes with pain that begins at the inner canthus.

注：見橫骨穴。

Explanation: see Héng Gǔ (KI-11).

Eighteenth Point of the Kidney Channel
Shí Guān – Stone Pass (KI-18)
腎經第十八穴石關

穴在陰都下一寸，去中行各一寸五分，挾下脘旁。《銅人》：鍼一寸，灸五壯。

This point is located 1 cùn below Yīn Dū (KI-19), at 1 cùn 5 fēn from the midline on each side, clasping the sides of Xià Wǎn (REN-10). *The Tóngrén* states, "Needle 1 cùn, and moxa 5 cones."[101]

---

[101] For "5 cones" *the Tóngrén* actually states "3 cones."

注：水皆下行，而腎水獨上行，以成水火既濟之象，腎之經至胃，下脘之旁曰幽門者，乃胃之下口，小腸之上口也，水遇土，有關之象焉。水穿土而上行，亦有關之象。不曰土關，而曰石關，蓋腎經由大腸部分而上行至此，則離大腸之金而入胃土，其曰石者，指陽明金大腸而言，腎之穴曰石關，任之穴曰石門，皆指大腸而言也。

Explanation: all water flows downwards, however, kidney water alone flows upwards, so that it forms the image of mutual assistance between fire and water.[102] When the kidney channel reaches the stomach, it is at Yōu Mén (KI-21)[103] to the sides of Xià Wǎn (REN-10),[104] which is the lower opening of the stomach and the upper opening of the small intestine. This is where water encounters earth,[105] [thus] it has the image of a Guān (Pass). As water passes through earth to ascend further, it also has the image of a Guān (Pass). [For the reason why] it is not called earth Guān (Pass) but Shí Guān (Stone Pass) instead, this is because the kidney channel ascends to reach here from the area of the large intestine, as such, it departs from metal of the large intestine to enter stomach earth; for this Shí (Stone), it is referring to the yángmíng metal large intestine. For this point of the kidney [channel] called Shí Guān (Stone Pass) and the point of the rèn [channel] called Shí Mén (REN-5, Stone Gate),[106] they are both referring to the large intestine.

腎之本病：脊强不利，多唾，腹痛氣淋，小便黃，大便不通，婦人無子，臟有惡血，腹痛不可忍。

Principal diseases of the kidneys: inhibitive stiffness of the spine, copious spittle, abdominal pain with qì strangury, yellow urine, constipation,[107] female childlessness, malign blood in the zàng-viscera, and insufferable abdominal pain.

---

[102] This "mutual assistance between fire and water 水火既濟" refers to hexagram 63 of the *Yijīng*, with water above and fire below, depicting an image of fire reaching downward and water reaching upward. As water has a natural tendency to flow downward and fire has a natural tendency to ascend, by their natures, they would only drift further apart from each other (as in hexagram 64, lack of mutual assistance); however, with this nature-defying movement of fire descent and water ascent, they interact with each other to create life. In the human body, this means the descent of the heart yáng and ascent of kidney yīn, and the interaction of heart fire and kidney water.

[103] KI-21 is also the location of the dark gate, one of the seven gates, synonymous with the pylorus.

[104] REN-10 is also the location of the lower stomach duct.

[105] I.e., kidney water encountering stomach earth.

[106] REN-5 is named Stone Gate.

[107] Also known as faecal stoppage.

注：腎之經自內行者，上股內後廉貫脊，屬腎絡膀胱，脊強不利，乃腎氣之滯也，取此穴以通貫脊之腎氣。唾者，腎之液也，多唾，乃腎氣之上逆，腎之直行者，上貫膈，入肺中，循喉嚨，挾舌本也，取此穴以降腎之濕氣。

Explanation: as the kidney channel travels in the interior, it ascends the rear ridge of the inner thigh, pierces the spine, adjoins to the kidneys and networks with the bladder; thus, for inhibitive stiffness of the spine, this is due to stagnation of kidney qì, choose this point in order to free the kidney qì that pierces the spine. Spittle is the humour of the kidneys; when there is copious spittle, this is due to the counterflow ascent of kidney qì; because the vertical pathway of the kidneys ascends to pierce the diaphragm, enters the lung, follows the throat, and clasps the root of the tongue; choose this point in order to descend the damp qì of the kidneys.

腹痛氣淋，乃腎有邪熱，留於氣分，而有是症，宜泄之。小便黃、大便不通，皆胃熱也，司二便者，腎也，泄之以去腎胃之熱。婦人無子，以臟有惡血，上衝腹，乃惡血在大腸，隨衝脈而衝腹焉，泄之以降逆上之氣，而下惡血。

Abdominal pain with qì strangury is due to the presence of evil heat in the kidneys, when it is lodged in the qì aspect, there will be this sign, it is appropriate to drain it. Yellow urine and constipation are in all cases stomach heat, as the kidneys are that which control the urine and stool, drain this [point] in order to eliminate the heat of the kidneys and stomach. Female childlessness is because of the presence of malign blood in the zàng-viscera, which is surging upwards into the abdomen; this malign blood is surely located in the large intestine, it follows the chōng vessel to surge into the abdomen; drain it in order to descend the ascending counterflow qì, so that the malign blood can be precipitated.

腎之脾病：噦噫嘔逆，心下堅滿。

Spleen diseases of the kidneys: retching and belching with vomiting counterflow, hardness and fullness below the heart.

注：噦噫嘔逆，衝脈逆上也，逆上至此而犯胃，遂有是症，宜泄之。心下堅滿，亦衝脈之逆也，取此穴之義，與上症同。

Explanation: retching and belching with vomiting counterflow is counterflow ascent of the chōng vessel; when the counterflow ascent reaches here, it will invade the stomach, which subsequently leads to this sign, it is appropriate to drain it. Hardness and fullness below the heart is also counterflow of the chōng vessel; as for the intention of choosing this point, it is the same as the previous sign.

Nineteenth Point of the Kidney Channel
Yīn Dū - Yīn Metropolis (KI-19)
腎經第十九穴陰都

一名食宮

Alternate name: Food Palace

穴在通谷下一寸，去腹中行各一寸五分，挾建里旁，足少陰、衝脈之會。《銅
人》：鍼三分，灸三壯。

**This point is located 1 cùn[108] below Tōng Gǔ (KI-20), 1 cùn 5 fēn on each side
of the abdominal midline, clasping the sides of Jiàn Lǐ (REN-11). It is the
meeting of the foot shàoyīn and chōng vessels. *The Tóngrén* states, "Needle 3
fēn, and moxa 3 cones."**

注：穴名陰都者，此陰乃足太陰脾也，部分乃足太陰所治之地，而少陰又
過之，故曰陰都。都者，會也。一名食宮，乃胃藏食之所，故曰食宮。

Explanation: regarding the point name Yīn Dū (Yīn Metropolis), this Yīn
(Yīn) refers to the foot tàiyīn spleen; as [this point's] area is precisely the region
governed by the foot tàiyīn, where the shàoyīn [channel] also traverses, thus it is
called Yīn Dū (Yīn Metropolis). Dū (Metropolis) is referring to a large city. An
alternate name is Shí Gōng (Food Palace), as this is where the stomach stores the
food, thus it is called Shí Gōng (Food Palace).

腎之脾病：身寒熱瘧病，心下煩滿，氣逆腸鳴。

**Spleen diseases of the kidneys: malaria disease with generalised chills and
fever, vexation and fullness below the heart, and qì counterflow with rumbling
intestines.**

注：無痰不作瘧，胃爲注痰之器，而少陰、衝脈過於其處，有寒邪，則胃
爲之寒，不能運化，至其中之經，按時而發，取此穴以去胃邪。心下煩滿，乃胃之
所也，衝脈上行而犯胃，故氣逆腸鳴，少陰有邪而胃弱，亦致此症，故取此穴，以
降逆氣。

Explanation: in the absence of phlegm, malaria cannot occur; the stomach is
the receptacle which phlegm pours into; in addition, the shàoyīn and chōng vessels
traverse that place; when there is a presence of cold evil, the stomach will become
cold and unable to transport and transform; when [the cold evil] affects this channel

---

[108] "1 cùn" was "5 fēn" in the primary manuscript. The editors of this manuscript, Zhāng and
Zhà, have amended it according to the secondary manuscript and the *Zhēnjiǔ Dàchéng*.

that is afflicted [with phlegm], [malaria] will manifest periodically, choose this point in order to eliminate the stomach evil.

Vexation and fullness below the heart occur at where the stomach is located, when the chōng vessel ascends to invade the stomach, there will be counterflow qì and rumbling intestines; in addition, when there is stomach weakness due to evil in the shàoyīn [channel], it will result in this sign, thus choose this point in order to descend the counterflow qì.

腎之肺病：肺脹氣搶。

Lung disease of the kidneys: distention of the lung with rushing qì.

注：腎經在內直行者入肺，衝脈氣盛而犯之，故有此症，宜泄之。

Explanation: as the internal vertical pathway of the kidney channel enters the lung, when the chōng vessel qì is exuberant, it will invade it, thus there will be this sign, it is appropriate to drain it.

腎之肝病：脇下煩滿，目赤痛自內眥始。

Liver diseases of the kidneys: vexation and fullness under the rib-sides, and reddening of the eyes with pain that begins at the inner canthus.

注：衝脈不昇而逆於肺，遂有熱滿之症，取此穴以昇氣。目赤痛自內眥始，註見橫骨穴。

Explanation: when the chōng vessel fails to ascend, there will be counterflow in the lung; as a result, there will be signs of heat and fullness, choose this point in order to ascend the qì. For reddening of the eyes with pain that begins at the inner canthus, see the explanation at Héng Gǔ (KI-11).

Twentieth Point of the Kidney Channel
Tōng Gǔ – Flowing Valley[109] (KI-20)
腎經第二十穴通谷

穴在幽門下一寸，去腹中行各一寸五分，挾中脘旁，足少陰、衝脈之會。《銅人》：鍼五分，灸五壯。《明堂》：灸三壯。

This point is located 1 cùn below Yōu Mén (KI-21), 1 cùn 5 fēn on each side of the abdominal midline, clasping the sides of Zhōng Wǎn (REN-12). It is the

---

[109] *Grasping the Wind* names it "Open Valley."

meeting of the foot shàoyīn and chōng vessels. *The Tóngrén states, "Needle 5 fēn, and moxa 5 cones." The Míngtáng states, "Moxa 3 cones."*

注：谷者，水所行之地，有虛象焉，穴以谷名，正胃中脘之旁，胃屬土而中虛，有谷象焉，足少陰自下而上行，同衝脈以過之，故曰通谷。

Explanation: for Gǔ (Valley), it is the terrain where water moves, it has the image of emptiness in it. For this point to include Gǔ (Valley) in its name, it is precisely because it is besides the central stomach duct,[110] as the stomach belongs to earth and is hollow in its centre, it has the image of a Gǔ (Valley). In addition, since the foot shàoyīn [channel] ascends from below and traverses [this point] with the chōng vessel, thus it is called Tōng Gǔ (Flowing Valley).

腎之本病：暴瘖不能言。

Principal disease of the kidneys: sudden loss of voice with inability to speak.

注：暴瘖，有腎氣不上交於舌本而致者，當取此穴，以通腎氣。

Explanation: for sudden loss of voice, this is a result from the failure of kidney qì to ascend and intersect with the tongue, one should choose this point in order to free the kidney qì.

腎之脾病：失欠口喎，食飲善嘔，結積留飲，痞癖，胸滿食不化，心恍惚善嘔。

Spleen diseases of the kidneys: yawning with deviation of the mouth, frequent retching of food and drink, bound accumulations with lodged rheum, strings and aggregations,[111] fullness in the chest with indigestion, and heart abstraction with frequent retching.

注：凡口喎之病，皆取胃經在面之穴，而又取此穴者，以去犯上之寒邪也。食飲善嘔者，氣逆也，宜泄之。結聚留飲、痞癖，乃胃中脘之所司也，此穴挾中脘旁，故取此穴，以去寒，蓋無寒不積也。胸滿，氣逆於胸也，取此穴以降胸中之逆氣，氣降則食化而下矣。心恍惚善嘔，皆氣逆之所致，亦取此穴，以降逆氣。

Explanation: for the disease of deviation of the mouth, in all cases, choose a point on the stomach channel located on the face; the reason to further include this point is to eliminate the cold evil that has invaded the above. Frequent retching of food and drink is due to counterflow qì, it is appropriate to drain it.

For bound accumulations with lodged rheum, strings and aggregations, these are [signs] controlled by the central stomach duct; as this point clasps the sides of Zhōng Wǎn (REN-12), thus choose this point in order to eliminate the cold, as without exception, all cold leads to accumulation.

---

[110] 中脘 Central Duct is also the name of REN-12.
[111] For "strings and aggregations," see footnote 28.

Fullness in the chest is because of qì counterflow in the chest, choose this point in order to descend the counterflow qì within the chest; once the qì descends, the food will be transformed and descended. Heart abstraction[112] with frequent retching is always a result of qì counterflow, also choose this point in order to descend the counterflow qì.

腎之肝病：目赤痛，自内眥始。

Liver disease of the kidneys: reddening of the eyes with pain that begins at the inner canthus.

注：解見横骨穴。

Explanation: see the explanation at Héng Gǔ (KI-11).

Twenty-First Point of the Kidney Channel
Yōu Mén – Dark Gate (KI-21)
腎經第二十一穴幽門

一名上門
Alternate name: Upper Gate

穴在巨闕旁各一寸五分陷中，足少陰、衝脈之會。《銅人》：鍼五分，灸五壯。

This point is located in the depression 1 cùn 5 fēn on each side of Jù Quē (REN-14). It is the meeting of the foot shàoyīn and chōng vessel. *The Tóngrén* states, "Needle 5 fēn, and moxa 5 cones."

注：腎經至此，將入胸中清淨之所，故曰幽門，言其深遠難測也。

Explanation: upon arriving at this point, the kidney channel is about to enter the place that is clear and pure within the chest,[113] thus it is called Yōu Mén (Dark Gate), which is referring to its profound depth that is difficult to fathom.

腎之本病：小腹脹滿，泄利膿血。

Principal diseases of the kidneys: distension and fullness in the lower abdomen, diarrhoea with pus and blood.

---

[112] According to *the Practical Dictionary*, abstraction is described as "inattention to present objects or surroundings, or low powers of mental concentration. It is a sign of heart disease."

[113] *Sùwèn* Chapter 2 states, "天氣，清淨光明者也 the heavenly qì is clear, pure, bright, and radiant."

注：腎脈至此，不上行則脹於下，故取此穴，以昇其鬱。泄利膿血，乃大腸之氣下脫也，取此穴以昇其下脫之氣。

Explanation: upon arriving here, if the kidney vessel fails to ascend further, there will be distension in the below, thus choose this point in order to lift[114] the depression. Diarrhoea with pus and blood is due to the qì sinking and desertion of the large intestine, choose this point in order to lift the sunken and deserted qì.

腎之脾病：嘔吐涎沫，喜唾，心下煩滿，胸中引痛，不嗜食，女子心中痛，逆氣善吐，食不下。

Spleen diseases of the kidneys: vomiting and retching of foamy drool, frequent spitting, vexation and fullness below the heart, pain that radiates into the chest, no pleasure in eating, pain in the heart in females, counterflow qì with tendency to vomit, and inability to ingest food.

注：嘔吐涎沫、喜唾，胃有濕邪也，取此穴以去胃之濕邪。心下煩滿、胸中引痛、不嗜食，氣逆所致也，取此穴以降逆氣。女子心痛、氣逆善吐、不下食，衝脈之逆也，取此穴以降衝脈之逆。

Explanation: for vomiting and retching of foamy drool, as well as frequent spitting, [both] are due to damp evil in the stomach, choose this point in order to eliminate the damp evil of the stomach. For vexation and fullness below the heart, pain that radiates into the chest, and no pleasure in eating, all of these are a result of counterflow qì, choose this point in order to descend the counterflow qì. For heart pain in females, qì counterflow with tendency to vomit, and inability to ingest food, [these are] because of counterflow of the chōng vessel, choose this point in order to descend the counterflow of the chōng vessel.

腎之肺病：裏急數咳。

Lung diseases of the kidneys: internal urgency with frequent coughing.

注：氣逆於內，故裏急，取此穴以通內逆之氣。數咳，氣之逆也，降其氣而咳自息。取此穴使氣不逆於肺。

Explanation: when there is qì counterflow in the interior, there will be internal urgency, choose this point in order to free the counterflow qì in the interior. Frequent coughing is due to counterflow of qì, descend the qì and coughing will naturally cease. Choose this point to prohibit the counterflow qì in the lung.

腎之心病：健忘。

Heart disease of the kidneys: forgetfulness.

---

[114] The character here, biàn 昪 (enliven, delight), is most likely a typo for shēng 昇 (raise, lift), as biàn 昪 is a rather rare character that may not completely fit the context.

注：健忘者，心血虛也，亦心氣不清所致也，取此穴以清心氣。

Explanation: forgetfulness is not only due to heart blood vacuity, but also a result of unclear heart qì, choose this point in order to clear the heart qì.

腎之肝病：目赤痛，自內眥始。

Liver disease of the kidneys: reddening of the eyes with pain that begins at the inner canthus.

注：見橫骨穴。

Explanation: see the [explanation] at Héng Gǔ (KI-11).

Twenty-Second Point of the Kidney Channel
Bù Láng – Corridor Steps[115] (KI-22)
腎經第二十二穴步廊

穴在神封下一寸六分，去胸中行各二寸，與中庭橫相值，仰面取之。《銅人》：鍼三分，灸五壯。《素》注：鍼四分。

This point is located 1 cùn 6 fēn below Shén Fēng (KI-23), 2 cùn on each side of the chest midline, in a horizontal line on par with Zhōng Tíng (REN-16); lie supine to locate it. *The Tóngrén* states, "Needle 3 fēn, and moxa 5 cones." *The Sùzhù* states, "Needle 4 fēn."

注：腎經至此而入胸，胸中爲清淨之府，有廊之象焉，與中行任之中庭橫值，庭在中，而廊在旁，自下而上，故曰步廊。

Explanation: upon arriving here, the kidney channel enters the chest; as the chest centre is the clear and pure mansion, [this point] has the image of a Láng (Corridor). It is in a horizontal line on par with Zhōng Tíng (REN-16, Centre Courtyard) of the rèn [vessel] on the midline; as this courtyard is located in the centre, Láng (Corridors) are located to its sides. Moreover, as [the kidney channel] ascends from below, thus it is called Bù Láng (Corridor Steps).

腎之肺病：胸脇支滿，痛引胸，鼻塞不通，呼吸少氣，咳逆嘔吐，不嗜食，喘息不得舉臂。

Lung diseases of the kidneys: propping fullness in the chest and rib-side, pain that radiates into the chest, cold nose that is obstructed, scantness of breath,

---

[115] *Grasping the Wind* names it "Corridor Walk."

cough and counterflow with retching and vomiting, no pleasure in eating, and panting with inability to lift the arm.

注：胸脇支滿，衝脈上逆也，痛引胸，亦衝脈上逆也，宜泄之。鼻寒不通，呼吸少氣，皆衝脈之邪上逆，而正氣不伸也，宜泄之。咳逆嘔吐，氣之逆也，不嗜食，氣逆食不下也，宜泄之。喘息不得舉臂，皆氣逆之症，久則傳爲痿，急泄此穴，以防痿。

Explanation: propping fullness in the chest and rib-side is counterflow ascent of the chōng vessel; for pain that radiates into the chest, it is also counterflow ascent of the chōng vessel, it is appropriate to drain it. For cold nose that is obstructed and scantness of breath, both are due to counterflow ascent of evil in the chōng vessel, which leads to the failure of the upright qì to spread, thus it is appropriate to drain it.

Cough and counterflow with retching and vomiting are counterflow of the qì; no pleasure in eating is counterflow qì with inability to ingest food, it is appropriate to drain it. Panting with inability to lift the arm is always a sign of qì counterflow; over an extended period of time, it will transmit and become wilting, urgently drain this point in order to prevent one from having wilting.

Twenty-Third Point of the Kidney Channel
Shén Fēng – Spirit Border[116] (KI-23)
腎經第二十三穴神封

穴在靈墟下一寸六分陷中，去中行各二寸，仰而取之。《素》注：鍼四分。《銅人》：鍼三分，灸五壯。

This point is located in the depression 1 cùn 6 fēn below Líng Xū (KI-24), at 2 cùn from the midline on each side; lie supine to locate it. *The Sùzhù* states, "Needle 4 fēn." *The Tóngrén* states, "Needle 3 fēn, and moxa 5 cones."

注：穴名神封者，蓋心藏神，此穴近心，乃神藏之所，封者，界也，故曰神封。又以神藏於內，故曰神封。

Explanation: regarding the point name Shén Fēng (Spirit Border), undoubtedly, the heart stores the spirit; as this point is nearby the heart, it is the location where the spirit is stored. Fēng (Border) is a boundary, thus it is called Shén Fēng (Spirit Border). In addition, as the spirit is stored in the interior, thus it is called Shén Fēng (Spirit Seal).

---

[116] *Grasping the Wind* names it "Spirit Seal."

腎之肺病：胸滿不得息，乳癰，洒淅惡寒，不嗜食。

Lung diseases of the kidneys: fullness in the chest with inability to catch the breath, mammary welling-abscess, aversion to cold as though after a soaking, and no pleasure in eating.

注：氣逆於胸則滿，滿則不得息，取此穴以散上逆之氣。乳癰雖爲陽明經症，而部分則在於胸，取此穴以散胸中之毒。

Explanation: when there is counterflow qì in the chest, there will be fullness; for fullness in the chest with inability to catch the breath, choose this point in order to disperse the counterflow qì ascent. Although mammary welling-abscess is a yángmíng channel sign, yet the area [of this channel] is also on the chest, choose this point in order to disperse the toxin within the chest.

洒淅惡寒、不嗜食，乃肺症也，肺主皮毛，肺有寒邪，因有此症，宜泄。

For aversion to cold as though after a soaking and no pleasure in eating, these are surely lung patterns; as the lung governs the skin and body hair, when there is cold evil in the lung, these signs will occur, it is appropriate to drain.

腎之脾病：咳逆，嘔吐。

Spleen diseases of the kidneys: cough and counterflow, retching and vomiting.

注：咳逆者，胃中之氣上衝，取此穴以散胃中上衝之氣。腎之穴凡在胸者，無不治咳逆，皆以散胸中之逆氣也。嘔吐者，亦胃中之氣上逆也，取此穴以散胃中之逆氣。

Explanation: cough and counterflow are due to the upsurge of qì within the stomach, choose this point in order to disperse the upsurging qì in the stomach. For the points of the kidney channel that are on the chest, without exception, all of them treat cough and counterflow; in all cases, they disperse the counterflow qì in the chest. Retching and vomiting are also the counterflow ascent of qì within the stomach, choose this point in order to disperse the counterflow qì in the stomach.

Twenty-Fourth Point of the Kidney Channel
Líng Xū – Divine Mound[117] (KI-24)

腎經第二十四穴靈墟

穴在神藏下一寸六分陷中，去中行各二寸，仰而取之。《素》注：鍼四分。《銅人》：鍼三分，灸五壯。

This point is located in the depression 1 cùn 6 fēn below Shén Cáng (KI-25), at 2 cùn from the midline on each side; lie supine to locate it. *The Sùzhù* states, "Needle 4 fēn." *The Tóngrén* states, "Needle 3 fēn, and moxa 5 cones."

注：穴名靈墟者，心之神最靈，此穴乃心神所致之所，故曰靈墟。

Explanation: this point is named Líng Xū (Divine Mound) because the spirit of the heart is the most Líng (Divine). As this point is indeed the location where the heart spirit reaches, thus it is called Líng Xū (Divine Mound).

腎之肺病：胸脇支滿，痛引膺，不得息。

Lung diseases of the kidneys: propping fullness in the chest and rib-side, pain that radiates into the breast, and inability to catch the breath.

腎之脾病：咳逆嘔吐，不嗜食。

Spleen diseases of the kidneys: cough and counterflow with vomiting and retching, and no pleasure in eating.

注：二條俱見前。

Explanation: for these two passages, see the previous explanations.

Twenty-Fifth Point of the Kidney Channel
Shén Cáng – Spirit Storehouse (KI-25)

腎經第二十五穴神藏

穴在或中下一寸六分陷中，去中行各二寸，仰而取之。《銅人》：鍼三分，灸五壯。《素》注：鍼四分。

This point is located in the depression 1 cùn 6 fēn below Yù Zhòng (KI-26), at 2 cùn from the midline on each side; lie supine to locate it. *The Tóngrén* states, "Needle 3 fēn, and moxa 5 cones." *The Sùzhù* states, "Needle 4 fēn."

---

[117] *Grasping the Wind* names it "Spirit Ruins."

注：此穴乃近心之所，而心之神藏於其內，故曰神藏。

Explanation: this point is indeed nearby where the heart is, moreover, the spirit of the heart is Cáng (Stored) inside of this [point], thus it is called Shén Cáng (Spirit Storehouse).

腎之脾病：嘔吐不嗜食，咳逆。

Spleen diseases of the kidneys: vomiting with no pleasure in eating, cough and counterflow.

腎之肺病：喘不得息，胸滿，不嗜食。

Lung diseases of the kidneys: panting with inability to catch one's breath, fullness in the chest, and no pleasure in eating.

注：二條解見前。

Explanation: for these two passages, see the previous explanations.

Twenty-Sixth Point of the Kidney Channel
Yù Zhōng – Lively Centre (KI-26)
腎經第二十六穴彧中

穴在腧府下一寸六分，去胸中行各二寸，仰而取之。《銅人》：鍼四分，灸五壯。《明堂》：灸三壯。

This point is located 1 cùn 6 fēn below Shù Fǔ (KI-27), 2 cùn on each side of the chest midline; lie supine to locate it. *The Tóngrén* states, "Needle 4 fen, and moxa 5 cones." *The Míngtáng* states, "Moxa 3 cones."

注：彧字之義，《説文》解同郁字。又小雅詩：黍稷彧彧，茂盛貌。皆與此穴無關。遍考無據，俟後再詳。

Explanation: For the meaning of this character, Yù (Lively), according to the explanation of *the Shuōwén*,[118] it is the same as the character of "lush."[119]

---

[118] *The Shuōwén Jiězì* 説文解字 (*Explaining Graphs and Analysing Characters*, 2nd century CE) is one of the oldest and most authoritative dictionaries of Chinese characters.

[119] Note: this character referred here is yù 郁 (lush, dense, gloomy), which is also a homophone to yù 彧. The pinyin is left off the main text in order to avoid confusion.

Furthermore, the poem of the Lesser Court Hymns reads,[120] "How lush and dense is the sorghum!" This depicts an appearance of lushness. All of which have nothing to do with this point. As I investigate everything but cannot obtain any basis [of argument], I shall return to elaborate it at a later time.

腎之肺病：喘息不能食，胸脇支滿。

Lung diseases of the kidneys: panting with inability to eat, and propping fullness in the chest and rib-sides.

注：見前。

Explanation: see the previous [explanations].

腎之脾病：咳逆，涎出多唾。

Spleen diseases of the kidneys: cough and counterflow, and ejection of drool with copious spittle.

注：咳逆，涎出多唾，乃腎之水氣上逆於胃也，宜泄此穴。

Explanation: for cough and counterflow, as well as ejection of drool with copious spittle, these are due to the counterflow ascent of water qì of the kidneys into the stomach, it is appropriate to drain this point.

Twenty-Seventh Point of the Kidney Channel
Shù Fǔ – Transport Mansion (KI-27)
腎經第二十七穴腧府

穴在巨骨下、璇璣旁，各二寸陷中，仰而取之。《素》注：鍼四分，灸五壯。《銅人》：鍼三分，灸五壯。

This point is located below the great bone,[121] besides Xuán Jī (REN-21), in the depression 2 cùn on each [side of the midline]; lie supine to locate it. *The Sùzhù* states, "Needle 4 fēn, and moxa 5 cones." *The Tóngrén* states, "Needle 3 fēn, and moxa 5 cones."

思蓮子議曰：腧者，輸也。足少陰之經自湧泉而上輸至此穴，腎經之穴已盡，故曰腧府。

---

120 From 詩經小雅信南山 the *Book of Poetry*, "Lesser Court Hymn: Mount Xìnnán" (c. 6th century BCE).
121 I.e., the clavicle.

Master Sīlián's opinion: Shù (Transport Point) means to transport.[122] From Yǒng Quán (KI-1), the channel of the foot shàoyīn transports upwards to arrive at this point, as this is the terminal point of the kidney channel, thus it is called Shù Fǔ (Transport Mansion).

腎之肺病：喘嗽久，胸中痛，久喘，腹脹不下飲食。

Lung diseases of the kidneys: chronic panting with cough, pain in the chest, chronic panting, and abdominal distension with inability to get food and drink down.

注：喘嗽、胸中痛，肺氣爲衝脈逆也，宜泄。久喘，亦肺氣爲衝脈逆也，宜泄，灸七壯，其效。肺與大腸爲表裏，肺有逆氣，故腹爲之脹，取此穴以泄逆上之氣。

Explanation: for panting and cough, pain in the chest, this is counterflow of the lung qì caused by the chōng vessel, it is appropriate to drain. For chronic panting, it is also due to counterflow of the lung qì caused by the chōng vessel, it is appropriate to drain; perform seven cones of moxa, it will be effective. The lung and large intestine are an exterior-interior [pair], when there is qì counterflow in the lung, the abdomen will become distended, choose this point in order to drain the counterflow ascent of qì.

腎之脾病：嘔吐。

Spleen disease of the kidneys: vomiting and retching.

注：見前。

Explanation: See the previous [explanation].

---

[122] Shù 腧, from the point name, should be translated as a point, or as a transport point. It is a close homophone with shū 輸 (transport) that is used here as "to transport." Along with another homophone, shù 俞, these three characters are often used interchangeably in acupuncture literature; however, shù 腧 would be more specifically indicating the acupuncture point, as it has the 月 flesh radical; shū 輸 would be more indicating the function of transportation, as it has the 車 cart radical; and shù 俞 would be the broadest and most ambiguous, as it has no radical to specify its meaning.

Extra Points Associated with the Foot Shàoyīn Kidney Channel
足少陰腎經奇穴

Transverse Bone (KI-11)[123]
Héng Gǔ – 橫骨

《千金翼》云：婦人遺溺，灸橫骨，當陰門七壯。又治癩疝，在橫骨兩旁，挾莖灸之。

The Qiānjīn Yì states, "For urinary incontinence in women, moxa Héng Gǔ (KI-11), [in addition], one should moxa 7 cones on Yīn Mén.[124] It also treats downfall mounting, on the two sides of Héng Gǔ (KI-11), perform moxa [in sites] where they clasp the penis."

Yīn Spring (UEX-CA 47)
Quán Yīn – 泉陰

在橫骨旁三寸，治癩疝偏大，灸百壯。陰囊下第一橫紋，治風氣，眼反，口噤，腹中切痛，灸二七壯。

It is located 3 cùn to the sides of Héng Gǔ (KI-11). To treat downfall mounting that is larger on one side, moxa 100 cones. At the first skin crease below the scrotum, to treat wind qì, upward-turned eyes, clenched jaw, and stabbing pain in the abdomen, moxa 14 cones.

Yīn Stem[125]
Yīn Jīng – 陰莖

當溺孔是穴，治卒癲病，灸三壯，小便通即瘥。又灸陰莖頭三壯。

This point is located right at the urinary meatus; to treat sudden epileptic disease, moxa 3 cones; once the urine flows freely, there will be recovery. In addition, moxa 3 cones at the head of Yīn Jīng.

---

[123] This point shares the same name as KI-11, and there is not a separate extra point for it in various point compendiums; as such, we still regard it as KI-11 but with an alternative location.

[124] Known as Yīn Door, which is synonymous with the vulva.

[125] This is the penis. There is no categorized point number for it.

Ghost Storehouse (UEX-CA 51)
Guǐ Cáng – 鬼藏

男陰下縫、女玉門頭是穴，灸三壯。《千金翼》云：第十一次下鍼。

This point is located at the crease below the male genitalia, at the female's vaginal opening, moxa 3 cones. *The Qiānjīn Yì* states, "This is the eleventh [ghost point] to be needled."

Abode of the Corporeal Soul (UEX-CA 34)
Hún Shè – 魂舍

在挾臍兩旁，相去一寸。《千金》云：主小腹泄利膿血，灸百壯，小兒減之。

This point clasps the umbilicus on both sides, with [the points] 1 cùn apart from each other. *The Qiānjīn* states, "It governs the lower abdomen and diarrhoea with pus and blood, moxa 100 cones; reduce the amount for children."

The Hand Juéyīn
Pericardium Network
Channel & Points

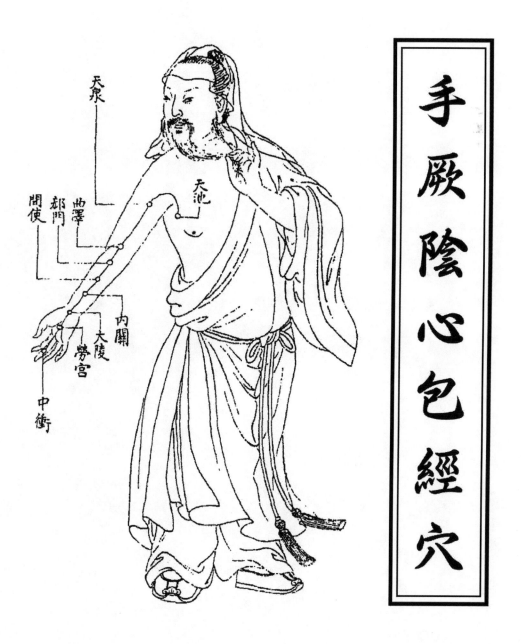

The Hand Juéyīn Pericardium Network Channel & Points
手厥陰心包絡經

Overview of the Hand Juéyīn Pericardium Network
手厥陰心包絡總論

思蓮子曰：心包絡，心之包也，爲手厥陰經，多血少氣。

Master Sīlián says, the pericardiac network is the wrapping of the heart, it is the hand juéyīn channel, its blood is copious and qì is scant.

起於胸中，出屬心下之包絡，受足少陰腎經之交，由是自膻中下膈，歷任之中脘穴，及臍下任脈之陰交穴，歷絡上、中、下之三焦；其支者，自屬心包處，上循胸出腋，下腋三寸，本經之天池穴，上行抵腋下，循臑內本經之天泉穴，以界乎手太陰肺經、手少陰心經兩經之中，

It commences within the chest, emerges where it adjoins at the wrapping network below the heart, which is the intersection that transfers from the foot shàoyīn kidney channel. From here, it descends from Dàn Zhōng (REN-17) to below the diaphragm, passing through Zhōng Wǎn (REN-12) of the rèn [vessel], and reaching Yīn Jiāo (REN-7) of the rèn vessel below the umbilicus. It passes through and networks with the upper, middle, and lower [jiāos] of the sānjiāo.

From the place where it adjoins to the pericardium, a branch ascends following the chest and emerges from the armpit, at Tiān Chí (PC-1) of this channel, which is 3 cùn below the armpit. It ascends to arrive at the armpit, following the inner flesh of the upper arm to Tiān Quán (PC-2) of this channel, which is situated at the boundary between the two channels of the hand tàiyīn lung channel and the hand shàoyīn heart channel.

入肘中本經之曲澤穴，又由肘中下臂，行臂兩筋之間，循本經之郄門穴及間使、內關、大陵等穴，遂入掌中，過本經之勞宮穴，循中指出其端之中衝穴；其支別者，循無名指出其端，而交於手少陽三焦經焉。

It enters the centre of the elbow at Qū Zé (PC-3) of this channel, continues from the middle of the elbow to descend the forearm, travelling in the space between the two sinews of the forearm, following Xī Mén (PC-4) of this

channel, reaching the points Jiān Shǐ (PC-5), Nèi Guān (PC-6), and Dà Líng (PC-7). Thereupon, it enters the centre of the palm, traverses Láo Gōng (PC-8) of this channel, and follows the middle finger to Zhōng Chōng (PC-9) at the tip. A branch diverges to follow the ring finger and emerges at the tip, where it intersects with the hand shàoyáng sānjiāo channel.

Diseases of the Hand Juéyīn Pericardium Network Channel
手厥陰心包絡經病

是動病則爲手心熱，以脈行掌中勞宮穴也。爲臂肘攣急，爲腋腫，皆脈所行處。甚則胸脇支滿，以脈循胸出脇也。爲心中憺憺大動，以脈出心包也。爲面赤，以赤爲心之正色也。爲目黃，心爲之精，心病則目黃。爲喜笑不休，以心在聲爲笑也。

When there are changes resulting in diseases, there will be heat in the centre of the palms, this is because the vessel travels to Láo Gōng (PC-8), which is at the centre of the palm. For hypertonicity of the arm and elbow,[126] as well as swelling of the armpit, both are places where the vessel travels. When it is severe, there will be propping fullness of the chest and rib-side, this is because the vessel follows the chest and emerges at the rib-side. For the intense and uncomfortable stirring sensation within the heart, this is because the vessel emerges from the pericardium. For red face, this is because red is the normal colour of the heart. For yellowing of the eyes, [the eyes are] the essence of the heart; thus, when the heart is diseased, there will be yellowing of the eyes. For incessant joyfulness and laughing, this is because the heart corresponds to laughter in sounds.

所生病爲煩心，爲心痛，爲掌中熱諸病。邪氣盛則泄之，正氣虛則補之。熱則泄之，疾去其鍼，寒則溫之，久留其鍼。脈陷下者，用艾灸之。若不盛不虛，則取本經，不必求手少陽三焦經也。

For diseases itself engenders, there is vexation of the heart, heart pain, and various types of heat diseases in the palms.

When the evil qì is exuberant, drain it; when the upright qì is vacuous, supplement it. When there is heat, drain it and quickly remove the needle; when there is cold, warm it and retain the needle.

---

126 The character here, "臂 upper arm," was originally "背 upper back" in the source text. It is not known if this is a typographical error or a scribal error from the two manuscripts. It has been amended in accordance with *Língshū* Chapter 10.

When the vessel is sunken, moxa it. When there is neither exuberance nor vacuity, then only choose this channel, as there is no need to use the hand shàoyáng sānjiāo channel.

如寸口較人迎之脈大者一倍而躁，則心包爲實宜泄，三焦爲虛宜補。若寸口較人迎之脈小者一倍而不躁，則心包爲虛宜補，三焦爲實宜泄也。

When the cùnkǒu pulse in comparison to the rényíng pulse is one times larger and agitated, the pericardium is replete, one ought to drain it; the sānjiāo is vacuous, one ought to supplement it. When the cùnkǒu pulse in comparison to the rényíng pulse is one times smaller and not agitated, the pericardium is vacuous, one ought to supplement it; the sānjiāo is replete, one ought to drain it.

The Hand Heart Governor Sinew Channel
手心主經筋

手心主之筋，起於手中指之中衝，與手太陰之筋並行，結於肘之內廉曲澤，上臂陰以結於腋下之天泉、天池，下散於在前、在後之挾脇處；其支者，則入於腋，散於胸中，爲胸痛，爲息賁。

The sinew channel of the hand heart governor commences at Zhōng Chōng (PC-9) of the middle finger, it travels together with the sinew [channel] of the hand tàiyīn, to knot at the inner aspect of the elbow at Qū Zé (PC-3). It ascends the upper arm to knot below the armpit at Tiān Quán (PC-2) and Tiān Chí (PC-1), it then descends and dissipates in the rib-side area that is clasped between the front and the back. A branch enters the armpit and dissipates within the chest. [When it is diseased,] there is chest pain and rushing respiration.

First Point of the Pericardium Network
Tiān Chí – Celestial Pool (PC-1)
心包絡第一穴天池

一名天會
Alternate name: Celestial Convergence

穴在腋下三寸，乳後一寸，着脇，直腋撅肋間，手厥陰心包、足厥陰肝經、足少陽膽經、手少陽三焦經相會之地。《銅人》：灸三壯，鍼二[127]分。《甲乙》：

---

[127] The Tóngrén actually states "2 cones" instead of "3 cones" listed above.

鍼七分。《千金》：治頸漏瘰癧，灸百壯。《素》注：在乳後同身寸之二寸。

This point is located 3 cùn below the armpit, 1 cùn to the side of the breast, on the rib-side, in a line between the armpit and the free rib, in the intercostal space.[128] It is the location where the hand juéyīn pericardium [channel], the foot juéyīn liver channel, the foot shàoyáng gallbladder channel, and the hand shàoyáng sānjiāo channel meet with one another. *The Tóngrén* states, "Moxa 3 cones, and needle 2 fēn." *The Jiǎyǐ* states, "Needle 7 fēn." *The Qiānjīn* states, "To treat exudative scrofula of the neck, moxa 100 cones." *The Sùzhù* states, "It is located 2 cùn of the body inch to the side of the breast."

注：此經之直者，既下膈歷絡三焦矣，而支者，自屬心包處，上循胸，橫出腋，結爲此穴。雖與膽經之淵腋、輒筋，俱下腋三寸，而此穴則近乳一寸，獨在前矣，乃本經初見之穴，而爲本經最高之處，有天之象焉。三焦主氣，此經主血，血之所行，有水象焉，故曰天池。

Explanation: the vertical [pathway] of this channel descends through the diaphragm, passes through and networks with the sānjiāo. From the place where it adjoins to the pericardium, a branch ascends and follows the chest to exit horizontally at the armpit, knotting at this point.

Although [this point] together with Yuān Yè (GB-22) and Zhé Jīn (GB-23) of the gallbladder channel, all of them are 3 cùn below the armpit, however, this point is 1 cùn nearby the breast. It alone is on the front [of the body], which is the first observable point of this channel; in addition, it is in the highest location of this channel [points], thus, it has the image of Tiān (The Celestial).

While the sānjiāo governs qì, this channel governs blood; as [this channel] is where the blood moves, it has the image of water within it; therefore, it is called Tiān Chí (Celestial Pool).

心包之肺病：胸中有聲，胸膈煩滿，上氣寒熱，熱病汗不出，頭痛，四肢不舉，腋下腫，痎瘧臂痛。

Lung diseases of the pericardium: sounds within the chest, vexation and fullness in the chest and diaphragm, qì ascent with chills and fever, febrile disease with absence of sweating, headache, inability to lift the four limbs, axillary swelling, and intervallic malaria with arm pain.

注：此經循胸中出，胸膈煩滿，而右尺脈洪，右寸脈亦洪，乃本經之氣滯於胸也，宜泄此穴，以泄胸中之熱。熱病汗不出、頭痛、四肢不舉，則周身皆受病

---

128 "肋間 Intercostal space" was originally "筋間 between the sinews" in the primary manuscript. The editors of this manuscript, Zhāng and Zhà, have amended it in accordance with *the Zhēnjiǔ Dàchéng, Jiǎyǐ Jīng*, and *Tóngrén*.

矣，而腋下獨腫，乃本經所行之部分也，上氣寒熱，而又近於少陽，此經與手少陽
爲表裏，故取此穴，以去周身之熱。痎瘧者，肺受暑也，臂者，本經所行之部分
也，宜泄此穴。

Explanation: this channel follows and emerges from within the chest; thus, there is vexation and fullness in the chest and diaphragm; as a result, the right chǐ pulse [position] will be surging, and the right cùn pulse [position] will also be surging, this is due to the stagnation of qì of this channel in the chest; it is appropriate to drain this point in order to drain the heat within the chest.

For febrile disease with absence of sweating, headache, and inability to lift the four limbs, the whole body has contracted disease; yet, only the armpit is swollen, as this is the area where this channel travels.

Qì ascent with chills and fever is similar to the shàoyáng [disease],[129] as this channel and hand shàoyáng are an exterior-interior [pair], thus choose this point in order to eliminate the heat from the whole body. Intervallic malaria is due to the lung contracting summerheat; for arm [pain], this is the area where this channel travels, it is appropriate to drain this point.

心包之肝病：目䀮䀮不明。

Liver disease of the pericardium: blurry dim vision.

注：目䀮䀮不明，乃火熱盛，泄此穴以降火。

Explanation: blurry dim vision is due to the exuberance of fire and heat, drain this point in order to descend fire.

Second Point of the Pericardium Network
Tiān Quán – Celestial Spring (PC-2)
心包絡第二穴天泉

一名天濕
Alternate Name: Celestial Dampness[130]

穴在曲腋下二寸，舉臂取之。《銅人》：鍼六分，灸三壯。

---

[129] Another way to read this line is, "For qì ascent with chills and fever, [as this point] is near the shàoyáng [channel]…" Nevertheless, this current translation is chosen as it seems to fit the context better.

[130] *Grasping the Wind* names it "Celestial Damp."

This point is located 2 cùn below the axillary fold, raise the arm to locate it. *The Tóngrén* states, "Needle 6 fēn, and moxa 3 cones."

注：此穴在本經初入臂而下行，自中衝而視之，乃最高焉。天池在胸，有停水之象，故曰天池。此穴乃注水而下行，故曰天泉。

Explanation: this point is where this channel enters the arm and begins its descent. When viewing [this point] from Zhōng Chōng (PC-9), this point is at the highest place. Tiān Chí (Celestial Pool, PC-1) is located on the chest, it has the image of water collecting, thus it is called Tiān Chí (Celestial Pool, PC-1). Because this point is where the water pours and descends, thus it is called Tiān Quán (Celestial Spring).

心包之心病：心病，胸脇支滿，咳逆，膺、背、胛間、臂内廉痛。

Heart diseases of the pericardium: heart disease, propping fullness in the chest and rib-side, cough and counterflow, pain of the breast, upper back, between the scapulae, and inner aspect of upper arm.

注：心病而至於胸脇支滿，咳逆，膺、背、胛間、臂内廉痛，皆此經所行之部分，心痛乃此經之正病，宜泄此穴，以泄胸中之逆氣。

Explanation: for heart disease that causes propping fullness in the chest and rib-side, cough and counterflow, pain of the breast, upper back, between the scapulae, and inner aspect of the upper arm, these are all areas where this channel travels. For heart pain, this a principal disease of this channel, it is appropriate to drain this point in order to drain counterflow qì within the chest.

心包之肝病：目眽眽不明，惡風寒。

Liver diseases of the pericardium: blurry dim vision, aversion to wind and cold.

注：目眽眽，肝病也；惡風寒者，肺有寒邪也。二者兼之，則寒久變而爲熱，宜泄此穴，以去火邪。

Explanation: for blurry vision, this is a liver disease. For aversion to wind and cold, this is due to the presence of cold evil in the lung. When [one contracts] these two [diseases] concurrently, after an extended period of time, the cold [evil] will transmute into heat, it is appropriate to drain this point in order to eliminate the fire evil.

Third Point of the Pericardium Network
Qū Zé – Marsh at the Bend (PC-3)
心包絡第三穴曲澤

穴在肘內廉陷中，大筋內側橫紋中，動脈是穴，屈肘得之，心包絡脈所入爲合水。《銅人》：灸三壯，鍼二分，留七呼。

This point is located in the depression on the inner aspect of the elbow, on the inside of the great sinew at the transverse crease. The point is at the pulsating vessel, bend the elbow to locate it. The pericardiac network vessel enters here, as the uniting and water point. *The Tóngrén* **states, "Moxa 3 cones, needle 2 fēn,[131] and retain for 7 respirations."**

注：水所聚者爲澤，此穴乃在肘臂曲折之處，故曰曲澤。又爲本經所入爲合水，亦爲澤象。

Explanation: a place where water accumulates is a Zé (Marsh); as this point is located at the place where the arm Qū (Bends) and extends, thus it is called Qū Zé (Marsh at the Bend). Also, it is where this channel enters as the uniting and water point, which also has the image of Zé (Marsh).

心包之心病：心痛善驚，身熱煩渴口乾，心下憺憺。

Heart diseases of the pericardium: heart pain with susceptibility to fright, generalised heat with vexation thirst and dry mouth, and stirring discomfort below the heart.[132]

注：心包受邪，則爲之痛，而善驚者，神不寧也，宜補心包之水穴，以治火。身熱煩渴口乾，火盛極矣，亦補此穴，以治火。心下憺憺，宜安靜而反動也，宜補此穴，以治火。

Explanation: when the pericardium contracts an evil, there will be pain, and it will lead to susceptibility to fright as the spirit is disquieted, it is appropriate to supplement the water point of the pericardium in order to treat fire.

For generalised heat with vexation thirst and dry mouth, this is due to extreme exuberance of fire, it is appropriate to supplement this point in order to treat fire. For stirring discomfort below the heart, it is appropriate to quiet and

---

[131] For "3 fēn" *the Tóngrén* actually states "2 fēn."

[132] According to *the Collated Explanations Zhēnjiǔ Dàchéng*, "憺憺 stirring discomfort" means, "胃脘部有翻動不適之感。憺憺，爲大水動貌。 stirring and uncomfortable sensation in the stomach duct; as for 憺憺, it [originally] means the appearance of a great river in movement."

tranquilise in order to counteract the stirring; it is appropriate to supplement this point in order to treat fire.

心包之肺病：身熱風疹，頭清汗出不過肩。

Lung diseases of the pericardium: generalised body heat with wind papules, and cool sensation in the head with sweating that does not extend past the shoulder.[133]

注：心火外凌皮毛，而生風疹。皮毛者，肺之合也。補心包之水，以治心火。汗出不過肩，乃氣滯不通也，宜泄此穴，以通肩背之氣。

Explanation: when heart fire intimidates the skin and body hair outside, this will lead to engenderment of wind papules. For skin and body hair, they are connected with the lung, supplement the water point of the pericardium in order to treat heart fire. For [cool sensation in the head with] sweating that does not extend past the shoulder, this is due to blockage caused by stagnation of qì, it is appropriate to drain this point in order to unblock the qì of the shoulder and upper back.

心包之脾病：逆氣嘔涎血，傷寒逆氣嘔吐。

Spleen diseases of the pericardium: counterflow qì with vomiting of drool and blood, cold damage with counterflow qì, and retching and vomiting.

注：涎者，血也，皆屬乎心者也，逆氣上而嘔之，心火熱極，宜補此穴，以治其火。傷寒逆氣嘔吐，此經下絡三焦，氣逆而有是症，宜泄此穴，以降其逆。

Explanation: regarding drool,[134] it is blood, both of which belong to the heart; counterflow qì ascent will lead to vomiting of them,[135] this is extreme heat of heart fire, it is appropriate to supplement this point in order to treat the fire. For cold damage with counterflow qì, retching and vomiting, as this channel descends to network with the sānjiāo, when there is counterflow qì [in this channel], there will be this sign, it is appropriate to drain this point in order to descend the counterflow.

心包之肝病：臂肘手腕，不時動搖。

Liver diseases of the pericardium: occasional shaking of the arms, elbows, hands, and wrists.[136]

---

[133] The *Zhēnjiǔ Dàchéng* has "漬 soaked" in place of "清 cool," which would instead read, "head soaked with sweat that does not extend past the shoulders."

[134] Note: According to *the Practical Dictionary*, "drool is one of the five humours that is associated with the spleen."

[135] I.e., drool and blood.

[136] The scribal manuscript had "不能 inability" in place of "不時 occasional", Zhāng and Zhà changed it in accordance with *the Zhēnjiǔ Dàchéng*.

注：此筋受風也，而部分乃爲本經所行之地，此穴又臂肘交折上下相連之
處，宜泄此穴，以去風。

Explanation: this is the contraction of wind by the sinews; in addition, these places are areas where the channel travels, and this point is also the place where the upper arm and elbow bend and where the upper [arm] and lower [arm] connect with each other, it is appropriate to drain this point in order to eliminate wind.

Fourth Point of the Pericardium Network
Xī Mén – Cleft Gate (PC-4)
心包絡第四穴郄門

穴在掌後去腕五寸，手厥陰心包絡脈郄。《銅人》：鍼三分，灸三[137]壯。

This point is located behind the palm, 5 cùn from the wrist. It is the hand juéyīn pericardiac network cleft point. *The Tóngrén* states, "Needle 3 fēn, and moxa 3 cones."

注：此穴乃手厥陰經之郄也，界在手少陰、手太陰兩脈之間，而有郄焉，
有門象，故曰郄門。

Explanation: this point is the Xī (Cleft) point of the hand juéyīn channel, it is situated between the two vessels, the hand shàoyīn and the hand tàiyīn, where there is a Xī (Cleft). Furthermore, it also has the image of a Mén (Gate), thus it is called Xī Mén (Cleft Gate).

心包之心病：心痛嘔噦，驚恐畏人，神氣不足。

Heart diseases of the pericardium: heart pain with retching and vomiting, fright and fear with fear of people, and insufficiency of the spirit qì.

注：心痛嘔噦，而至於驚恐畏人，神氣爲之不足，此正氣不足，而邪氣有
餘也，宜先補正氣，而後泄邪氣。

Explanation: for heart pain with retching and vomiting, it will lead to fright and fear with fear of people, as the spirit qì has become insufficient, this is insufficiency of the upright qì, in addition to the superabundance of evil qì; it is appropriate to initially supplement the upright qì, then subsequently drain the evil qì.

心包之肺病：衄血。

Lung disease of the pericardium: nosebleeds.

---

[137] For "5 fēn" *the Tóngrén* actually states "3 fēn."

注：心火上凌肺金，血自鼻出，宜泄此穴，以降心火。

Explanation: when heart fire ascends to intimidate lung metal, blood will spontaneously eject from the nose, it is appropriate to drain this point in order to descend heart fire.

心包之脾病：嘔血。

Spleen disease of the pericardium: retching of blood.

注：嘔血者，胃有積血也，本經歷絡三焦，中焦乃其所歷也，宜泄此穴，以降胃中之逆。

Explanation: for retching of blood, there is an accumulation of blood in the stomach; as this channel passes through and networks with the sānjiāo, as such, the middle jiāo is where it passes through, so it is appropriate to drain this point in order to descend the counterflow within the stomach.

Fifth Point of the Pericardium Network
Jiān Shǐ – Intermediary Courier (PC-5)
心包絡第五穴間使

穴在掌後三寸，兩筋間陷中，心包絡所行爲經金。《素》注：鍼六分，留七呼。《銅人》：鍼三分，灸五壯。《明堂》：灸七壯。《甲乙》：灸三壯。

This point is located behind the palm, 3 cùn [from the wrist], in the depression between the two sinews. The pericardiac network flows here, as the river and metal point. *The Sùzhù* states, "Needle 6 fēn, and retain for 7 respirations." *The Tóngrén* states, "Needle 3 fēn, and moxa 5 cones." *The Míngtáng* states, "Moxa 7 cones." *The Jiǎyǐ* states, "Moxa 3 cones."

注：此穴在兩陰經之間，而本經乃心主臣使之官，故曰間使。有病則其脈至，無病則其脈止。

Explanation: this point is located in the Jiān (Intermediary) between the two yīn channels; moreover, this channel is the heart governor, which is the official acting as minister and Shǐ (Courier),[138] thus it is called Jiān Shǐ (Intermediary Courier). When there is a presence of disease, a pulse will appear here; when there is an absence of disease, the pulse will disappear.

---

[138] From *Sùwèn* Chapter 8.

心包之心病：卒心痛，多驚，掌中熱。

Heart diseases of the pericardium: sudden heart pain, frequent fright, and heat in the palms.

注：心痛多驚，邪勝正也，宜先補其正，而後泄其邪。掌中熱，乃本經所行之部分也，熱乃火動，宜泄此穴，以去熱。

Explanation: for heart pain and excessive fright, this is because of evil prevailing over the upright [qì], it is appropriate to initially supplement the upright [qì], then subsequently drain the evil. For heat in the palms, this is because it is the area is where this channel travels; furthermore, the heat is due to fire stirring, it is appropriate to drain this point in order to eliminate the heat.

心包之肺病：傷寒結胸，心中如饑，卒狂，胸中憺憺，惡風寒，嘔沫。

Lung diseases of the pericardium: cold damage with chest bind, a sensation of scarcity in the heart,[139] sudden mania, stirring discomfort in the chest, aversion to wind and cold, and vomiting of foam.

注：胸者，肺之室。本經起於胸中，胸有邪，則致諸症，急泄此穴，以降胸中之逆。

Explanation: the chest is the chamber of the lung. As this channel commences within the chest, when there is evil within the chest, there will be these various signs, urgently drain this point in order to descend the counterflow within the chest.

心包之脾病：寒中少氣，鬼邪霍亂，乾嘔。

Spleen diseases of the pericardium: cold in the centre with scantness of breath,[140] ghost evil with sudden turmoil, and dry retching.

注：中者，中脘也。寒中少氣，乃不足也，宜補此穴，以生中氣。中氣亂，而後有霍亂之症，宜泄此穴，以分消其霍亂。

Explanation: the centre refers to the middle stomach duct.[141] For cold in the centre with scantness of breath, this is due to insufficiency, it is appropriate to supplement this point in order to engender the centre qì. When the centre qì is in chaos, subsequently there will be the sign of sudden turmoil, it is appropriate to drain this point in order to separate and dissolve the sudden turmoil.

---

[139] Here "in the heart" is likely synonymous with "in the chest," as this is listed under lung diseases rather than heart diseases.

[140] "Cold in the centre" could also be interpreted as "cold strike," we have chosen the former in accordance with his explanation.

[141] This is also the name for Zhōng Wǎn (REN-12).

心包之肝病：中風氣逆，涎上昏危，瘖不得語，咽中如梗，腋腫肘攣，小兒客忤，婦人月水不調，血結成塊。

Liver diseases of the pericardium: wind strike with counterflow qì, rising drool and critical clouding, loss of voice with inability to speak, sensation of blockage in the pharynx, swelling of the armpit and hypertonicity of the elbow, child visiting hostility, irregular menstruation, and bound blood that forms into clots.

注：本經歷絡上、中、下三焦，今氣上逆而涎隨之，所以昏危不語，涎不得上，所以如梗，宜泄此穴，以降三焦之氣。本經循胸出腋入肘，皆其所行部分，腫而攣，皆本經鬱滯之邪也，宜泄此穴，以通其滯。小兒客忤，乃正氣之虛，而邪氣乘之，宜先補正氣，而後泄邪氣。足厥陰、手厥陰，皆司血者，本經之氣鬱，上、中、下三焦不暢，而足厥陰之經亦鬱，故有血結之病，宜泄此穴，以通三焦之氣，而破其結，則經自調矣。

Explanation: this channel passes through and networks with the upper, middle, and lower [jiāos] of the sānjiāo; presently, there is counterflow qì ascent that is followed by drool, which will result in critical clouding with inability to speak; if the drool is unable to be ejected, it will result in the sensation of blockage, it is appropriate to drain this point in order to descend the qì of the sānjiāo.

This channel follows the chest to emerge at the armpit and enter the elbow, all of these are areas where the channel travels, thus for swelling and hypertonicity, both of these are due to depression and stagnation of evil in this channel, it is appropriate to drain this point in order to free the stagnation.

For child visiting hostility,[142] this is due to vacuity of the upright qì, which the evil qì overwhelms; initially supplement the upright qì, then subsequently drain the evil qì.

Both the foot juéyīn and the hand juéyīn control the blood, when there is depression of qì in this channel, the upper, middle, and lower [jiāos] of the sānjiāo will be inhibited, leading also to the depression of the channel of foot juéyīn, thus resulting in a disease of the bound blood; it is appropriate to drain this point in order to free the qì of the sānjiāo, so that the bound [blood] can be broken, as such, the menstruation will naturally become regulated.

---

[142] According to the *Practical Dictionary*, child visiting hostility is described as "crying, fright, disquietude, or even changes in complexion in infants brought on by seeing a stranger or strange sight, or being exposed to unfamiliar surroundings or circumstances."

Sixth Point of the Pericardium Network
Nèi Guān – Inner Pass (PC-6)
心包絡第六穴內關

穴在掌後，去腕二寸兩筋間，與三焦經外關穴相抵，手心主之絡，別走手少陽三焦經。《銅人》：鍼五分，灸三壯。

This point is located behind the palm, 2 cùn [from the wrist], and between the two sinews; it is a counterpart to Wài Guān (SJ-5) of the sānjiāo channel. It is the network point of the hand heart governor, it diverges to the hand shàoyáng sānjiāo channel. *The Tóngrén* **states, "Needle 5 fēn, and moxa 3 cones."**

注：穴名內關者，第四穴名郤門，而間使穴在於其中，既過門，而復有關焉。內者，與外相對也，皆離肘而入掌骨節交經之處，有關象焉，故曰關。又手厥陰別走手少陽之絡，亦有關象。《內經》云：手心主之別，名曰內關，去腕二寸，出於兩筋之間循經以上系於心包絡，心系實則心痛，虛則爲頭強，取之本穴。

Explanation: regarding the point name Nèi Guān (Inner Pass), the fourth point is called Xī Mén (PC-4, Cleft Gate), and Jiān Shǐ (PC-5, Intermediary Courier) is located between them; such that, after [the courier] has gone past the gate, there is another Guān (Pass) ahead. Nèi (Inner) is the counterpart of Outer,[143] both of which are at the location where the channels intersect as they depart the elbow to enter the bone joints of the palm; as such, they both have the image of a Guān (Pass), thus they are called Guān (Pass).

In addition, as it is the network-vessel of the hand juéyīn that diverges to the hand shàoyáng, it also has the image of a Guān (Pass). *The Nèijīng* states, "The divergence of the hand heart governor, it is called Nèi Guān (Inner Pass); it is 2 cùn from the wrist, it emerges in the space between the two sinews and follows the channel in order to ascend and connect with the pericardiac network. When the heart connector is replete, there will be heart pain; when it is vacuous, there will be stiffness of the head; [in either case], choose this point."[144]

心包之心病：失志心痛，實則心暴痛，虛則頭強。

Heart diseases of the pericardium: loss of will with heart pain, when replete there is sudden heart pain, and when vacuous there is stiffness of the head.

---

[143] Wài 外 (Outer) here likely refers to Wài Guān (SJ-5).

[144] From *Língshū* Chapter 10; however, the original line from Chapter 10 concludes with "取之兩筋間也 choose it (i.e., the point) between the two sinews."

注：失志，則心氣鬱而不暢，故心痛焉，急泄此穴，以通其鬱。實則心痛宜泄，凡心痛，皆先責此穴，以此穴爲三焦之絡，泄此穴則氣暢於上下，而痛立止。氣虛則不能至於頭，而頭爲之強，故補此穴，而生上行之氣。

Explanation: when there is a loss of will, heart qì is depressed and has become impeded, thus there is heart pain, urgently drain this point in order to free the depression. When there is repletion, there is heart pain, it is appropriate to drain [this point]. For any type of heart pain, always seek this point first, as this point serves as the network-vessel to the sānjiāo, so drain this point and the qì will become unimpeded in the above and below, and the pain will immediately stop.

When the qì is vacuous and is unable to reach the head, the head will become stiff, thus supplement this point and it will engender the ascending qì.

心包之肝病：目赤，支滿，肘攣，手中風熱。

Liver diseases of the pericardium: red eyes, propping fullness, hypertonicity of the elbow, and wind-heat in the hands.

注：目赤者，心火盛，泄此穴以散心火。支滿者，氣鬱也，泄之。肘攣者，氣不至肘也，補之。手中風熱，皆心火盛也，宜泄此穴，而去掌中之風熱。此穴在八法，與奇經陰維相通，而下又與脾之公孫，主客相應。

Explanation: red eyes is exuberant heart fire, drain this point in order to dissipate the heart fire. Propping fullness is due to qì depression, drain this [point]. Hypertonicity of the elbow is because the qì fails to reach the elbow, supplement it. For wind-heat in the hands, in all cases, it is due to exuberant heart fire, it is appropriate to drain this point and the wind heat in the palms will be eliminated.

Among the Eight Confluent [points],[145] this point and the yīnwéi [vessel] communicate with each other; in the below, [this point] and Gōng Sūn (SP-4) of the spleen [channel] correspond to each other as the host and guest, respectively.[146]

---

[145] This literally refers to the "eight methods," which is the eightfold method of the sacred tortoise and the eightfold soaring method from *the Dàchéng*, where the eight confluent points came from.

[146] From *the Dàchéng* vol. 7, where PC-6 is said to govern diseases of the heart, gallbladder, spleen, and stomach; SP-4 would serve as the assistant point.

Seventh Point of the Pericardium Network
Dà Líng – Great Mound (PC-7)
心包絡第七穴大陵

穴在掌後骨兩筋間，手厥陰心包所注爲腧土，心包絡實則泄之。《銅人》：鍼五分。《素》注：鍼六分，留七呼，灸三壯。

This point is located behind the palm, in the space between the bones and the two sinews. The hand juéyīn pericardium pours here, as the stream and earth point. When the pericardiac network is replete, drain it. *The Tóngrén* states, "Needle 5 fēn." *The Sùzhù* states, "Needle 6 fēn, retain for 7 respirations, and moxa 3 cones."

注：陵者，土也，以此穴爲本經之腧穴，故曰陵。又其穴在掌後骨下，其上骨肉豐隆，而穴在其下，故曰大陵。

Explanation: Líng (Mound) is earth, as this point is the stream point[147] of this channel, thus it is Líng (Mound). In addition, this point is located behind the palm and below the bone; above this [point], the flesh and blood are bountiful and bulging, as this point is located at the base of it, thus it is called Dà Líng (Great Mound).

心包之心病：熱病汗不出，手心熱，肘臂攣痛，腋腫，善笑不休，煩心，心懸若饑，心痛掌熱，善悲泣驚恐，嘔啘無度，狂言不樂，瘑瘡疥癬。

Heart diseases of the pericardium: febrile disease with absence of sweating, heat in the centre of the palms, hypertonicity and pain of the arm and elbow, swelling of the armpit, frequent incessant laughing, vexation of the heart, heart that feels suspended as if one is famished, heart pain with heat in the palms, frequent sorrowful weeping with fright and fear, uncontrollable dry retching, manic ravings and unhappiness, and metacarpophalangeal sores with scabs and lichen.[148]

注：因熱病汗不出，而有下數症，皆本經之症也，宜泄本經之子穴，以出其汗，而症自息。心痛掌熱，掌乃本經所行之處，乃本經之氣有餘也，善悲泣驚

[147] I.e., the earth point.

[148] For metacarpophalangeal sores, according to *the Yīzōng Jīnjiàn* 醫宗金鑒 (*the Golden Mirror of Medical Ancestry*, 1742 CE), "瘑瘡每發指掌中,兩手對生茱萸形,風濕癢痛津汁水,時好時發久生蟲 metacarpophalangeal sores always break out in the fingers and palm, simultaneously on both hands, [sores] in the shape of [Shan] Zhu Yu appear/are engendered; it is wind-damp with itchiness, pain, exudation of thin fluid, which disappears and reoccurs occasionally. Over an extended period of time, insects will grow in it."

恐，皆正氣虛而邪盛之症，宜泄本經之子穴。嘔啘無度，心氣上逆也，狂言不樂，心火盛也，亦宜泄其子穴。瘑瘡疥癬，皆屬乎火，宜泄火之子。

Explanation: because of the febrile disease with absence of sweating, it will lead to the other subsequent signs [listed above]; all of them are signs of this channel, it is appropriate to drain the child point of this channel in order to eject the sweat, then the [above] signs will naturally cease.

For heart pain with heat in the palms, as the palms are where this channel travels, it is because there is a superabundance of qì in this channel. For frequent sorrowful weeping with fright and fear, it is always a pattern of upright qì vacuity with exuberance of evil qì, it is appropriate to drain the child point of this channel.

Uncontrollable dry retching is due to counterflow ascent of heart qì; manic ravings with unhappiness is due to exuberance of heart fire, it is also appropriate to drain the child point. Metacarpophalangeal sores, scabs and lichen are all ascribed to fire, it is appropriate to drain the child [point] of fire.[149]

心包之肺病：喉痺口乾，身熱頭痛短氣，胸脇滿。

Lung diseases of the pericardium: throat impediment with dry mouth, generalised heat with headache and shortness of breath, fullness of the chest and rib-side.

注：喉痺而至於口乾，肺受心火上凌也，泄火之子，所以降心火也。胸脇皆本經所行部分，身熱頭痛短氣，而證之以胸脇痛，則知爲本經之邪，宜泄其子，以去其邪。

Explanation: for throat impediment that causes dry mouth, this is because the lung is intimated by the ascent of heart fire, drain the child [point] of fire so as to descend the heart fire.

The chest and rib-side are both areas where this channel travels; where there is generalised heat with headache and shortness of breath, one needs to further verify that there is [also] chest and rib-side pain; in doing so, one knows that it is caused by the evil of this channel, it is appropriate to drain the child [point] in order to eliminate the evil.

心包之肝病：目赤目黃，小便如血。

Liver diseases of the pericardium: red eyes with yellowing of the eyes, and urine that appears bloody.

---

[149] This line is reminiscent of *Sùwèn* Chapter 74, which contains the nineteen pathomechanisms and states "諸痛癢瘡, 皆屬於心 all diseases of pain, itching and sores are ascribed to the heart."

注：目赤目黃，皆心火盛也，而又證之小便如血，則心火移於小腸矣，宜泄火之子，以弱心火。

Explanation: for red eyes with yellowing of the eyes, both are due to exuberance of heart fire; in addition, for the pattern of urine that appears bloody, heart fire has been transferred to the small intestine, drain the child [point] of fire in order to weaken the heart fire.

Eighth Point of the Pericardium Network
Láo Gōng – Palace of Toil (PC-8)
心包絡第八穴勞宮

一名五里
Alternate name: Five Li[150]

一名掌中
Alternate name: Centre of the Palm

穴在掌中之後，屈中指、無名指二指至手掌，二指之間，動脈是穴。心包絡所溜爲滎火。《素》注:鍼二分，留六呼。《銅人》：灸三壯。《明堂》：鍼二分，得氣即泄，只一度，鍼過二度，令人虛，禁灸，灸令人瘜肉日加。《千金》：心中懊憹痛，刺五分，補之。

This point is located behind the centre of the palm; bend the middle finger and the ring finger to touch the palm; in the space between the two fingers, at the pulsating vessel, that is the point. The pericardiac network gushes here, as the brook and fire point. The Sùzhù states, "Needle 2 fēn,[151] and retain for 6 respirations." The Tóngrén states, "Moxa 3 cones." The Míngtáng states, "Needle 2 fēn, obtain qì then promptly drain; only [needle] once, if needled twice this will cause the person to become vacuous. Moxibustion is contraindicated, as moxibustion will cause a polyp to gradually increase in size." The Qiānjīn states, "For anguish pain in the heart, pierce 5 fēn, and supplement it."

注：人勞於思，則此穴之脈大動，蓋以此穴爲本經之火，心勞則火動，火動則脈大動於此穴，故曰勞宮。禁灸者，以火濟火，而心火愈熾也。

Explanation: when a person Láo (Toils) oneself in contemplation, there will be great pulsations at this point, because this point is the fire [point] of this channel.

---

[150] Note: "Lǐ 里" is a measure of length, approximately one third of a mile.
[151] For "3 fēn" the Sùzhù actually states "2 fēn."

When the heart is Láo (Toiled), fire will be stirred up; when the fire is stirred, there will be a great pulsation of the vessel at this point, thus it is called Láo Gōng (Palace of Toil). Moxibustion is prohibited, as this is fire assisting fire, which will make the heart fire ever more intense.

心包之心病：熱病汗不出，怵惕，脇痛不可轉側，大、小便血，衄血不止，氣逆嘔噦，煩渴，食飲不下。

Heart diseases of the pericardium: febrile disease with absence of sweating, apprehensiveness, rib-side pain with inability to turn to the sides, blood in the stool and urine, incessant nosebleeds, qì counterflow with retching and belching, vexation and thirst, inability to get food and drink down.

注：熱病而汗不出者，數日，邪漸入內，怵惕者，神亂也，脇痛不可轉側，乃本經之由腋行者氣逆也，大小便血、衄血，本經屬火，血被火逆，上下俱出，氣逆嘔噦，內不容邪也，煩渴，食飲不下，皆火逆於內所致，急泄火之子，以降火。

Explanation: for febrile disease that leads to absence of sweating, this is because the evil gradually enters the interior over the span of several days. Apprehensiveness is due to derangement of the spirit. For rib-side pain with inability to turn to the sides, this is caused by counterflow qì in [the branch] of this channel that travels from the armpit.

For blood in the stool and urine, as well as incessant nosebleeds, since this channel belongs to fire, when fire causes counterflow in blood, [blood] will eject from both the above and below. For counterflow qì with retching and belching, the evil cannot be contained inside; for vexation and thirst, inability to get food and drink down, both are a result of counterflow fire in the interior, urgently drain the child [point] of fire in order to descend fire.

心包之脾病：大小人口中腥臭，口瘡，黃疸目黃，小兒齗爛。

Spleen diseases of the pericardium: fishy odour of the mouth in adults or children, mouth sores, jaundice with yellowing of the eyes, and erosion of gums in children.

注：胃火盛而口臭及口生瘡，皆胃有火也。然本經歷絡三焦，中焦乃所必過之處，泄本經之火穴，以解中焦之火。胃有濕熱而黃疸生，目亦爲之黃，泄此穴以解胃中之熱也。小兒齗爛，亦胃火盛也，取此穴與前症意同。

Explanation: exuberance of stomach fire will lead to [fishy] odour in the mouth and engenderment of mouth sores, in both cases, this is fire in the stomach; however, as this channel passes through and networks with the sānjiāo, the middle jiāo is a location which it must traverse, thus drain the fire point of this channel in order to resolve the fire of the middle jiāo.

Damp heat in the stomach will lead to the engenderment of jaundice, the eyes will also become yellow, drain this point in order to resolve the heat within the stomach. Erosion of gums in children is also due to the exuberance of stomach fire; the reason for choosing this point is identical to the previous sign.

心包之肝病：中風，善怒、悲，笑不休，手痺，胸脇支滿。

Liver diseases of the pericardium: wind strike, frequent bouts of anger and sorrow, incessant laughing, impediment of the hand, and propping fullness in the chest and rib-side.

注：中風而至且怒、且悲、且笑不休，則神亂矣，急取心之火穴而泄之，以定其神。手爲之痺者，乃本經所過之部分，以是徵之，而知邪在此經，故泄此穴。胸脇支滿，雖爲肝病，而亦取此穴者，以本經亦爲厥陰，在下而胸脇亦爲本經所行之部故也。

Explanation: after [contracting] wind strike, it further develops incessant anger, sorrow, and laughing, this is indicative of the derangement of spirit, urgently choose the fire point of the heart [governor] and drain it in order to stabilise the spirit. For the impediment of the hand, as this is the area where this channel traverses, consequently, it will manifest like this and indicate that the evil is located in this channel, thus drain this point.

For propping fullness in the chest and rib-side, although this is a liver disease, this point can also be chosen, as this channel is also juéyīn; in addition, the chest and rib-side are also areas where this channel travels.

Ninth Point of the Pericardium Network
Zhōng Chōng – Middle Surge[152] (PC-9)
心包絡第九穴中衝

穴在手中指端，去爪甲如韭葉陷中，心包絡所出爲井木，心包絡虛則補之。《銅人》：鍼一分，留三呼。《明堂》：灸一。

This point is located on the tip of the middle finger, in the depression at one chive leaf's width from the nail. The pericardium network emerges here, as the well and wood point. When the pericardium network is vacuous, supplement it. *The Tóngrén* states, "Needle 1 fēn, and retain for 3 respirations."[153] *The Míngtáng* states, "Moxa 1 [cone]."

---

[152] *Grasping the Wind* names it "Central Hub."
[153] "Retain for 3 respirations" is absent in *the Tóngrén*.

注：穴名中衝者，以中指而得名，言心包之脈，在兩陰之間，而直衝於手中指之端也，故曰中衝。

Explanation: regarding the point name Zhōng Chōng (Middle Surge), it is named after the Zhōng (Middle) finger. This also indicates the vessel of the pericardium is located between the two yīn [vessels]; moreover, it Chōng (Surges) straight to the tip of the Zhōng (Middle) finger, therefore it is called Zhōng Chōng (Middle Surge).

心包之心病：熱病煩滿，汗不出，掌中熱，身如火，心痛煩滿，舌强。

Heart diseases of the pericardium: febrile disease with vexation and fullness, absence of sweating, heat in the palms, body feels like it is on fire, heart pain with vexation and fullness, and stiff tongue.

注：熱病煩滿，火鬱於中也，再以掌中熱徵之，又身如火，急泄心包之木穴，以弱其火。心痛煩滿、舌爲之强，乃本經之火鬱於下，而上及於心之竅也，泄其木穴，而心火散矣。

Explanation: for febrile disease with vexation and fullness, this is because of depressed fire in the centre; if there is further manifestation of heat in the palms and if the body feels like it is on fire, urgently drain the wood point of the pericardium in order to weaken the fire. For heart pain with vexation and fullness, as well as the stiffening of the tongue, this is due to depressed fire of this channel in the lower, which has now ascended to reach the heart's orifice; drain the wood point and then heart fire will be dissipated.

Extra Points Associated with the Hand Pericardium Network Channel

手心包絡經奇穴

The Points Behind the Palm on the Arm (UEX-UE 8)

Shǒu Zhǎng Hòu Bì Jiān Xué – 手掌後臂間穴

《千金》云：治疔腫，灸掌後橫紋後五指許，男左女右，七壯即驗。又治風牙痛，以繩量自手中指頭至掌後第一橫紋，折爲四分，乃復自橫紋比量向後於臂盡處，兩筋間是穴，灸三壯，隨左右灸之，兩患者灸兩臂，甚驗。

***The Qiānjīn* states, "To treat clove sores and swelling, moxa the transverse creases about five finger widths behind the palm; for males on the left, for females on the right, 7 cones and it will be immediately effective.**

It also treats wind toothache; measure with a thin rope the length between the [tip of] middle finger to the first transverse crease behind the palm, and fold the rope into four equal portions; from the [first] transverse crease, extend such measured length rearwards the other end of the arm, [at the end of the folded rope] in the space between the two sinews, it is this point. Moxa 3 cones, moxa the left or right accordingly; when one suffers from [wind toothache] on both sides, moxa both arms, it is extremely effective."

Fist Tip (UEX-UE 26)
Quán Jiān – 拳尖

穴在中指本節前骨尖上，屈指得之。捷法云：穴在手腕中上側兩筋間陷中，灸二七壯，蓋此以陽谿言也，觀者辨之，主治五隔反胃。

This point is located on the middle finger, at the bony tip in front of the base joint,[154] bend the finger to locate it.

The Jié Fǎ states, "This point is located on the upper side of the wrist, in the depression between the two sinews, moxa 14 cones." Nevertheless, this is actually speaking about Yáng Xī (LI-5). The observant one can differentiate them. The [latter point][155] governs the treatment of the five isolations and stomach reflux.

Point [in the Depression After] the First Joint (UEX-UE 26)
Shǒu Zhōng Zhǐ Dì Yī Jié Xué – 手中指第一節穴

《千金》云：牙齒痛，灸手中指背，第一節前有陷處。灸七壯，下火立愈。

The Qiānjīn states, "[To treat] toothache, moxa the back of the middle finger, in the depression in front of the first joint. Moxa 7 cones to descend fire and there will be immediate recovery."

---

154 I.e., the third metacarpophalangeal joint.
155 I.e., Yáng Xī (LI-5).

The Hand Shàoyáng Sānjiāo Channel & Points

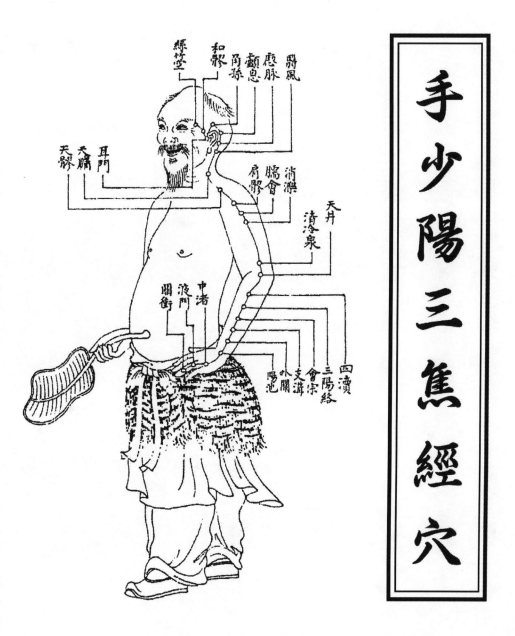

The Hand Shàoyáng Sānjiāo Channel & Points
手少陽三焦經

Overview of the Hand Shàoyáng Sānjiāo
手少陽三焦經總論

思蓮子曰：此經有形有名，所治之部分，膈之上爲上焦，乃心、肺之所居也；膈之下爲中焦，乃胃、脾之所居也；臍之下爲下焦，乃腎、肝、大、小腸及膀胱之所治也。故曰：上焦如霧，言氣之所蒸也；中焦如漚，言物之所化也；下焦如瀆，言一化之物所出也，此三焦所治之部分。凡腹中上下空處，皆三焦之氣所到處，則皆三焦治及之處，而尚非三焦所居之位、成形之所也。《内經》云：三焦者，決瀆之官，氣化則能出矣。

Master Sīlián says, this channel has a form and a name;[156] for the areas it manages, above the diaphragm, it is the upper jiāo, which is where the heart and lung reside; below the diaphragm, it is the middle jiāo, which is where the stomach and spleen reside; below the umbilicus, it is the lower jiāo, which manages the kidneys, liver, large and small intestines, and bladder.

Thus, it is said that "the upper jiāo is like a mist," which is speaking of the steaming of the qì; for "the middle jiāo is like foam," it is speaking of the transformation of substances by [the qì]; for "the lower jiāo is like a sluice," it

---

[156] Note: this is a major point of theoretical contention. As *Nànjīng* Difficulties 25 and 38 states that the sānjiāo "有名而無形 has a name but lacks a form;" however, not all commentators agree with this point. Mǎ Shì, whom Yuè Hánzhēn often cited in this work, wrote an extensive commentary to argue that the sānjiāo must have a form in his annotation of *the Nànjīng, Nànjīng Zhèngyì* 難經正義 (*the Orthodox Concept of the Nànjīng*, c. 16th century CE). He first noted that such a concept of the sānjiāo "無形 lacking a form" cannot be found anywhere in the *Nèijīng*; furthermore, based on the writing of the *Nèijīng*, though it is not explicitly stated, however, various passages do suggest the anatomy and various physical functions of the sānjiāo; in addition, he cited an anatomical account by Xú Duàn 徐遁 and writing by Lǐ Dōngyuán 李東垣 as further evidences for his claim; therefore, he concluded that the sānjiāo must have a form. Here, we speculate that this statement by Yuè Hánzhēn comes from his extensive influence by Mǎ Shì.

is speaking of where the substances exit once they are transformed.[157] These are the areas that the sānjiāo manages.

For any cavities within the abdomen, upper and lower, all of them are places that are reached by the qì of the sānjiāo; as a result, all of them are places managed by the sānjiāo; however, [these places] are still not the location where the sānjiāo resides, nor are they the places where [the sānjiāo] takes shape. *The Nèijīng* states, "The sānjiāo is the official of dredging the sluices; when there is qì transformation, it is able to emanate."[158]

瀆所藏水，決所出水，不能藏則散而不收，不能出則滯不能通矣。三焦所居之位，在兩腎之下，中有脂大如掌，前對氣海，此氣一鼓，大小便方能出。

Whereas the sluices are what store water, dredging is what releases the water; when there is no storage, it will disperse without collecting; when there is no release, it will stagnate and be unable to flow. The location where the sānjiāo resides is below the two kidneys, within it, there is a [piece of] fat that is as large as the palm of a hand, which is the counterpart to the sea of qì[159] in front. Once this qì is invigorated, then the urine and stool can be passed.

三焦所治之部，則膈之上，臍之上下，凡有空處，皆其所治之部分也。外應毫毛腠理，其厚薄、緩急、結止，與膀胱同。

For the areas where the sānjiāo manage, whether it is above the diaphragm, above or below the umbilicus, wherever there are any cavities, all of them are areas managed by it. Externally, it corresponds to the fine hairs and the interstices, their thickness, tenseness, and boundness are the same as the bladder.[160]

其經起於手小指次指之端外側，去爪甲如韭葉之關衝穴，上行至小指次指歧骨間，握拳取之之液門穴，又上行至手小指、次指本節後陷中之中渚穴，又上行至手表腕中之陽池穴，遂出臂外兩骨之間，至腕後二寸兩骨間之外關穴，又上腕後臂外三寸兩骨間之支溝穴，

---

[157] The opening clauses of each sentence are from *Língshū* Chapter 18, with additional commentary by Yuè Hánzhēn himself.

[158] From *Sùwèn* Chapter 8; however, in the original passage, the first line regarding the function of the sānjiāo is followed by "水道出焉 the waterways emanate from it," and "氣化則能出 when there is qì transformation, it is able to emanate" actually follows after the bladder at the end of the paragraph. Though this may seem to be a misquote, however, some *Nèijīng* commentators have argued that the second line, "when there is qì transformation, it is able to emanate," does not only apply to the bladder but in fact applies to all zàng-viscera and fǔ-bowels in this passage as well. Here, it is possible that Yuè Hánzhēn adopted such an interpretation.

[159] Also the name of REN-6.

[160] From *Língshū* Chapter 47.

The channel commences at Guān Chōng (SJ-1) on the outside at the tip of the ring finger,[161] at one chive leaf's width from the nail corner. It ascends to arrive at Yè Mén (SJ-2), at the space where the bones of the ring and little finger bifurcate, which is located by forming a fist. It continues to ascend to arrive at Zhōng Zhǔ (SJ-3), which is within the depression behind the base joint, between the ring and little finger.

It ascends to arrive at Yáng Chí (SJ-4) on the outside of the wrist. It continues and emerges in the space between the two bones on the outside of the arm, and it arrives at Wài Guān (SJ-5), which is between the two bones and 2 cùn behind the wrist. It continues in the space between the two bones to Zhī Gōu (SJ-6), which is 3 cùn behind the wrist.

又上行腕後三寸，中空一寸之會宗穴，又上行過臂上大交脈，支溝上一寸之三陽
絡穴，又上行過肘前五寸，外廉陷中之四瀆穴，又上行肘外大骨後，肘上一寸，
輔骨兩筋間之天井穴，遂從天井上行，循臂臑之外，歷肘上二寸，伸肘舉臂取之
清冷淵穴，

It continues to travel to Huì Zōng (SJ-7), which is 3 cùn behind the wrist, 1 cùn [from the centre] in the hollow. It ascends and traverses the great intersection of the vessels on the arm, which is Sān Yáng Luò (SJ-8) at 1 cùn above Zhī Gōu (SJ-6). It continues and traverses to Sì Dú (SJ-9), which is 5 cùn in front of the elbow, in the depression on the outer ridge.

It travels to behind the great bone on the outside of the elbow to Tiān Jǐng (SJ-10), which is 1 cùn above the elbow, between the two sinews on the assisting bone. Upon passing Tiān Jǐng (SJ-10), it ascends the outer ridge of the upper arm, passes through Qīng Lěng Yuān (SJ-11) at 2 cùn above the elbow, which is located by extending the elbow and raising the arm.

又歷肩下臂外間，腋斜肘分下之消濼穴，行手太陽之裏，手陽明之外，上肩前
廉，在肩後三寸宛宛中，與奇經陽維所會之臑會穴，又上肩端臑上陷中，斜取之
肩髎穴，又上缺盆中𣙜骨際，陷中央有空起肉上，與手、足少陽、陽維所會之天
髎穴，

It passes through the space outside the upper arm and below the shoulder, to Xiāo Luò (SJ-12) that is below the midpoint of the slanted line between the armpit and the elbow. It travels on the inside of the hand tàiyáng [channel] and on the outside of the hand yángmíng [channel], ascends the front ridge of the shoulder, to Nào Huì (SJ-13) in the depression 3 cùn behind the shoulder, where it meets with the extraordinary channel yángwéi.

---

[161] Lit. the finger next to the little finger.

It ascends to Jiān Liáo (SJ-14) within the depression above the upper arm at the edge of the shoulder, which is located by raising the arm at an angle. It ascends the border of the hidden bone[162] within Quē Pén (ST-12), to Tiān Liáo (SJ-15) at the centre of the depression where the flesh rises, where it meets with the hand and foot shàoyáng [channels], and yángwéi [vessel].

遂交出足少陽膽經之後，過手太陽小腸經，在本經天髎穴外，肩上肩顒後，舉臂有空之秉風穴，足少陽膽經肩上陷中，缺盆上，大骨前之肩井穴，下入缺盆後，由足陽明胃經之外，而交會於膽經之上焦，散布絡繞於心包絡，乃下膈入絡膀胱，以約下焦，附右腎而生；

Thereupon, it intersects and emerges behind the foot shàoyáng gallbladder channel, traverses Bǐng Fēng (SI-12) of the hand tàiyáng small intestine channel, which is outside of Tiān Liáo (SJ-15) of this channel and behind Jiān Yú (LI-15)[163] on the shoulder, where a hollow appears by raising the arm. [It traverses] Jiān Jǐng (GB-21) of the foot shàoyáng gallbladder channel, which is in the depression on the shoulder, above Quē Pén (ST-12), and in front of the great bone.[164] It descends to enter the upper jiāo, which is behind Quē Pén (ST-12), outside of the foot yángmíng stomach channel, where it intersects and meets with the gallbladder channel; thereupon, it disseminates and networks to encircle the pericardial network. Here, it continues and descends the diaphragm to enter and network to the bladder, where it binds with the lower jiāo; it further attaches to the right kidney,[165] where it is engendered.

其支行者，從膻中而出缺盆之外，上項過大椎，而與足太陽、足少陽、手太陽會，又却而循本經天牖穴，上耳後尖角陷中，按之引耳中痛之翳風穴，又上耳後，雞足青絡之瘈脈穴，又上耳後間，青絡脈中之顱息穴，

From Dàn Zhōng (REN-17), a branching pathway emerges at the outside of Quē Pén (ST-12), ascends the neck and traverses Dà Zhuī (DU-14), where it meets with the foot tàiyáng, foot shàoyáng, and hand tàiyáng. It then retreats to follow Tiān Yǒu (SJ-16) of this channel.

It ascends to Yì Fēng (SJ-17), which is in the depression behind the rear-tip of the ear, where pain radiates into the ear upon pressing. It ascends to Chì Mài (SJ-18), which is behind the ear, at the blue-green network vessels that

---

162 I.e., the superior angle of the scapula.
163 Could also refer to head of the shoulder.
164 This is likely the spine of the scapula.
165 This is likely the mìngmén as *Nànjīng* Difficulty 36 stated, "the right [kidney] is the mìngmén... where the source qì is connected to." Also, *Nànjīng* Difficulty 66 stated, "the sānjiāo is the divergence and courier of the source qì... the source, it is the honorific name of the sānjiāo."

resembles a chicken foot. It continues to ascend to Lú Xī (SJ-19), which is in the space behind the ear, at the blue-green network vessels.

直上出耳上角，至耳廓中間，開口有空之角孫穴，而與手太陽小腸經、足少陽膽經會，遂斜上過足少陽膽經懸釐、頷厭二穴，又橫過眉上，足少陽膽經之陽白穴，下至足太陽之睛明穴，曲屈至耳煩，至頰自下頤，會顴髎之分；

It ascends vertically to emerge at Jiǎo Sūn (SJ-20), which is located around the apex of the ear, at the centre of the auricle,[166] where a hollow appears upon opening the mouth; here, it meets with the hand tàiyáng small intestine channel and foot shàoyáng gallbladder channel. It then ascends obliquely to traverse the two points, Xuán Lí (GB-6) and Hàn Yàn (GB-4) of the shàoyáng gallbladder channel.

It continues horizontally, traversing Yáng Bái (GB-14) of the foot shàoyáng gallbladder channel above the eyebrow. It descends to arrive at Jīng Míng (BL-1) of the tàiyáng [channel]. It then curves around the ear to arrive at the cheeks; further, from the forehead, it descends through the bridge of the nose; [both pathways] then meet in the area of Quán Liáo (SI-18).

其又支者，從耳後翳風穴入耳中，過手太陽在耳中珠子大如赤小豆之聽宮穴，歷本經耳前起肉，當耳缺之耳門穴，却出直上斜至目銳眥，而與足少陽膽經，會於膽經之瞳子髎穴，又上眉後陷中本經絲竹空，又與足少陽膽經會也。

From Yì Fēng (SJ-17), another branch enters the ear, traverses Tīng Gōng (SI-19) of the hand tàiyáng [channel] at the pearl in the ear, which resembles the size of a rice bean. It passes through to Ěr Mén (SJ-21) at the fleshy protuberance in front of the ear, exactly at the notch of the ear. It retreats to re-emerge and ascend obliquely in a straight line to arrive at the outer canthus, where it meets with the foot shàoyáng gallbladder channel at Tóng Zi Liáo (GB-1) of the gallbladder channel. It continues to ascend to Sī Zhú Kōng (SJ-23)[167] of this channel at the depression behind the eyebrow, where it meets again with the foot shàoyáng gallbladder channel.

然三焦之脈，雖行於手，其腑則附右腎而生，故其所附之下腧，又在於足，其脈在足小指之前，即足太陽膀胱經脈氣所行，又足少陽膽經脈氣之後，出於膕中外廉，名曰委陽穴，乃足太陽之穴，正其絡脈所別，正爲手少陽三焦經之下腧也。

---

[166] According to the entry for SJ-20, Yuè Hánzhēn himself does not understand the meaning of "耳廓中間 at the center of the auricle" either. For this very line, *the Qiānjīn Yì* and *the Wàitái* has one extra character, "耳廓中間[上] [above] the center of the auricle," which is in line with the modern definition and should makes more sense.

[167] We have kept the modern designation of these points, SJ-21 and SJ-23; however, do note that they are the twenty-third and twenty-first points in reverse in their individual entries of this chapter.

Regarding the vessel of sānjiāo, although it travels on the hand, its fǔ-bowel is attached to the right kidney, where it is engendered; thus, for its attached lower transport point, it is located on the leg. The vessel is located in front of the little toe, it is where the vessel qì of the foot tàiyáng bladder channel flows; in addition, it is behind the vessel qì of the foot shàoyáng gallbladder; as such, it emerges [in the space between the two sinews][168] on the lateral ridge of the back of the knee, it is named Wěi Yáng (BL-39), as a point of the foot tàiyáng [channel]. This is exactly where its network-vessel diverges to, which is precisely the lower transport point of the hand shàoyáng sānjiāo channel.

此三焦者，乃足少陽膽經，及足太陽膀胱之所將，將者，相將而行也。委陽穴既爲足太陽經別行之穴，而外踝上五寸，足少陽膽經之絡穴光明者，三焦經又與之別入貫腨腸，共出於委陽穴，乃並足太陽經正脈，入內絡於膀胱，同約束下焦。實則爲病閉癃，閉癃者，水道不利也，當泄之。虛則病遺溺，當補之，此又手少陽之別行在下者也。《內經》云：三焦合於委陽者，此之謂也。

For this sānjiāo [lower pathway], it is that which supports the foot shàoyáng gallbladder channel and the foot tàiyáng bladder [channel]. What is meant by "support" here? It means that [these channels] support one another in their functions.[169]

Wěi Yáng (BL-39) is not only the point where the foot tàiyáng channel diverges;[170] moreover, the sānjiāo channel also joins with the divergence from Guāng Míng (GB-37),[171] which is the network point of the foot shàoyáng gallbladder channel at 5 cùn above the outer ankle [bone]; thereupon, they enter to pass through the calf intestine,[172] and emerge together at Wěi Yáng (BL-39), where they combine with the principal vessel of the foot tàiyáng channel, enter internally to network with the bladder, and bind together in the lower jiāo.

When it is replete, one will suffer from dribbling urinary blockage; dribbling urinary blockage is due to the inhibition of the water ways, one ought to drain

---

[168] Inserted here from the entry of BL-39 from the first volume of this work.

[169] This paragraph and the following two paragraphs come directly from Mǎ Shì's annotation of Língshū Chapter 2.

[170] Do note this is neither the network-vessel found in Língshū Chapter 10 nor the channel-divergence found in Língshū Chapter 11. This is simply a pathway noted in Língshū Chapter 2 and Chapter 4 for the treatment of the sānjiāo.

[171] This one is the network-vessel of gallbladder found in Língshū Chapter 10. In the Nèijīng, both luòmài 絡脈 (network-vessel) and jīng bié 經別 (channel-divergence) are noted simply as "別 divergence;" thus, it is important to take note of the context and consult these relevant chapters to determine which channel system is being mentioned.

[172] According to Grasping the Wind (p184) "the area at the top of the back of the lower leg as 'calf intestine.'"

it.[173] When it is vacuous, one will suffer from enuresis, one ought to supplement it. In addition, this [point] is the divergent pathway of the hand shàoyáng [channel] in the below. This is what is meant by the statement of *the Nèijīng*, "The sānjiāo unites at Wěi Yáng (BL-39)."[174]

取委陽穴之法，屈其體以覓承扶之陰紋，伸其體以度委陽之分寸，委陽在承扶下六寸，承扶在尻臀下陷紋之中，故《内經》云：取委陽者，屈伸而索之也。

For the method of locating Wěi Yáng (BL-39), bend the torso forward to look for Chéng Fú (BL-36) in the indented crease; afterwards, extend the torso backward to measure the distance from Wěi Yáng (BL-39), as Wěi Yáng (BL-39) is located 6 cùn below Chéng Fú (BL-36), and Chéng Fú (BL-36) is located in the depression on the crease below the buttocks; thus, *the Nèijīng* states, "To locate Wěi Yáng (BL-39), bend [the torso] forward and backward, so that one can find it."[175]

滎腧治外，經合治内，治三焦之内者，當取其合之委陽焉。何以爲内？閉癃、遺溺者，三焦之内病也。

The brook and stream points treat the exterior, while the river and uniting points treat the interior;[176] to treat the interior of the sānjiāo, one should choose the uniting point that is Wěi Yáng (BL-39). What should one regard as the interior [patterns of sānjiāo]? Dribbling urinary blockage and enuresis are internal diseases of the sānjiāo.[177]

Diseases of the Hand Shàoyáng Sānjiāo Channel

手少陽三焦經病

是動病則爲耳聾渾渾然、焞焞然，甚覺不聰，以本經之脈，從耳後入耳中，出走耳前，或出本經，或由合經也。

When there are changes, it will result in diseases such as deafness where it is as though one feels muddle-headed and dimmed, when one has a severe inability to perceive any sound, because the vessel of this channel enters inside of the ear from behind the ear; it then emerges to go to the front of the

---

[173] I.e., Wěi Yáng (BL-39).

[174] From *Língshū* Chapter 4. Nevertheless, do note that *the Nèijīng* does not offer a precise description of sānjiāo channel that goes from the torso to Wěi Yáng (BL-39).

[175] From *Língshū* Chapter 4.

[176] Paraphrased from *Língshū* Chapter 4.

[177] From the diseases treated by Wěi Yáng (BL-39) found in *Língshū* Chapter 4.

ear, where it either emerges at the principal channel or joins with other channels.[178]

所生病爲汗出，以汗爲心液，本經爲心包絡之表也。爲目銳眥痛，本經之脈至目銳眥也。爲煩腫，以本經之脈交煩也。爲耳後肩臑肘臂外皆痛，乃本經所行部分也。爲手小指次指不能舉用，乃本經之所出也。

For disease itself engenders, there is sweating, this is because sweat is the liquid of the heart, and this channel is the exterior of the pericardiac network. For pain of the outer canthus, this is because the vessel of this channel arrives at the outer canthus. For swelling of the cheeks, this is because the vessel of the channel intersects with the cheeks. For pain behind the ear, in the shoulder, upper arm, elbow, and outer arm, this is because all of these are areas where this channel travels. For inability to use the ring finger, this is because it is where the channel emerges.

正虛則當補，邪實則當泄，脈陷下則當灸，不盛不虛，則再求之本經，而不必求之心包絡。

When the upright is vacuous, one ought to supplement it; when the evil is replete, one ought to drain it. When the vessel is sunken, moxa it. When there is neither exuberance nor vacuity, again seek this channel; moreover, it is unnecessary to seek the pericardiac network [channel].

人迎較寸口之脈大一倍而躁疾者，則當泄本經穴，而補手厥陰心包絡經穴，人迎較寸口之脈小一倍而不躁疾者，則當補本經穴，而泄手厥陰心包絡之經穴也。

When the rényíng pulse in comparison to the cùnkǒu pulse is one times larger as well as agitated and racing, one ought to drain this channel's points, and supplement the hand juéyīn pericardiac network channel's points. When the rényíng pulse in comparison to the cùnkǒu pulse is one times smaller without being agitated and racing, one ought to supplement this channel's points, and drain the points of the hand juéyīn pericardiac network channel.

Meeting and Diverging Points
與別經會穴

外關穴，手少陽絡，別走心主。臑會穴，奇經陽維與本經會於此穴。天髎穴，足少陽膽經、奇經陽維，與本經會於此穴。角孫穴，手太陽小腸經、足少陽膽經，

---

[178] I.e., the primary pathway and branch pathway mentioned in the previous section.

與本經會於此穴。絲竹空，足少陽膽經與本經會於此穴。和髎穴，太陽小腸經、
足少陽膽經，與本經會於此穴。

Wài Guān (SJ-5) is the hand shàoyáng network point, it diverges to the heart governor [channel]. For Nào Huì (SJ-13), the extraordinary vessel yángwéi and this channel meet at this point. For Tiān Liáo (SJ-15), the foot shàoyáng gallbladder channel, the extraordinary vessel yángwéi, and this channel meet at this point.

For Jiǎo Sūn (SJ-20), the hand tàiyáng small intestine channel, the foot shàoyáng gallbladder channel, and this channel meet at this point. For Sī Zhú Kōng (SJ-23), the foot shàoyáng gallbladder channel and this channel meet at this point. For Hé Liáo (SJ-22), the tàiyáng small intestine, the foot shàoyáng gallbladder, and this channel meet at this point.

The Hand Sānjiāo Sinew Channel
手少陽經筋

手少陽筋，起於手小指之次指，即第四指之端關衝穴，由液門、中渚，結於手表
腕上之陽池穴，上循臂之外關、支溝、會宗、三陽絡，以結於肘之四瀆、天井，
上繞臑之外廉，即臑會穴，以上肩端之肩髎、天髎，走於頸之天牖，以合於本經
之太陽；

The sinew [channel] of the hand shàoyáng commences on the finger next to the little finger, precisely at Guān Chōng (SJ-1) on the tip of the fourth finger. Following Yè Mén (SJ-2) and Zhōng Zhǔ (SJ-3), it knots at Yáng Chí (SJ-4) on the surface of the wrist. It ascends following Wài Guān (SJ-5), Zhī Gōu (SJ-6), Huì Zōng (SJ-7), and Sān Yáng Luò (SJ-8) on the arm, to knot at Sì Dú (SJ-9) and Tiān Jǐng (SJ-10) at the elbow.

It ascends the outer aspect of the upper arm, precisely at Nào Huì (SJ-13). From there, it ascends to Jiān Liáo (SJ-14) and Tiān Liáo (SJ-15) at the edge of the shoulder. It goes toward Tiān Yǒu (SJ-16) at the neck, where this channel unites with the tàiyáng [channel].

又其支者，當曲頰前，以入系於舌本；又其支者，上於曲牙，循於耳前之角孫、
耳門、和髎，以屬目外眥之絲竹空，且上乘於頜，結於角。及其爲病，則凡筋所
經過者，即爲肢轉筋，爲舌卷。

Right in front of the corner of the jaw, a branch enters to connect with the root of the tongue. Another branch ascends the mandible bone,[179] following Jiǎo

---

[179] Also an alternate name for ST-6.

Sūn (SJ-20), Ěr Mén (SJ-23), and Hé Liáo (SJ-22) in front of the ear, where it adjoins to Sī Zhú Kōng (SJ-21) at the outer canthus; moreover, it further ascends over the cheek to knot at the corner [of the head].

When it becomes diseased, wherever the sinews traverse, there will be cramping of the limbs and curled tongue.

First Point of the Sānjiāo Channel
Guān Chōng – Surging Pass[180] (SJ-1)
三焦經第一穴關衝

穴在手小指之次指外側，去爪甲如韭葉，手少陽三焦經所出爲井金。《銅人》：鍼一分，留三呼，灸一壯。《素》注：灸三壯。

This point is located on the outside of the ring finger, at one chive leaf's width from the nail. The hand shàoyáng sānjiāo channel emerges here, as the well and metal point. *The Tóngrén* states, "Needle 1 fēn, retain for 3 respirations,[181] and moxa 1 cone." *The Sùzhù* states, "Moxa 3 cones."

注：三焦經行手太陽、手陽明兩脈之中，有關象焉，衝而上行，故曰關衝，以與包絡之中衝者對，彼以在手太陰、手少陰之中，故曰中衝。

Explanation: as the sānjiāo channel travels between the two vessels, the hand tàiyáng and the hand yángmíng, it has the image of a Guān (Pass); in addition, as it surges to ascend, thus it is called Guān Chōng (Surging Pass), so that it serves as a counterpart to Zhōng Chōng (Middle Surge, PC-9) of the pericardium network; the latter of which is located in the Zhong (Middle) between the hand tàiyīn and the hand shàoyīn [channels], thus it is called Zhōng Chōng (Middle Surge, PC-9).

關衝之本病：喉痺喉閉，胸中氣噎，不嗜食，肘臂病不可舉，目生翳膜，視物不明，舌卷口乾，頭痛。

Principal diseases of Guān Chōng: throat impediment with throat blockage, qì dysphagia within the chest, no desire to eat, suffering from being unable to raise elbow and arm, generation of membranous eye screens, dim vision, curled tongue with dry mouth, and headache.

注：脈下交頰，所以有喉痺喉閉之病，脈下膻中，所以有胸中氣噎之病，臂肘皆本經所行部分，氣滯則痛，瞳子髎，本經會膽經之處，本經又爲火，故有目視物不明之病，皆宜取本經井穴泄之。舌者，心之竅，本經與膽經爲表裏，故有舌

---

[180] *Grasping the Wind* names it "Passage Hub."
[181] "Retain for 3 respirations" is absent in *the Tóngrén*.

卷之病，口乾者，火盛也，亦宜泄此穴。本經之脈，曲折上頭，而有頭痛之病，故亦泄此穴。

Explanation: the vessel descends to intersect the cheek, as a result, there is the disease of throat impediment with throat blockage. The vessel descends the chest centre,[182] as a result, there is the disease of qì dysphagia within the chest. Both the arm and elbow are areas where the channel travels, when qì stagnation occurs, there will be pain. Tóng Zǐ Liáo (GB-1) is the location where this channel meets with the gallbladder channel; in addition, this channel is also categorised as fire, thus there is the disease of dim vision; for all cases, it is appropriate to choose the well point of this channel and drain it.

The tongue is the orifice of the heart, as this channel and the gallbladder channel[183] are an exterior-interior [pair], thus there is the disease of curled tongue; dry mouth is due to exuberance of fire, it is also appropriate to drain this point. The vessel of this channel winds as it ascends the head, hence there is the disease of headache, thus drain this point.

關衝之本腑病：霍亂。

Principal fǔ-bowel disease of Guān Chōng: sudden turmoil.

注：本經下膈入絡膀胱，氣亂遂有霍亂之症，取井穴以散其亂氣。

Explanation: as this channel descends the diaphragm to network with the bladder, when the qì is in chaos, consequently, there will be the signs of sudden turmoil,[184] choose the well point in order to dissipate the chaotic qì.

Second Point of the Sānjiāo Channel
Yè Mén – Humour Gate (SJ-2)
三焦經第二穴液門

穴在小指次指歧骨間陷中，握拳取之，手少陽三焦脈所溜爲滎水。《銅人》：鍼二分，留二呼，灸三壯。《千金》：治耳聾不得眠，刺三分，補之。

This point is located in the depression where the bones of the ring and little finger bifurcate, make a fist to locate it. The hand shàoyáng sānjiāo vessel

---

182 Also the name of REN-17.

183 Note: Based on the context, this "gallbladder channel" is likely a scribal error in the manuscript and should be the "pericardiac network" instead, as the latter is the exterior-interior counterpart of the sānjiāo channel. Due to the intimate relationship between the heart and the pericardiac network, by being able to treat the pericardiac network, the sānjiāo channel can treat the heart as well.

184 Note: "亂 Chaos" is part of the compound of "霍亂 sudden turmoil."

gushes here, as the brook and water point. *The Tóngrén* **states, "Needle 2 fēn, retain for 2 respirations,[185] and moxa 3 cones."** *The Qiānjīn* **states, "To treat deafness and insomnia, pierce 3 fen, and supplement it."**

注：液者，水之稱也，主經爲火而主氣，本穴乃水穴也，則亦液而已，在歧骨之間，有門象焉，故曰液門。

Explanation: Yè (Humour) signifies water; [this point] governs manifestations of fire in this channel and governs qì,[186] because this point is the water point, which also refers to Yè (Humour). As it is located in the space where the bones bifurcate, it has the image of a Mén (Gate), thus it is called Yè Mén (Humour Gate).

液門之本病：咽外腫，寒厥，手臂痛不能自上下，目赤澀，頭痛，暴得耳聾，齒齦痛，寒熱痎瘧，驚悸妄言。

Principal diseases of Yè Mén: swelling on the outside of the pharynx, cold reversal, hand and arm pain with inability to raise and lower them, red dry eyes, headache, sudden deafness, pain in the teeth and gums, intervallic malaria with chills and fever, and fright palpitations with raving.

注：本經脈由頰下喉，火盛則咽腫，故泄此穴。手臂皆本經部分，寒中則有痛不能自上下之症，當灸此穴，以去本經之寒。目赤痛，火盛，補水穴以治本經之火。本經之脈入耳，暴得耳聾，乃火也、氣也，宜泄此穴。本經脈繞頰而下，齒有病，亦火盛也，故責之。少陽之病主寒熱，故瘧，責火經之水穴，所以治其寒熱也。驚悸妄言，三焦火盛也，宜補水穴，以治火。

Explanation: since this channel's vessel descends from the cheek to the throat, when fire is exuberant, there will be swelling of the pharynx, thus drain this point. The hand and arm are both areas of this channel, when there is cold strike, there will be pain with inability to raise and lower them, one ought to moxa this point in order to eliminate the cold in this channel.

Red painful eyes are due to exuberant fire, supplement the water point in order to treat the fire of this channel. As the vessel of this channel enters the ear, sudden deafness is due to fire and qì [stagnation], it is appropriate to drain this point.

---

[185] "Retain for 2 respirations" is absent in *the Tóngrén*.

[186] For "主經爲火而主氣 it governs fire manifestations in this channel and governs qì," the editors of this manuscript, Zhāng and Zhà, have amended it to "本經爲火而主氣 this channel is fire and governs qì." However, besides stating a factual attribute about the channel, this edit makes little sense in the context of this paragraph, thus we have reverted back to the original passage, which we feel to be more illuminating.

As this channel's vessel encircles the cheek and then descends, when there is a disease in the teeth, it is exuberant fire, thus seek this [point]. The disease of shàoyáng governs chills and fever,[187] thus for malaria, seek the water point of the fire channel so as to treat the chills and fevers. Fright palpitations with raving is due to exuberant fire of the sānjiāo, it is appropriate to supplement the water point in order to treat fire.

Third Point of the Sānjiāo Channel
Zhōng Zhǔ – Middle Pond[188] (SJ-3)
三焦經第三穴中渚

穴在手小指次指本節後陷中，在液門下一寸，手少陽三焦脈所注爲腧木，三焦虛補之。《素》注：鍼二分，留三呼。《銅人》：灸三壯，鍼三分。《明堂》：灸二壯。

This point is located in the depression behind the base joints of the ring and little finger, it is located 1 cùn behind Yè Mén (SJ-2). The hand shàoyáng sānjiāo vessel pours here, as the stream and wood point. When the sānjiāo is vacuous, supplement it. _The Sùzhù_ states, "Needle 2 fēn, and retain for 3 respirations." _The Tóngrén_ states, "Moxa 3 cones, and needle 3 fēn."[189] _The Míngtáng_ states, "moxa 2 cones."

注：渚者，水所留之稱也，中乃三焦之脈，行乎兩經之中也，故曰中渚。

Explanation: for Zhǔ (Pond), it signifies a collection of water; for Zhōng (Middle), because the vessel of the sānjiāo travels in the Zhōng (Middle) between the other two channels, thus it is called Zhōng Zhǔ (Middle Pond).

中渚之本病：目眩頭痛，耳鳴，目生翳膜，咽腫，肘臂痛，手五指不得屈伸，熱病汗不出。

Principal Diseases of Zhōng Zhǔ: dizzy vision with headache, tinnitus, generation of membranous eye screens, swelling of the pharynx, pain in the elbow and arm, inability to bend and stretch the five fingers, and febrile disease with absence of sweating.

---

[187] This likely refers to the formula Xiǎo Cháihú Tāng 小柴胡湯 (Minor Bupleurum Decoction) from _the Shānghán Lùn_, which primarily treats shàoyáng disease that features chills and fevers.

[188] _Grasping the Wind_ names it "Central Islet." Note: based on the following explanation, Yuè Hánzhēn seems to interpret zhǔ 渚 (islet) as its homophone, zhū 瀦 (pond, pool, accumulation); the two characters can be used interchangeably at times.

[189] For "3 fēn," _the Tóngrén_ actually states "2 fēn."

注：此乃本經木穴，木生火者，目眩頭痛，耳聾耳鳴，目翳咽腫，皆火病也，泄其母穴，所以解其熱也。肘臂痛，非氣滯，則風寒，乃宜灸之。熱病汗不出，則宜補之。

Explanation: this point is this channel's wood point, as wood engenders fire, for dizzy vision with headache, deafness, tinnitus, generation of membranous eye screens, and swelling of the pharynx, all of these are fire diseases, drain the mother point so as to resolve the heat. For pain in the elbow and arm, if it is not [caused by] qì stagnation, then it is cold and wind, thus it is appropriate to moxa it. For febrile disease with absence of sweating, it is appropriate to supplement it.

Fourth Point of the Sānjiāo Channel
Yáng Chí – Yáng Pool (SJ-4)
三焦經第四穴陽池

穴在手表腕上陷中，從指本節直摸下至腕中心，手少陽三焦脈所過爲原，三焦虛實皆拔之。《素》注：鍼二分，留六呼，灸三壯。《銅人》：禁灸。鍼透抵大陵穴，不可破皮，不可搖手，恐傷鍼轉曲。

This point is located in the depression on the surface of the wrist, which can be palpated at the centre of the wrist in a straight line below the base joint of the [ring] finger. The hand shàoyáng sānjiāo vessel traverses here, as the source point. Whether the sānjiāo is vacuous or replete, it will uproot [the disease]. _The Sùzhù_ states "Needle 2 fēn, retain for 6 respirations, and moxa 3 cones." _The Tóngrén_ states, "Moxibustion is contraindicated." Also, "The needle can pass through to reach Dà Líng (PC-7), but one must not break theskin; in addition, [the patient] must not move the hand, this is due to fear of needle injury as well as twisting and bending [the needle]."[190]

---

[190] Though _the Zhēnjiǔ Dàchéng_ attributes this statement to _the Zhǐ Wēifù_ 指微賦 (_Ode of Pointing to the Subtleties,_ c. 12th century CE), this quote cannot be found in today's copy of it, nor is it found in the very same ode cited by _the Zhēnjiǔ Dàchéng_ itself. Upon brief research, the same quote is found only in a later work, _the Gǔfǎ Xīnjiě Huìyuán Zhēnjiǔ Xué_ 古法新解會元針灸學 (_the New Interpretation of Ancient Method of Acupuncture Study,_ 1937 CE), which repeats the exact quote and reference; yet, it cannot be found in any other major acupuncture literature before Yuè Hánzhēn's time. As Yuè Hánzhēn used _the Zhēnjiǔ Dàchéng_ as the source text for this work, we speculate that he was fully aware of this reference made by _the Zhēnjiǔ Dàchéng_. He may have intentionally removed the reference to _Ode of Pointing to the Subtleties_ as this claim could not be verified.

注：水之所聚者爲池，此穴上自關衝，至腕陷中，有聚象，故曰池，陽指三焦而言也。

Explanation: a place where water accumulates is known as a Chí (Pool); as this point ascends from Guān Chōng (SJ-1) to arrive at this depression on the wrist, there is an image of accumulation, thus it is called Chí (Pool); Yáng (Yáng) is indicating the sānjiāo.

陽池之本病：或因折傷手腕，捉物不得，肩臂痛不得舉，消渴口乾，煩悶寒熱瘧。

Principal diseases of Yáng Chí: inability to grasp objects due to fracture and injury of the wrist, shoulder and arm pain with inability to raise it, dispersion-thirst with dry mouth, vexation and oppression, and malaria with chills and fever.

注：折傷而取此穴，恐腕中有積氣留血也。肩臂痛，乃三焦所行部分也。消渴口乾，三焦有熱積於中也。少陽之症，多爲寒熱也。均宜責此穴，所謂虛實皆拔之也。

Explanation: choose this point for fracture and injury [of the wrist], this is due to the fear of the accumulation of qì and retained blood within the wrist. For shoulder and arm pain, it is because they are the areas where the sānjiāo [channel] travels. Dispersion-thirst with dry mouth is due to the sānjiāo accumulating heat in the centre. The signs of shàoyáng [disease] are predominantly chills and fever. In all instances, it is suitable to seek this point, this is what is meant by [the statement], "whether [the sānjiāo] is vacuous or replete, it will uproot [the disease]."

Fifth Point of the Sānjiāo Channel
Wài Guān – Outer Pass (SJ-5)
三焦經第五穴外關

穴在腕後二寸兩骨間，與手厥陰經內關相對，手少陽絡別走心主。《銅人》：鍼三分，留七呼，灸三壯。《明堂》：灸三壯。

This point is located in the space between the two bones, 2 cùn behind the wrist; it is a counterpart to Nèi Guān (PC-6) of the hand juéyīn channel. It is the hand shàoyáng network point that diverges to the heart governor. *The Tóngrén* states, "Needle 3 fēn, retain for 7 respirations, and moxa 3 cones. *The Míngtáng* states, "Moxa 3 cones."

注：外關者，對內關而言也，此穴在八法中，以爲通帶脈，而與足少腸膽經之臨泣穴通陽維，爲男女主客相應。

Explanation: for Wài Guān (Outer Pass), it is speaking of the counterpart to Nèi Guān (Inner Pass, PC-6). Amongst the eight confluent [points],[191] this point communicates with the dài vessel; as such, it serves as a correspondence of male and female, host and guest, with [Zú] Lín Qì (GB-41) of the foot shàoyáng gallbladder channel, which communicates with the yángwéi vessel.[192]

外關之本病：耳聾，渾渾焞焞無聞，五指盡痛，不能握物。

Principal diseases of Wài Guān: deafness, inability to hear with muddle-headedness and dimness, and pain in all five fingers with inability to grasp objects.

注：前症乃本經上下所行部分，正症也，宜責此穴。

Explanation: the above signs [occur] in the areas where this channel travels above and below, thus, these are the principal signs [of this channel], it is appropriate to seek this point.

Sixth Point of the Sānjiāo Channel
Zhī Gōu – Branch Ditch (SJ-6)
三焦經第六穴支溝

一名飛虎
Alternate name: Flying Tiger

穴在腕後臂外三寸，兩骨間陷中，手少陽脈所行爲經火。《銅人》：鍼二分，灸二七壯。《明堂》：灸五壯。《素》注：鍼二分，留七呼，灸三壯。

This point is located on the outside of the arm, 3 cùn behind the wrist, in the depression between the two bones. The hand shàoyáng vessel flows here, as the river and fire point. *The Tóngrén* states, "Needle 2 fēn, and moxa 14 cones." *The Míngtáng* states, "Moxa 5 cones." *The Sùzhù* states, "Needle 2 fēn, retain for 7 respirations, and moxa 3 cones."

---

[191] This literally refers to the "eight methods," which is namely the eightfold method of the sacred tortoise and the eightfold soaring method from *the Dàchéng*, where the eight confluent points came from.

[192] Note: this passage needs clarification. Whereas Wài Guān (SJ-5) serves as the confluent point for the yángwéi vessel, [Zú] Lín Qì (GB-41) serves as the confluent point for the dài vessel. The two points are usually paired together as host (primary point) and guest (assisting point) upon applying treatment to the yángwéi vessel and dài vessel; as such, it is possible that Yuè Hánzhēn interprets that the yángwéi vessel and dài vessel communicate with each other; thus, Wài Guān (SJ-5) as the confluent point of the yángwéi vessel also communicates with the dài vessel, and vice versa for [Zú] Lín Qì (GB-41).

注：溝者，水之所行也，此穴在手臂之外，如木有枝，故曰支溝。

Explanation: regarding Gōu (Ditch), it is a place where water flows; as this point is located on the outside of the arm, it is like a Zhī (Branch) of a tree, thus it is called Zhī Gōu (Branch Ditch).

支溝之本病：熱病汗不出，肩背痠重，脇腋痛，四肢不舉，口噤不開，暴瘖不能言，傷寒結胸，痫瘡疥癬，婦人妊脈不通，産後血暈，不省人事。

Principal diseases of Zhī Gōu: febrile disease with absence of sweating, aching and heaviness of the shoulder and upper back, pain of the rib-side and armpit, inability to lift the four limbs, clenched jaw that cannot open, sudden loss of voice with inability to speak, cold damage with chest bind, metacarpophalangeal sores with scabs and lichen, obstruction of the pregnancy vessel[193] in women, postpartum dizziness due to blood [loss], and loss of consciousness.

注：熱病汗不出，泄其火穴而汗自出。肩背乃本經所行部分，有氣滯焉，而有痠重不舉之症，宜泄其火，而行本經之氣。口噤不開、暴瘖，皆三焦之氣閉也，宜泄其火，而昇其氣。傷寒結胸，以本經之脈下行膻中也，故責之。瘡癬者，火症也，本經爲火，本穴爲火，宜泄其火。三焦之氣滯，而妊脈不通，泄此穴所以通其氣也，氣行則血行矣。産後血暈，火有餘也，泄三焦之火穴，以定其暈。

Explanation: for febrile disease with absence of sweating, drain the fire point and sweating will naturally occur. The shoulder and upper back are areas where this channel travels, so when there is qì stagnation within it, there will be signs of aching and heaviness[194] with inability to lift [the limbs], it is appropriate to drain the fire point to move the qì of this channel.

For clenched jaw with inability to speak, as well as sudden loss of voice, both are due to blockage of qì in the sānjiāo, it is appropriate to drain the fire in order to ascend the qì. Cold damage with chest bind is because the vessel of this channel descends through Dàn Zhōng (REN-17), thus seek it. Scabs and lichen are fire signs; as this channel is fire, this point is also fire, it is appropriate to drain the fire.

When there is qì stagnation of the sānjiāo, it will result in obstruction of the pregnancy vessel, drain this point so as to free the qì; once the qi moves, the blood will move. Postpartum dizziness due to blood [loss] indicates superabundance of fire, drain the fire point of the sānjiāo in order to stabilise the dizziness.

---

[193] I.e., the 任脈 rèn vessel, as the two characters 任 (rèn) and 妊 (pregnancy) are homophones and interchangeable.

[194] The scribal manuscript has "痛 pain" here in place of "重 heaviness." The editors of this manuscript, Zhāng and Zhà, have changed in accordance with the previous paragraph.

支溝之內症：霍亂嘔吐，心悶不已，卒心痛，鬼擊。

Internal signs of Zhī Gōu: sudden turmoil with vomiting and retching, incessant oppression of the heart, sudden heart pain, and attack by ghosts.[195]

注：三焦之氣逆於內，所以有霍亂之症，責此穴者，以散三焦之火也。脈下膻中，有滯焉而心爲之悶，泄其火穴，而悶自散。卒心痛，心包絡之氣逆也，泄其表之火，所以治其裏。鬼擊之症，乃人神昏也，神昏者，火旺也，宜泄其本穴之火，以定其神。

Explanation: when there is qì counterflow of the sānjiāo in the interior, it will result in the sign of sudden turmoil, seek this point in order to disperse the fire of the sānjiāo. As the vessel [of this channel] descends through Dàn Zhōng (REN-17), when there is stagnation within it, the heart will become oppressed, drain the fire point and the oppression will naturally dissipate.

Sudden heart pain is due to qì counterflow of the pericardiac network, drain the fire from exterior [fǔ-bowels] so as to treat the interior [zàng-viscus]. For the sign of ghost attack, this is due to the clouded spirit of a person; when there is clouded spirit, this is the effulgence of fire, it is appropriate to drain the fire of the principal point in order to stabilise the spirit.

Seventh Point of the Sānjiāo Channel
Huì Zōng – Convergence and Gathering (SJ-7)
三焦經第七穴會宗

穴在腕後三寸五分。《銅人》：灸七壯。《明堂》：灸五壯，禁鍼。

This point is located 3 cùn 5 fēn[196] behind the wrist. *The Tóngrén* states, "Moxa 7 cones." *The Míngtáng* states, "Moxa 5 cones, and needling is contraindicated."

注：後此之穴爲三陽絡，三陽者，手太陽、少陽、陽明也，僅離支溝一寸，而此穴乃在去腕三寸五分之中，三陽絡在腕後四寸之中，與此穴僅去五分，則三陽之絡，俱會於三陽絡之穴，而此穴乃其將會之穴，故曰會宗。

Explanation: the point succeeding this is Sān Yáng Luò (Three Yáng Network, SJ-8), where the "three yáng" refers to the hand tàiyáng, shàoyáng and

---

[195] For "attack by ghosts," it means sudden manifestation of swelling, distension, blood stasis, or loss of consciousness due to unknown causes.

[196] For "3 cùn 5 fēn behind the wrist," both *the Zhēnjiǔ Dàchéng* and *the Tóngrén* has "腕後三寸空中一寸 3 cùn behind the wrist and 1 cùn apart from the centre" instead.

yángmíng; in addition, [Sān Yáng Luò (SJ-8)] is only 1 cùn from Zhī Gōu (SJ-6), whereas this point (SJ-7) is located 3 cùn 5 fēn from the wrist. Sān Yáng Luò (SJ-8) is located 4 cùn behind the wrist, which is only 5 fēn apart from this point (SJ-7); thus, when all network-vessels of the three yáng Huì (Converge) at the point of Sān Yáng Luò (SJ-8), as this point (SJ-7) is the point where they are about to Huì (Converge), thus it is called Huì Zōng (Convergence and Gathering).

會宗之本病：五癇，肌膚痛，耳聾。

Principal diseases of Huì Zōng: the five epilepsies,[197] skin and muscle pain, and deafness.

注：癇之作也，未有不由火作者，三焦爲火之經，必三焦之火俱發，而後有癇，所以責此穴，以爲三陽絡會之所也。耳聾乃本經之正病，俱宜灸此穴，以散其火。

Explanation: regarding the onset of epilepsy, it is unprecedented that it is not caused by fire; as the sānjiāo is a channel of fire, the fire of the sānjiāo must effuse first before epilepsy can occur; as a result, seek this point, as it is the place where the three yáng network-vessels meet. Deafness is indeed a principal disease of this channel, without exception, it is always appropriate to moxa this point in order to disperse the fire.

Eighth Point of the Sānjiāo Channel
Sān Yáng Luò – Three Yáng Network[198] (SJ-8)
三焦經第八穴三陽絡

一名通門
Alternate name: Connecting Gate

穴在臂上大交脈，支溝上一寸。《銅人》：灸七壯。《明堂》：灸五壯，禁鍼。

This point is located at the great intersection of the vessels on the arm, 1 cùn above Zhī Gōu (SJ-6). *The Tóngrén* states, "Moxa 7 cones." *The Míngtáng* states, "Moxa 5 cones, and needling is contraindicated."

---

[197] The term "五癇 five epilepsies" comes from the paediatric work, *Xiǎo'ér Yàozhèng Zhíjué 小兒藥證直訣* (*the Key to Diagnosis and Treatment of Children's Diseases*, 1119 CE) by Qián Yǐ 錢乙. The five epilepsies are namely, liver epilepsy, heart epilepsy, spleen epilepsy, lung epilepsy, and kidney epilepsy based on the pathology; in addition, they can also be categorized as the dog epilepsy, goat epilepsy, cow epilepsy, chicken epilepsy, and pig epilepsy based on the sound patient produces during the onset of epilepsy.

[198] *Grasping the Wind* names this point "Three Yáng Connection."

注：手太陽、陽明俱有絡，與本經會於此穴，故曰三陽絡。

Explanation: both the hand tàiyáng and yángmíng [channels] have Luò (Networks) that meet with this channel at this point, thus it is called Sān Yáng Luò (Three Yáng Network).

三陽絡之本病：暴瘖瘡耳聾，嗜臥，四肢不欲動搖。

Principal diseases of Sān Yáng Luò: sudden loss of voice with sores and deafness, somnolence, and no desire to move the four limbs.

注：瘖、聾，手太陽小腸及本經皆有之症，四肢不欲動者，乃合手太陽、陽明及本經，三經俱有之症也，故責此穴。

Explanation: loss of voice and deafness are signs of both the hand tàiyáng small intestine and this channel. No desire to move the four limbs is indeed a sign that manifests in all three of the hand tàiyáng, yángmíng, and this channel, thus seek this point.

Ninth Point of the Sānjiāo Channel
Sì Dú – Four Rivers (SJ-9)
三焦經第九穴四瀆

穴在肘前五寸，外廉陷中。《銅人》：灸三壯，鍼六分，留七呼。

This point is located 5 cùn in front of the elbow, in the depression on the outer ridge. *The Tóngrén* states, "Moxa 3 cones, needle 6 fēn, and retain for 7 respirations."

注：三陽加手厥陰與本經相爲表裏，故曰四瀆。瀆者，通水之名也。.

Explanation: there are the three yáng [channels], as well as the hand juéyīn [channel] that is an exterior-interior [pair] with this channel, thus it is called Sì Dú (Four Rivers). Dú (River) is a name for where water flows.

四瀆之本病：暴氣耳聾，下齒齲痛。

Principal diseases of Sì Dú: sudden qì deafness, and lower tooth decay with pain.

注：耳聾齒痛，皆本經氣脈所行之處，故均責之。

Explanation: both deafness and tooth decay [occur] in locations where the vessel qì of this channel travels, thus in both instances seek this [point].

Tenth Point of the Sānjiāo Channel
Tiān Jǐng – Celestial Well (SJ-10)
三焦經第十穴天井

穴在肘外大骨後，肘上一寸，輔骨上兩筋叉骨罅中，屈肘拱胸取之，手少陽三焦
脈所入爲合土，三焦實泄之。《素》注：鍼一分，留七呼。《銅人》：鍼三分，
灸三壯。

This point is located behind the great bone on the outside of the elbow, 1 cùn above the elbow, in the bony gap where the two sinews diverge on the assisting bone; bend the elbow and place it on the chest to locate it. The hand shàoyáng sānjiāo vessel enters here, as the uniting and earth point. When the sānjiāo is replete, drain it. *The Sùzhù* **states, "Needle 1 fēn, and retain for 7 respirations."** *The Tóngrén* **states, "Needle 3 fēn, and moxa 3 cones."**

注：此穴以本經自關衝而上，入於是穴，以爲合土，水入焉，有井象，其
位在乎上也，故曰天井。

Explanation: for this point, the channel has ascended from Guān Chōng (SJ-1) to enter this point, as the uniting and earth point; it is as though water is entering it, thus it has the image of a Jǐng (Well). As its position is located in the above, thus it is called Tiān Jǐng (Celestial Well).

天井之本病：耳聾，嗌腫，喉痺，汗出，目銳眥痛，頰腫痛，耳後、臑、背痛，
捉物不得，振寒，頸項痛，風痺，脚氣上攻。

Principal diseases of Tiān Jǐng: deafness, swollen pharynx, throat impediment, sweating, pain of the outer canthus, swelling and pain of the cheeks, pain behind the ears, in the upper arm and upper back, inability to grasp objects, quivering with cold, neck and nape pain, wind impediment, and leg qì attacking upwards.

注：前症皆本經所行部分，有邪客之，或風、或寒、或火，故作痛焉，而
取此穴，乃實則泄其子之義。脚氣者，下焦之病也，上攻則及上焦矣，此三焦俱有
之病，故泄本經之合土穴，以散三焦之滯。

Explanation: the above signs are all areas where this channel travels; when there is evil lodged in [these areas], whether by wind, cold, or fire, it will cause pain, so choose this point, because this is the very meaning of draining the child [point] in the presence of repletion. Leg qì is a disease of the lower jiāo; when it attacks upwards, it means that it has now reached the upper jiāo; as such, this is a disease of the entire sānjiāo, thus drain the uniting and earth point of the principal channel in order to dissipate the stagnation of the sānjiāo.

天井之内病：心胸痛，咳嗽上氣，短氣不得語，唾膿不嗜食，寒熱，悽悽不得臥，驚悸瘈瘲，癲疾五癎，嗜臥，大風默默不知所痛，悲傷不樂。

Internal diseases of Tiān Jǐng: heart and chest pain, cough with qì ascent, shortness of breath with inability to speak, spitting pus with no desire to eat, chills and fever, hunger[199] with inability to lie down, fright palpitations with tugging and slackening, epileptic disease and the five types of episodic epilepsies,[200] somnolence, great wind with taciturnity and lack of awareness to pain,[201] and sorrow with unhappiness.

注：心胸痛，邪滯於上焦也，唾膿不嗜食，上焦有火也，三焦爲少陽，少陽之症多寒熱，驚悸瘈瘲、癲癎，皆三焦有火也，三焦者，火盛則神昏，神昏則嗜臥也，大風默默不知所痛，三焦內外俱病也，悲傷，三焦火盛，上凌於肺也，皆三焦之在內者有餘也，故泄本經之子穴。

Explanation: pain in the heart and chest is due to stagnation of evil in the upper jiāo; spitting of pus with no desire to eat is presence of fire in the upper jiāo; as the sānjiāo is shàoyáng, there are signs of shàoyáng, which are predominantly chills and fever; fright palpitations with tugging and slackening, as well as epilepsy are all due to presence of fire in the sānjiāo. Regarding the sānjiāo, when fire is exuberant, there will be clouding of the spirit; when the spirit is clouded, there will be somnolence; great wind with taciturnity and lack of awareness to pain is a sānjiāo disease of both the interior and exterior; sorrow is exuberant fire of the sānjiāo, which ascends to intimidate the lung, in all cases, this is superabundance of the sānjiāo in the interior, thus drain the child point of this channel.

天井之外病：撲傷腰髖痛。

Exterior disease of Tiān Jǐng: pain of the lumbus and hip due to striking injury.

注：撲傷腰髖痛，下焦有瘀血也，責此穴者，散之之義也。

Explanation: pain of the lumbus and hip due to striking injury will cause stasis of blood in the lower jiāo; thus, the reason for seeking this point is to disperse it.

---

[199] "Hunger 悽悽" here may also be interpreted as the feelings of sorrow and misery.
[200] For "five types of episodic epilepsies," see footnote 197.
[201] For "great wind with taciturnity and no awareness to pain," see footnote 42.

Eleventh Point of the Sānjiāo Channel
Qīng Lěng Yuān – Clear Cold Abyss (SJ-11)
三焦經第十一穴清冷淵

穴在肘上二寸，伸肘舉臂取之。《銅人》：鍼二分，灸三壯。

This point is located 2 cùn above the elbow; extend the elbow and raise the arm to locate it. *The Tóngrén* states, "Needle 2 fēn,[202] and moxa 3 cones."

注：此經主火者也，而於是穴，謂之清冷淵者，其以本經過天井之後，火氣稍息歟？抑以在肘之外，常爲風寒所襲歟？尚俟高明。

Explanation: this channel governs fire; however, for this point to be called Qīng Lěng Yuān (Clear Cold Abyss), could it be that as this channel traverses behind Tiān Jǐng (SJ-10), the fire qì has diminished slightly? Or perhaps, could it be that as it is located on the outside of the elbow, it is often assailed by wind and cold? [The name of this point] will require [resolution by] future people of brilliance and knowledge.

清冷淵之本病：肩臂痛，臂臑不能舉，不能帶衣。

Principal diseases of Qīng Lěng Yuān: shoulder and arm pain, inability to raise the shoulder and upper arm, and inability to put on clothes.

注：所治皆本經風寒之症，則命名爲清冷之義可得矣，寒者熱之，則宜灸也。

Explanation: what [this point] treats are all signs of wind and cold of this channel; thus, from this, one can be ascertain the reasoning behind bestowing the name as clear and cold. When there is cold, warm it, hence it is appropriate to moxa.

Twelfth Point of the Sānjiāo Channel
Xiāo Luò – Dispersing Riverbed (SJ-12)
三焦經第十二穴消濼

穴在肩下臂外間，腋斜肘分下。《銅人》：鍼一分，灸三壯。《明堂》：鍼六分。《素》注：鍼五分。

This point is located in the space between the shoulder and outside of the upper arm, below the midpoint of the slanted line between the armpit and the

---

[202] For "2 fēn", *the Tóngrén* actually states "3 fēn."

elbow. *The Tóngrén* states, "Needle 1 fēn,[203] and moxa 3 cones." *The Míngtáng* states, "Needle 6 fēn." *The Sùzhù* states, "Needle 5 fēn."

注：消濼，此寒冷之義也，火經而以此名穴，命名之義，想有所指，尚俟高明。

Explanation: regarding Xiāo Luò (Dispersing Riverbed), this carries the meaning of frigidity. For this point on the fire channel to be named as such, I believe there to be a certain purpose for the reasoning behind bestowing this name; however, it still requires [resolution by] future people of brilliance and knowledge.

消濼之本病：風痹，頸項強急，腫痛，寒熱頭痛，癲疾。

Principal disease of Xiāo Luò: wind impediment, stiffness of the neck and nape, [generalised] swelling and pain, chills and fever with headache, and epileptic disease.

注：本經由頸項而入面，風中之，病強急，宜灸以溫之。寒熱乃少陽之本病也，頭痛則風寒客之也，皆宜灸之。癲疾雖爲陰症，然必三焦有氣與痰滯之，而始有是症，宜灸之以通其滯。

Explanation: as this channel enters the face from the neck and nape, when it is struck by wind, there will be the disease of stiffness; it is appropriate to moxa in order to warm it. Chills and fever indeed indicate the principal disease of the shàoyáng, and headache is caused by wind and cold lodging in it, in both cases, it is appropriate to moxa it. Although epileptic disease is a yīn sign, there must first be stagnation of qì and phlegm in the sānjiāo, before this sign can manifest; thus, it is appropriate to moxa it in order to free the stagnation.

---

[203] For "1 fēn", *the Tóngrén* actually states "6 fēn." Note: we speculate this to be an error in the manuscript, as the depth is too shallow; in addition, most sources, including *the Dàchéng*, have "6 fēn" as well.

Thirteenth Point of the Sānjiāo Channel
Nào Huì – Upper Arm Convergence[204] (SJ-13)
三焦經第十三穴臑會

一名臑交

Alternate name: Upper Arm Intersection

穴在肩前廉，去肩頭三寸宛宛中，手少陽、奇經陽維之會。《素》注：鍼五分，灸五壯。《銅人》：鍼七分，留十呼，得氣即泄，灸七壯。

This point is located on the front ridge of the shoulder, in the depression 3 cùn from the head of the shoulder. It is the meeting of the hand shàoyáng and extraordinary channel yángwéi [vessel]. *The Sùzhù* states, "Needle 5 fēn, and moxa 5 cones." *The Tóngrén* states, "Needle 7 fēn, retain for 10 respirations, obtain qì then promptly drain, and moxa 7 cones."

注：肘之內爲臑，此穴所在，雖爲肩之外廉，有肉斜生，勢與臑會，而又奇經陽維自足下起，上會本經，經於此穴，故曰臑會。

Explanation: the inside of the elbow is called the Nào (Upper Arm). Although the location of this point is on the outer ridge of the shoulder, there, a flesh slants [downwards], which will certainly Huì (Converge) with the Nào (Upper Arm). Moreover, the extraordinary channel yángwéi begins from below the foot, ascends to Huì (Converge) with this channel, and passes through this point, thus it is called Nào Huì (Upper Arm Convergence).

臑會之本病：臂痰無力，痛不能舉，肩腫引胛中痛，項瘦氣瘤，寒熱。

Principal diseases of Nào Huì: aching of the arm with lack of strength, pain with inability to raise it, swelling of the shoulder with pain that radiates to the scapula, goitres and qì tumours on the neck, chills and fever.

注：肩、臂、瘦，皆本經所致部分，或風或寒，或氣或火，客而滯之，所致之症，故泄此穴，以將上肩也。寒熱，則陽維之病也，以陽維會於此穴，故病寒熱者責之。

Explanation: the shoulder, arm, and goitre [of the neck], are all areas where this channel reaches; whether by wind, cold, qì or fire, when any of them lodges and causes stagnation in [these areas], these signs will occur as a result, thus drain this point as it [is where this channel] is about to ascend the shoulder. Chills and fever

---

[204] While the character, huì 會, is typically translated as "meeting," we are keeping the original translation from *Grasping the Wind*, which translates it as "convergence," as we find it to be fitting with the context provided in the following explanation.

are a disease of the yángwéi [vessel], as the yángwéi [vessel] meets at this point, thus for the disease of chills and fever, seek this [point].

Fourteenth Point of the Sānjiāo Channel
Jiān Liáo – Shoulder Bone-Hole (SJ-14)
三焦經第十四穴肩髎

穴在肩端臑上陷中，斜舉臂取之。《銅人》：鍼七分，灸三壯。《明堂》：灸五壯。

This point is located in the depression at the edge of the shoulder on the upper arm, raise the arm at an angle to locate it. *The Tóngrén* states, "Needle 7 fēn, and moxa 3 cones." *The Míngtáng* states, "Moxa 5 cones."

注：此穴雖在肩之端，而尚在肩下臑上，取此穴者察之。

Explanation: although this point is located at the edge of the shoulder, it is still located below the shoulder and on the upper arm; when locating this point, one should be aware of it.

肩髎之本病：臂痛，肩重不能舉。

Principal diseases of Jiān Liáo: arm pain, and heaviness in the shoulder with inability to raise it.

注：正本經本穴部分中風之症也。鍼宜深而灸宜多。

Explanation: these are exactly the signs of wind strike [that occur] in the area around this point of this channel. It is appropriate to needle deeply and to moxa copiously.

Fifteenth Point of the Sānjiāo Channel
Tiān Liáo – Celestial Bone-Hole (SJ-15)
三焦經第十五穴天髎

穴在肩缺盆上，毖骨際陷中須缺盆處，上有突起肉上是穴，手、足少陽、陽維之會。《銅人》：鍼八分，灸三壯。當缺盆陷上突起肉上鍼之，若誤鍼之，傷人五臟氣，令人卒死。

This point is located on the shoulder, above Quē Pén (ST-12), in the depression at the border of the hidden bone,[205] around the location above Quē Pén (ST-12) where the flesh rises highest, that is the point. It is the meeting of the hand and foot shàoyáng [channels], and yángwéi [vessel]. *The Tóngrén* states, "Needle 8 fēn, and moxa 3 cones. One ought to needle exactly at where the flesh rises highest above the depression of Quē Pén (ST-12); if one needles it inaccurately, it will damage the qì of the five zàng-viscera and cause a person to die suddenly."

注：穴在缺盆之上，自腹中視之，固爲高處，即以本經自關衝來者，上肩則亦爲高處矣，故曰天髎。足少陽之會於此穴也，乃過天牖手少陽之脈，前下至肩井，却左右交出之際，而與本經會於此穴也。陽維之會本經於此也，乃陽維過肩下前，與手少陽會於臑會、天髎，而與本經會於此穴也。天髎在裏之上，肩井在外之下，所以有陷中之戒。

Explanation: as this point is located above Quē Pén (ST-12), when one looks [upwards] from the abdomen, it is undoubtedly at an elevated position; in addition, for this channel to arrive here from Guān Chōng (SJ-1), it has ascended the shoulder, which is likewise considered as an elevated position; therefore, it is called Tiān Liáo (Celestial Bone-Hole).

For the foot shàoyáng [channel] to meet at this point, prior, it traverses Tiān Yǒu (SJ-16) of the hand shàoyáng vessel, and then [continues] forwards to arrive at Jiān Jǐng (GB-21); after it pulls back from the region where its left and right [pathways] intersect and re-emerge,[206] [the foot shàoyáng channel] meets with this channel at this point (SJ-15).

For the yángwéi [vessel] to meet this channel here, prior, the yángwéi [vessel] traverses the shoulder and descends to its front, meeting with the hand shàoyáng at Nào Huì (SJ-13) and Tiān Liáo (SJ-15); as such, it meets with this channel at this point (SJ-15). Whereas Tiān Liáo (SJ-15) is located above on the inside, Jiān Jǐng (GB-21) is located below on the outside, this is the reason why it has the contraindication [of needling] the depression.

天髎之本病：肩臂痠痛，缺盆中痛，項筋急。

Principal diseases of Tiān Liáo: aching pain in the shoulder and arm, pain in the supraclavicular fossa, and tension of the sinews at the nape.

---

[205] I.e., the superior angle of the scapula.
[206] I.e., DU-14 where the left and right pathways of the gallbladder channel intersect.

注：前症皆本經所行部分之病，故責之。

Explanation: the above signs are all diseases which are in areas where the principal channel travels, thus seek this [point].

天髎之陽維病：寒熱汗不出，胸中煩滿。

Yángwéi diseases of Tiān Liáo: chills and fever with absence of sweating, and vexation with fullness in the chest.

注：此陽維及少陽在身側應有之症，故責之。

Explanation: these are corresponding signs of the yángwéi [vessel] and shàoyáng [channel] on the sides of the body, thus seek this [point].

Sixteenth Point of the Sānjiāo Channel
Tiān Yǒu – Celestial Window (SJ-16)
三焦經第十六穴天牖

穴在頸大筋外，缺盆上，天容後，天柱前，完骨下，髮際上。《銅人》：鍼一寸，留七呼，不宜補，不宜灸，灸即令人面腫眼合，先取譩譆，後取天容、天池即瘥。不鍼譩譆即難療。《明堂》：鍼五分，得氣即泄，泄盡更留三呼，不宜補。《素》注：灸三壯。《資生》：灸一壯。

This point is located on the outside of the great sinew on the neck, above Quē Pén (ST-12), behind Tiān Róng (SI-17), in front of Tiān Zhù (BL-10), below Wán Gǔ (GB-12), and above the hairline. *The Tóngrén* states, "Needle 1 cùn, retain for 7 respirations, it is inappropriate to supplement and inappropriate to moxa; if one uses moxa, it will promptly cause the face to swell and the eyes to shut; in that case, initially choose Yī Xī (BL-45), then subsequently choose Tiān Róng (SI-17) and Tiān Chí (PC-1),[207] and there will be recovery. Without needling Yī Xī (BL-45), it will be difficult to cure." *The Míngtáng* states, "Needle 5 fēn, and obtain qì then promptly drain; after draining its entirety, further retain for 3 respirations, it is inappropriate to supplement." *The Sùzhù* states, "Moxa 3 cones." *The Zīshēng* states, "Moxa 1 cone."

注：天者，言其高也，凡各經之穴在頸者，多以天名之。以其在頸之側，則以牖名之，如室之有牖，乃在室之側也。天柱者，太陽穴也，穴在挾項後髮際，大筋外廉陷中。天容者，手太陽小腸經穴也，在耳下曲頰。完骨者，足少陽膽經穴也，在耳後入髮際四分。

---

[207] The second group of point selection here, SJ-17 and PC-1, are actually SJ-16 and GB-20 in *the Tóngrén*.

Explanation: Regarding Tiān (Celestial), it is speaking of the height; in general, for points of each channel that are located on the neck, many are named as Tiān (Celestial). As this [point (SJ-16)] is located on the side of the neck, thus it is named Yǒu (Window), just like Yǒu (Windows) of a room are surely located on the sides of a room.

For Tiān Zhù (Celestial Pillar, BL-10), it is a tàiyáng point, it is located in the depression on the outside ridge of the great sinew that clasps the nape at the posterior hairline. For Tiān Róng (Celestial Countenance, SI-17), it is a point of the hand tàiyáng small intestine channel, it is located below the ear at the corner of the jaw.[208] For Wán Gǔ (GB-12), it is a point of the foot shàoyáng gallbladder channel, it is located 4 fēn into the hairline behind the ear.

則此穴，上直完骨之下，平直天柱之前，前直曲頰下天容之後，在胃經之缺盆則尚遠，無須考焉。此穴在上三穴之中，取之可矣。

As for this point (SJ-16), it is below Wán Gǔ (GB-12) that is directly above it, it is in front of Tiān Zhù (BL-10) that is in a horizontal line with it, and it is behind Tiān Róng (SI-17) that is directly in front and below the corner of the jaw; yet, it is quite far from the Quē Pén (ST-12) of the stomach channel, thus it is unnecessary to refer to that [point (ST-12)]. This point is located in the middle of these three points [discussed] above, locate them first, then [Tiān Yǒu (SJ-16)] can be located.

天池，乃手厥陰心包絡穴也。譩譆，乃足太陽次行穴也。天容見前。本經原爲火經，又在頸之側，誤灸之害在後取太陽之譩譆泄於後，在下在前取手厥陰之天池泄於前在下。而又取手太陽之天容泄之於上，以散其火之害。則取此穴者，可不慎哉。

For Tiān Chí (Celestial Pool, PC-1), it is a point of the hand juéyīn pericardium network. For Yī Xī (BL-45), it is a tàiyáng channel point on the second line. Tiān Róng (SI-17) is explained above. This channel is by its nature a fire channel, additionally, it is also located on the side of the neck; thus, for the harm of mistakenly using moxibustion, in the rear, choose Yī Xī (BL-45) of the tàiyáng [channel] to drain it from behind; in the below and in the front, choose Tiān Chí (PC-1) of the hand juéyīn [channel] to drain it from the front and from the below; furthermore, choose Tiān Róng (SI-17) of the hand tàiyáng [channel] to drain it from the above, so that the harm caused by the fire can be dispersed. When choosing this point, one cannot afford to be careless!

---

[208] In the entry of SI-17 (found in Vol. 1 of our translation), the location is described as "穴在耳下曲頰後 This point is located behind the corner of the jaw and below the ear."

天牖之本病：暴氣聾，目不明，耳不聰，目中痛，頭風面腫，項強不得回顧，夜夢顛倒，面青黃無顏色。

Principal diseases of Tiān Yǒu: sudden qì deafness, dim vision, deafness, pain within the eyes, head wind with facial swelling, stiffness of the nape with inability to look behind, deranged dreams at night, blue-green and yellow face with lack of colour in the complexion.

注：前症皆本經所主頭、耳、目部分應有之症也，夜夢顛倒，皆火之所爲也，宜泄此穴。

Explanation: all of the above signs are corresponding signs in the head, ear, and eye, the areas of which are governed by this channel; for deranged dreams at night, in all cases, it is caused by fire, it is appropriate to drain this point.

Seventeenth Point of the Sānjiāo Channel
Yì Fēng – Wind Screen (SJ-17)
三焦經第十七穴翳風

穴在耳後尖角陷中，按之引耳中痛，先以錢二十文，令患人咬之，尋取穴中，手、足少陽之會。《素》注：鍼三分。《銅人》：鍼七分。《明堂》：灸三壯，鍼、灸俱令咬銅錢開口。

This point is located in the depression behind the tip of the ear; upon pressing it, pain will radiate into the ear. First, make the patient bite on [a stack of] twenty pieces of coin, so that the point can be sought. It is the meeting of the hand and foot shàoyáng [channels]. *The Sùzhù* **states, "Needle 3 fēn."** *The Tóngrén* **states, "Needle 7 fēn."** *The Míngtáng* **states, "Moxa 3 cones." For both needling and moxibustion, make [the patient] bite on the copper coins [to ensure] the mouth is open.**

注：此穴在耳之下後，乃無物遮蔽之所，風之自後者，如風池、風府之穴，皆常中風之所也，故曰翳風。

Explanation: this point is located below and behind the ear, it is indeed a place that is covered by nothing. As Fēng (Wind) comes from the rear, points like Fēng Chí (Wind Pool, GB-20) and Fēng Fǔ (Wind Mansion, DU-16) are all places that are commonly struck by wind, thus [this point] is called Yì Fēng (Wind Screen).

翳風之本病：耳鳴耳聾，口眼喎邪，脫頷煩腫，口吃牙車急，口噤不開，不能言，小兒善欠。

Principal disease of Yì Fēng: tinnitus and deafness, deviation of the mouth and eyes [due to] evil,[209] dislocation of the chin with swelling of the cheeks, stuttering with tension of the jaw, clenched jaw that cannot open, inability to speak, and frequent yawning in children.

注：前症皆本經本穴所被風寒應得之症，故泄此穴，以散風寒，而後灸以溫之。

Explanation: all of the above signs are corresponding signs due to contraction of wind and cold at this point of this channel, thus drain this point in order to disperse wind and cold, and subsequently moxa in order to warm it.

Eighteenth Point of the Sānjiāo Channel
Chì Mài – Tugging Vessel (SJ-18)
三焦經第十八穴瘈脈

一名資脈
Supporting Vessel

穴在耳本後，鷄足青絡脈。《銅人》：刺出血如豆汁，不宜多出，鍼一分，灸三壯。

This point is located behind the base of the ear, at the blue-green network-vessel that resembles a chicken foot. *The Tóngrén* states, "Pierce to let blood that resemble soy milk, it is inappropriate [to let] an excessive amount, needle 1 fēn, and moxa 3 cones."

注：瘈瘲之症，在下則肝膽之經爲之，在上則手厥陰、手少陽爲之，以四經皆木火相生之經，而瘈瘲之症，非火不作，穴名瘈脈者，言此乃瘈瘲本也。

Explanation: regarding the sign of Chì (Tugging) and slackening, when it manifests in the below, it is caused by the channels of the liver and gallbladder; when it manifests in the above, it is caused by the hand juéyīn and hand shàoyáng [channels], because these four channels are the channels of wood and fire that mutually engender one another. Moreover, for the sign of Chì (Tugging) and slackening, without fire, it cannot manifest; therefore, regarding this point name Chì

---

209 Alternatively, as xié 邪 (evil) is homophone with xié 斜 (slanted), this line can simply be read as "deviation of the mouth and eyes."

Mài (Tugging Vessel), it is indicating that this [channel] is surely the root of Chì (Tugging) and slackening.

瘛脈之本病：小兒驚癇瘛瘲，頭風耳鳴，嘔吐泄利，無時驚恐，目睛不明，眵 瞢。

Principal diseases of Chì Mài: fright epilepsy with tugging and slackening in children, head wind with tinnitus, retching and vomiting with diarrhoea, sporadic episodes of fright and fear, dim vision, and eye discharge[210] with blurry eyesight.

注：前症皆本經受風之症也，故出此穴之血，以泄其火，但不亦多耳。

Explanation: all of the above signs are signs of wind contraction by this channel, thus let blood from this point in order to drain the fire; however, one should not do so too excessively.

Nineteenth Point of the Sānjiāo Channel

Lú Xí – Skull Breathing[211] (SJ-19)

三焦經第十九穴顱息

穴在耳後間青絡脈中。《銅人》：灸七壯，禁鍼。《明堂》：灸三壯，鍼一分，不得多出血，多出血殺人。

This point is located on the blue-green network-vessel in the space behind the ear. *The Tóngrén* states, "Moxa 7 cones, and needling is contraindicated." *The Míngtáng* states, "Moxa 3 cones, needle 1 fēn, and one must not bleed it too excessively, as excessive bleeding will cause death."

注：耳之竅，皆頭顱出息之所也，此穴在耳後青絡脈，正顱中與耳相通之 處，故曰顱息，氣之往來曰息。

Explanation: for the orifices of the ears, they are where the Xī (Breaths) of the head and Lú (Skull) exit. This point is located on the blue-green network-vessel behind the ear, exactly at the place where the Lú (Skull) and ear connect together, thus it is called Lú Xī (Skull Breathing), as the coming and going of qì is known as Xī (Breathing).

---

[210] "眵 eye discharge" was originally "多 excessive" in the scribal manuscript, the editors of this manuscript, Zhāng and Zhà, have changed it according to *the Zhēnjiǔ Dàchéng*.

[211] *Grasping the Wind* names it "Skull Rest."

顱息之本病：耳中痛，喘息，小兒嘔吐涎沫，瘈瘲發癇，胸脅相引，身熱頭痛，不得臥，耳腫及膿汁。

Principal diseases of Lú Xí: pain in the ear, panting, vomiting of spittle in children, tugging and slackening with epileptic episodes, pain that radiates between the chest and rib-side, generalised heat [effusion] with headache, inability to lie down, and swelling of the ear with pus.

注：本經所治多耳病，以本經入耳出耳，乃其正症也，且此穴緊在耳後，故耳症取之。小兒瘈瘲，又本經之所主也，故取此穴。

Explanation: what this channel predominantly treats are ear diseases;[212] as this channel enters and exits the ear, [ear diseases] are surely its primary signs; moreover, this point is located close to the behind of the ear, thus for ear signs choose it. For childhood tugging and slackening, it is also what the principal channels governs, thus choose this point.

Twentieth Point of the Sānjiāo Channel
Jiǎo Jūn – Angle Vertex (SJ-20)
三焦經第二十穴角孫

穴在耳廓中間，開口有空，手太陽、足少陽與本經相會之處。《銅人》：灸三壯。

This point is located at the centre of the auricle, where a hollow appears upon opening the mouth. It is the meeting place of the hand tàiyáng, the foot shàoyáng, and this channel. *The Tóngrén* states, "Moxa 3 cones."

注：此穴雖云耳廓中間，尚未詳明。耳之外輪為廓，按圖則應在耳廓中之上，若只云耳廓中間，何以為底據也。名角孫者，當在耳角之下也。手太陽之會於此穴也，乃支行者，從缺盆循頸之天窗、天容，上頰抵顴髎，上至目銳眥，過瞳子髎，却入耳中，循聽宮而與本經會也。足少陽之會於此穴者，乃支行者，自耳後顳顬間，過翳風之分，入耳中，過聽宮，至目銳眥者，而與本經會於此穴也。

Explanation: although this point is said to be "located at the centre of the auricle," [the location] is yet to be fully explained.[213] The outer wheel of the ear is the auricle; according to the illustrations, [this point] should be above the centre of the auricle; for it to simply state that it is "at the centre of the auricle," how does one

---

[212] Side note: Coincidentally, according to *Yīnyáng Shíyīmài Jiǔjīng* 陰陽十一脈灸經 (*Moxibustion Canon of Yin-Yang Eleven Channels*, c. 2nd century BCE) of the Mǎwángduī excavation, today's SJ channel was called the "耳脈 ear vessel."

[213] See footnote 166 in the pathway section.

utilize it as the basis of one's reference? It is named Jiǎo Sūn (Angle Vertex), thus it should be located below the Jiǎo (Angle) of the ear.

For the hand tàiyáng [channel] to meet at this point, prior, from the supraclavicular fossa, a branch pathway follows the neck, passing through Tiān Chuāng (SI-16)[214] and Tiān Róng (SI-17), ascends the cheek to reach Quán Liáo (SI-18); it continues ascending to arrive at the outer canthus of the eye, traverses Tóng Zǐ Liáo (GB-1), returns to enter the ear, passes through Tīng Gōng (SI-19), and then meets with this channel.

For the foot shàoyáng [channel] to meet at this point, prior, from the space in the temple region[215] behind the ear, a branch pathway traverses in the area of Yì Fēng (SJ-17), enters the ear, traverses Tīng Gōng (SI-19), arrives at the outer canthus of the eye, and then meets with this channel at this point.

角孫之本病：目生膚翳，齒齦腫，唇吻強，齒牙不能嚼物，齲齒，頭項強。

Principal diseases of Jiǎo Jūn: generation of skin screens in the eye, swelling of the gums, stiff lips, inability to chew objects with teeth, tooth decay, and stiffness of the head and nape.

注：以上諸病，皆本經所行之部分也，頭、面、齒、目，受風火之邪，致有此症，故宜取此穴，以泄風火之邪。

Explanation: for the various diseases above, they all occur in areas where this channel travels; when the head, the face, the teeth, or the eyes contract evils such as wind or fire, these signs will manifest as the result; thus, choose this point in order to drain the evil of wind or fire.

Twenty-first Point of the Sānjiāo Channel
Sī Zhú Kōng – Silk Bamboo Hole (SJ-23)[216]
三焦經第二十一穴絲竹空
一名目髎
Alternate name: Eye Bone-Hole

---

[214] "Tiān Chuāng (SI-16)" was originally "Tiān Tú 天突 (REN-22)" in the scribal manuscript, the editors of this manuscript, Zhāng and Zhà, have amended it as the hand tàiyáng does not pass through REN-22.

[215] I.e., another name for GB-19.

[216] As the numbering scheme of this work differs from the modern standard, to avoid confusion, the modern point numbers are always given in channel abbreviation and Arabic number (e.g., SJ-23), whereas the numbering scheme of this work is given in spelled out writing (e.g., Twenty-first Point of the Sānjiāo Channel).

穴在眉後陷中，手、足少陽脈氣所發。《素》注：鍼三分，留六呼。《銅人》：禁灸，灸之不幸，使人目小及盲，鍼三分，留三呼，宜泄不宜補。

This point is located in the depression behind the eyebrow. The hand and foot shàoyáng vessel qì effuses here. *The Sùzhù* states, "Needle 3 fēn, and retain for 6 respirations." *The Tóngrén* states, "Moxibustion is contraindicated; in unfortunate circumstances, moxibustion will cause a person's eyesight to diminish[217] and even become blind; needle 3 fēn, retain for 3 respirations; and it is appropriate to drain, but not appropriate to supplement.

注：此穴雖在目旁，而實通耳之竅，以聽聲者，故曰絲竹空。足少陽亦過於此處而上行，故曰足少陽脈氣所發。

Explanation: although this point is located beside the eye, in reality, it connects with the orifice of the ear; as it is associated with what hears the sound, it is called Sī Zhú Kōng (Silk Bamboo Hole).[218] The foot shàoyáng [vessel] also traverses this place before it further ascends, thus it is said that the foot shàoyáng vessel qì effuses here.

絲竹空之本病：目赤，視物眻眻不明，目眩頭痛，眼睫毛倒，偏正頭痛，惡風寒，風癇，目戴不識人，發狂吐涎，發即無時。

Principal diseases of Sī Zhú Kōng: red eyes, blurred dim vision, dizzy vision with headache, ingrown eyelash, hemilateral and frontal headache, aversion to wind or cold, wind epilepsy, upcast eyes with inability to recognise people, and mania with vomiting of drool that occur at sporadic times.

注：本穴近目，故所治多目病，目病皆火爲之，故不宜補。頭痛非風即火，亦不宜補。風癇、發狂，乃本經正病也，宜泄不宜補。吐涎，不識人，本經風痰上逆也，豈可補乎。

Explanation: this point is close to the eye, thus what it treats are predominantly eye diseases; as [these] eye diseases are always caused by fire, thus it is inappropriate to supplement. For headache, if it is not due to wind, then it is caused by fire, thus it is also inappropriate to supplement. Wind epilepsy and mania are principal diseases of this channel, for these, it is also appropriate to drain but inappropriate to supplement. For vomiting of drool and inability to recognise people, these are due to counterflow ascent of wind and phlegm in this channel, how is it acceptable to supplement?

---

[217] Literally, "[make] the eyes smaller."

[218] Silk and bamboo refer to traditional Chinese stringed and woodwind instruments and the music they produce, hence the connection with hearing.

Twenty-Second Point of the Sānjiāo Channel
Hé Liáo – Harmony Bone-Hole (SJ-22)
三焦經第二十二穴和膠

穴在耳前銳髮下，橫動脈中是穴，足少陽、手太陽與本經相會之處。《銅人》：鍼七分，灸三壯。

This point is located in front of the ear, below the sidelock, at the horizontal pulsating vessel, that is the point. It is the meeting place of the foot shàoyáng, the hand tàiyáng, and this channel. *The Tóngrén* **states, "Needle 7 fēn, and moxa 3 cones."**

注：此穴當在足少陽曲鬢穴之下，動脈中是穴，即以動脈取穴，則必於其上下四旁，擇其動脈者爲真。和膠之義未詳。

Explanation: this point is located below Qū Bìn (GB-7) of the foot shàoyáng, at the pulsating vessel, that is the point; thus, when locating this point by the pulsating vessel, one must seek the pulsating vessel at the four sides [of the point] above and below, that is the true [location]. The meaning of Hé Liáo (Harmony Bone-Hole) is still unknown.

和膠之本病：牙車引急，頸項腫，耳中嘈嘈，瘰癧口癖，頭重痛，鼻涕，面風寒，鼻準上腫，癰痛，招搖視瞻。

Principal diseases of Hé Liáo: radiating tension in the tooth carriage,[219] swelling of the neck, noisy tumult in the ears, tugging and slackening with deviation of the mouth, heaviness and pain in the head, nasal snivel, wind-cold in the face, swelling at the tip of the nose, painful abscess, and indistinct wavering vision.

注：耳也，牙車也，頸項也，鼻也，瘰癧也，口癖也，皆本經在面所行部分，如有風寒火邪客之，皆能致症，故取此穴。

Explanation: the ear, the tooth carriage, the neck, the nose, tugging and slackening, deviation of the mouth, these are all areas where this channel travels on the face; if there is wind, cold, or fire evil that has lodged in them, it can always result in these diseases, thus choose this point.

---

[219] I.e., the lower palatal bone.

Twenty-Third Point of the Sānjiāo Channel
Ěr Mén – Ear Gate (SJ-21)
三焦經第二十三穴耳門

穴在耳前起肉，當耳缺者陷中。《銅人》：鍼三分，留三呼，灸三壯。《下經》：禁灸，病宜灸者，不過三壯。

This point is located at the fleshy protuberance in front of the ear,[220] in the depression exactly at the notch of the ear.[221] *The Tóngrén* states, "Needle 3 fēn, retain for 3 respirations, and moxa 3 cones." *The Xiàjīng* states, "While moxibustion is [generally] contraindicated, when there is a disease that is appropriate to moxa, do not exceed 3 cones."

注：以穴在耳門旁，故曰耳門。

Explanation: because this point is located beside the Ěr Mén (Ear Gate), thus it is called Ěr Mén (Ear Gate).

耳門之本經病：耳鳴如蟬聲，聤耳膿出汁，耳生瘡，重聽無所聞，齒齲，唇吻強。

Principal channel diseases of Ěr Mén: ringing in the ears like the sound of cicadas, purulent ear with production of pus fluid, engenderment of ear sores, hearing impairment and inability to hear anything, tooth decay, and stiff lips.

注：此穴近耳，故治耳病，近頰，故治唇齒病，不宜灸者，耳之病多火，再以火益之，則不可也。古人有二火在面者，不可灸。二火謂太陽小腸火、手少陽三焦火也。

Explanation: this point is close to the ear, thus it treats ear diseases; it is [also] close to the cheek, thus it [also] treats diseases of the lips and teeth. Regarding the inappropriateness to moxa [this point], the diseases of the ear are predominantly due to fire, to further exacerbate it with fire, it is not acceptable. The ancients had [a saying that] since there are two entities of fire on the face, one cannot moxa it;[222] the "two entities of fire" are said to be the tàiyáng small intestine fire and the hand shàoyáng sānjiāo fire.

---

[220] I.e., the tragus, which is also known as Ěr Mén, the name of this point.
[221] I.e., the intertragic notch.
[222] We cannot find the origin of this quote.

The Foot Shàoyáng
Gallbladder Channel & Points

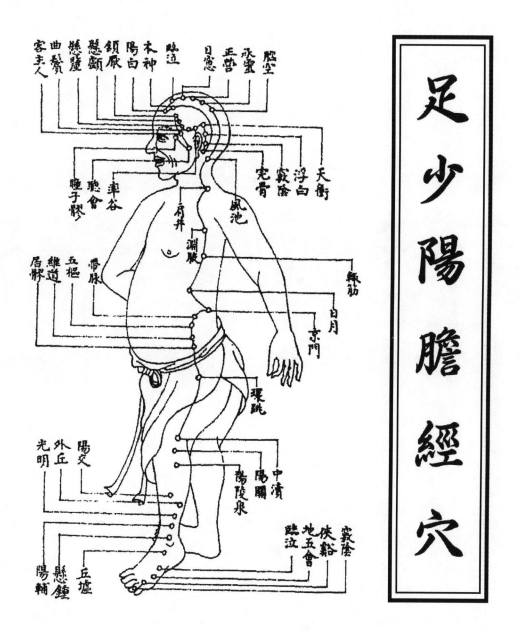

The Foot Shàoyáng Gallbladder Channel & Points
足少陽膽經

Overview of the Foot Shàoyáng Gallbladder Channel
足少陽膽經總論

思蓮子曰：足少陽膽經，多氣少血。其經之在外者，起於目銳眥之瞳子髎，斜下行至耳前陷中之聽會穴，反折上至耳前起骨，開口有空之上關穴中，又直上行至曲角下之頷厭穴，又斜行向下，過懸顱、懸釐二穴，又斜過耳上髮際隅中之曲鬢穴，

Master Sīlián says, the foot shàoyáng gallbladder channel has copious qì and scant blood.

For the external [pathway] of this channel, it commences at Tóng Zi Liáo (GB-1) by the outer canthus. It descends obliquely to Tīng Huì (GB-2) in the depression in front of the ear. It turns upwards and ascends to Shàng Guān (GB-3), which is in front of the ear, at prominent bone, where a hollow appears upon opening the mouth. It ascends vertically to arrive at Hàn Yàn (GB-4) below the corner [of the head]. Then it travels obliquely to descend, traversing the two points of Xuán Lú (GB-5) and Xuán Lí (GB-6). It continues to traverse obliquely to Qū Bìn (GB-7) at the border of the hairline above the ear.

又橫過耳上寸半之率谷穴，又彎而上過耳後髮際之天衝穴，又下折而後，入髮一寸之浮白穴，又下過完骨上，枕骨下，動搖有空之竅陰穴，又行耳後入髮際四分之完骨穴，至此遂反折而上至本經之本神穴，此穴在督經中行之神庭穴旁三寸，入髮一寸，猶當在耳上，

It traverses horizontally to Shuài Gǔ (GB-8) half a cùn above the ear. It bends and ascends to traverse to Tiān Chōng (GB-9), which is at the border of the hairline and behind the ear. It descends and turns to the rear, and [arrives] at Fú Bái (GB-10) 1 cùn into the hairline.

It descends to traverse [Tóu] Qiào Yīn (GB-11), which is above the completion bone,[223] below the occipital bone, where a hollow appears upon moving and shaking [the head]. It travels to Wán Gǔ (GB-12), which is 4 fēn into the

---

[223] This is the same as the point name Wán Gǔ (GB-12), yet in this instance it appears to be talking about bone instead.

hairline and behind the ear. Upon reaching here, it turns back and ascends to reach Běn Shén (GB-13) of this channel; this point is located 3 cùn to the side of Shén Tíng (DU-24) of the dū channel on the midline, 1 cùn into the hairline; alternatively, it is directly above the ear.

又下行至眉上一寸之陽白穴，與太陽會於睛明穴，至此又折而上，直目上入髮際五分陷中之臨泣穴，又上過入髮一寸之當陽穴，此穴圖不載，又上過入髮寸半之目窗穴，

It descends to arrive at Yáng Bái (GB-14) at 1 cùn above the eyebrow. It further meets the tàiyáng [channel] at Jīng Míng (BL-1). After arriving here, it turns and ascends to [Tóu] Lín Qì (GB-15), which is directly above the eye, in the depression 5 fēn into the hairline. It ascends and traverse to Dāng Yáng (EX-HN 2)[224] at 1 cùn into the hairline; this point is not recorded in the illustration. It continues and traverses to Mù Chuāng (GB-16) at 1 cùn and a half into the hairline.

又上過入髮三寸之正營穴，又上過入髮四寸之承靈穴，又上過入髮五寸半之腦空穴，遂折而下入於耳後髮內陷中之風池穴，以上少陽之在頭側者二十穴，凡三折。

It continues and traverses to Zhèng Yíng (GB-17) at 3 cùn into the hairline. It continues and traverses to Chéng Líng (GB-18) at 4 cùn into the hairline. It continues and traverses to Nǎo Kōng (GB-19) at 5 and a half cùn into the hairline. It then turns and descends to Fēng Chí (GB-20), which is in the depression inside of the hairline and behind the ear. The above twenty points are those of the shàoyáng on the side of the head, in total there are three turns.

自瞳子髎至完骨爲第一折，一瞳子髎，二聽會，三客主人，四頷厭，五懸顱，六懸釐，七曲鬢，八率谷，九天衝，十浮白，十一竅陰，十二完骨，初折共十二穴。

From Tóng Zi Liáo (GB-1) to Wán Gǔ (GB-12) are within the first turn; first is Tóng Zi Liáo (GB-1), second is Tīng Huì (GB-2), third is Kè Zhǔ Rén (GB-3),[225] fourth is Hàn Yàn (GB-4), fifth is Xuán Lú (GB-5), sixth is Xuán Lí (GB-6), seventh is Qū Bìn (GB-7), eighth is Shuài Gǔ (GB-8), nineth is Tiān Chōng (GB-9), tenth is Fú Bái (GB-10), eleventh is [Tóu] Qiào Yīn (GB-11), twelfth is Wán Gǔ (GB-12), there are twelve points in total within the first turn.

自完骨外折，而上至額止，一本神，二陽白，二折共二穴。又自陽白外折而上，一臨泣，二目窗，三正營，四承靈，五腦空，六風池，三折共六穴。此少陽在頭側曲折作穴之數，並曲折三疊之形，宜細心究焉。

---

[224] See the third extra point associated with the gallbladder channel.
[225] Yuè Hánzhēn appears to use both Shàng Guān and Kè Zhǔ Rén to refer to GB-3.

From Wán Gǔ (GB-12), it turns to the outside and ascends to stop at the forehead; the first is Běn Shén (GB-13) and the second is Yáng Bái (GB-14); the second turn has a total of two points.

Finally, from Yáng Bái (GB-14), it turns outside and ascends; first is [Tóu] Lín Qì (GB-15), second is Mù Chuāng (GB-16), third is Zhèng Yíng (GB-17), fourth is Chéng Líng (GB-18), fifth is Nǎo Kōng (GB-19), and sixth is Fēng Chí (GB-20); the third turn has a total of six points.

These are the numbers of points in these turns of the shàoyáng[226] [channel] located on the side of the head, as well as its three-fold shape with bends and turns. One should investigate these meticulously.

本經入風池之後，遂入頸，手少陽三焦經之頸大筋外，缺盆上，手太陽小腸經耳之下，曲頰之後，天容穴之後，足太陽經挾項後髮際，大筋外廉陷中，天柱穴之前，完骨下，髮際上，天牖穴之裏，前有天容，後有天牖，此脈下行於其中，下至本經，循本經之肩井穴，又下直下卻左右交出於少陽之後，橫過督經之大椎穴，太陽經之大杼穴，手太陽秉風之前，入足陽明胃經缺盆之外，而下行於腹。

After entering Fēng Chí (GB-20), this channel then enters the neck, traveling at the interior of Tiān Yǒu (SI-16) of the hand shàoyáng sānjiāo channel, which is outside of the great sinew, above Quē Pén (ST-12), below Wán Gǔ (GB-12), and above the hairline; furthermore, [Tiān Yǒu (SI-16)] is behind Tiān Róng (SI-17) of the hand tàiyáng small intestine channel, which is below the ear and behind the corner of the jaw; moreover, it is in front of Tiān Zhù (BL-10) of the foot tàiyáng channel, which clasps the nape at the posterior hairline, in the depression on the outer ridge of the great sinew.[227]

With Tiān Róng (SI-17) in front and Tiān Yǒu (SI-16) behind, this vessel traverses downward in between them, descends to arrive at the principal channel, and follows it to Jiān Jǐng (GB-21) of this channel.

---

[226] The manuscript had "xiǎoyáng 小陽 (minor yáng)" here instead of shàoyáng 少陽, which is likely a typographical error and has been amended.

[227] Note: This paragraph has been heavily rearranged for the sake of reading experience, as the original paragraph is filled with clustered inline annotations that render it almost incomprehensible, even in the Chinese source text. It is very likely that the original line was simply, "遂入頸，天牖穴之裏 [this channel] then enters the neck, traveling at the interior of Tiān Yǒu (SI-16);" however, the description of point location from SI-16 entry was added; in addition, as the SI-16 entry mentions two other points, ST-12 and BL-10, the location description of the latter two were further added to this supposed "one short sentence;" as a result, it becomes a rather bloated paragraph that is rather difficult to decipher. Sadly, the manuscript we have today does not differentiate between the main text and inline annotations; thus, we cannot simply introduce radical changes to the paragraph structure (e.g., using bolded font to designate the main text and/or parenthesis to specify annotations), as we could create something unintended by its original author. So, we can only aim to make it as readable as possible by rearranging sentences.

It continues to descend vertically, pulls back from the left and right, intersects and re-emerges behind the shàoyáng [channel], after having horizontally traversed past Dà Zhuī (DU-14) of the dū channel and Dà Zhù (BL-11) of the tàiyáng channel. In front of Bǐng Fēng (SI-12) of the tàiyáng [channel], it enters the outside of Quē Pén (ST-12) of the foot yángmíng stomach channel; thereupon, it descends to the abdomen.

但本經頭上二十穴，其曲折部分已載於前，而與各經交結所過之所，更宜詳焉。

For these twenty points of this channel on the head, the passage regarding their bends and turns has already been conveyed prior; yet, one should examine the places where each of the channels traverses and intersects even more thoroughly.

一穴瞳子髎穴，乃與手太陽小腸經、手少陽三焦經、足少陽膽經三脈交會之處。二聽會穴，不與各經會。三客主人穴，乃手少陽三焦、手陽明大腸、足陽明胃經與本經相會之處。四頜厭穴，手少陽三焦、手陽明大腸、足陽明胃與本經相會之地。

The first point, Tóng Zi Liáo (GB-1), is the location where [this channel] intersects and meets with three vessels, the hand tàiyáng small intestine channel, hand shàoyáng sānjiāo channel, and foot shàoyáng gallbladder channel. The second point, Tīng Huì (GB-2), does not meet with any other channels.

The third point, Kè Zhǔ Rén (GB-3), is the location where this channel meets with the hand shàoyáng sānjiāo, hand yángmíng large intestine, and foot yángmíng stomach channels. The fourth point, Hàn Yàn (GB-4), is the place where this channel meets with the hand shàoyáng sānjiāo, hand yángmíng large intestine, and foot yángmíng stomach channels.

五懸顱穴，亦手、足少陽、陽明相會之處。六懸釐穴，亦手、足少陽、陽明相會之處。七曲鬢穴，乃足太陽與本經相會之處，乃足太陽之絡，橫至耳者也。八率谷，亦足太陽與本經相會之處。九天衝穴，亦足太陽與本經相會之處。十浮白，亦足太陽與本經相會之處。

The fifth point, Wǔ Xuán Lú (GB-5), is also a location where [this channel] meets with the hand and foot shàoyáng and yángmíng [channels]. The sixth point, Xuán Lí (GB-6), is also a location where [this channel] meets with the hand and foot shàoyáng and yángmíng [channels]. The seventh point, Qū Bìn (GB-7), is the location where this channel meets with the foot tàiyáng, which is the network of the foot tàiyáng that [travels] horizontally to arrive at the ear.

The eighth [point], Shuài Gǔ (GB-8), is also a location where this channel meets with the foot tàiyáng [channel]. The ninth point, Tiān Chōng (GB-9), is likewise a location where this channel meets with the foot tàiyáng [channel].

The tenth point, Fú Bái (GB-10), is similarly a location where this channel meets with the foot tàiyáng [channel].

十一竅陰穴，乃足太陽、手少陽與本經相會之處。十二完骨穴，亦足太陽與本經相會之處。十三本神穴，乃奇經陽維與本經相會之處。十四陽白穴，乃足陽明胃經、手陽明大腸、手少陽三焦、奇經陽維與本經相會之處。

The eleventh point, [Tóu] Qiào Yīn (GB-11), is the location where this channel meets with the foot tàiyáng and hand shàoyáng [channels]. The twelfth point, Wán Gǔ (GB-12), is also a location where this channel meets with the foot tàiyáng [channel].

The thirteenth point, Běn Shén (GB-13), is the location where this channel meets with the extraordinary channel yángwéi [vessel]. The fourteenth point, Yáng Bái (GB-14), is the location where this channel meets with the foot yángmíng stomach channel, hand yángmíng large intestine, hand shàoyáng sānjiāo [channels], and extraordinary channel yángwéi [vessel].

十五臨泣穴，乃足太陽、奇經陽維與本經相會之處。十六目窗、十七正營、十八承靈、十九腦空，二十風池五穴，皆奇經陽維與本經相會之地。以上在頭及頸之二十穴與各經相會之所也。

The fifteenth point, [Tóu] Lín Qì (GB-15), is the location where this channel meets with the foot tàiyáng [channel] and extraordinary channel yángwéi [vessel]. The [next] five points are the sixteenth point Mù Chuāng (GB-16), seventeenth point Zhèng Yíng (GB-17), eighteenth point Chéng Líng (GB-18), nineteenth point Nǎo Kōng (GB-19), and twentieth point Fēng Chí (GB-20); they are all locations where this channel meets with the extraordinary channel yángwéi [vessel].

The above are the twenty points located on the head as well as the locations where [this channel] meets with other channels.

其支者，自耳後顳顬，即本經腦空穴間，過三焦經翳風穴之分，入耳過小腸聽宮穴後，自聽宮至目銳眥，至本經瞳子髎之處，而支者止。

A branch begins at the temple region behind the ear, this is namely in the space of Nǎo Kōng (GB-19) of this channel. It traverses the area of Yì Fēng (SJ-17) of the sānjiāo channel, enters the ear, and traverses behind Tīng Gōng (SI-19) of the small intestine [channel]. From Tīng Gōng (SI-19), it arrives at the outer canthus, [continues and] arrives at the location of Tóng Zi Liáo (GB-1) of this channel, where this branch terminates.

其支者，別又自目外瞳子髎穴，而下足陽明胃經大迎穴，合手少陽三焦經於頬，乃當手太陽小腸經顴髎穴之分，下臨胃經之頬車穴，

A branch also diverges from Tóng Zǐ Liáo (GB-1) on the outside of the eye, descends to Dà Yíng (ST-5) of the foot yángmíng stomach channel, and unites with the hand shàoyáng sānjiāo channel at the facial prominence, which is exactly the area of Quán Liáo (SI-18) of the hand tàiyáng small intestine channel; thereupon, it descends to reach Jiá Chē (ST-6) of the stomach channel.

始下頸循本經之前與左右相交入缺盆者相合，而下胸中，過手厥陰心包絡經天池之外而下貫膈，即足厥陰經期門穴之所，乃絡肝，而下至本經日月穴之下，而屬於膽也，

[At Jiá Chē (ST-6)], it begins to descend the neck and joins together with the aforementioned [pathway] of this channel that intersects from the left and right and enters Quē Pén (ST-12). It then descends into the chest, traverses outside of Tiān Chí (PC-1) of the hand juéyīn pericardiac network channel, and descends to pierce the diaphragm, exactly at the place of Qì Mén (LR-14) of the foot juéyīn channel, where it networks to the liver. Thereupon, it descends to arrive below Rì Yuè (GB-24) of this channel, and adjoins to the gallbladder.

自屬膽處，循脇內足厥陰肝經章門穴之裏，至陽明胃經氣衝穴，乃達毛際，遂橫入髀厭者之環跳穴；

From this location where it adjoins to the gallbladder, it follows the interior of Zhāng Mén (LR-13) of the foot juéyīn liver channel on the medial rib-side, arrives at Qì Chōng (ST-30) of the yángmíng stomach channel, and reaches the pubic hair region. Upon arriving here, it travels horizontally to enter Huán Tiào (GB-30) at the hip joint.

其在外之直行者，自肩井處，從缺盆下腋循胸，歷本經腋下三寸之淵液穴，又下直下復前一寸，而過本經三肋端，橫直蔽骨旁七寸五分，平直兩乳之輒筋穴，此穴乃本經之募，足太陽與本經會於此處，

As for the vertical pathway located on the outside, from the location of Jiān Jǐng (GB-21), it [travels through] Quē Pén (ST-12) to descend the armpit and follows the chest, passing through Yuān Yè (GB-22), which is 3 cùn below the armpit.

It continues to descend vertically and further move 1 cùn to the front, traversing to Zhé Jīn (GB-23) of this channel, which is located at the edge of the third rib, 7 cùn 5 fēn horizontally to the side of the sheltered bone,[228] and in line with the nipples; this point is the collecting point of this channel, and it is the location where this channel meets with the foot tàiyáng [channel].

---

[228] Likely the xiphoid process.

又下過肝經期門穴下之日月穴，此穴乃足太陰脾經、奇經陽維與本經相會之處，
遂斜下過季脇，至腰中之骨名監骨，下腰中季脇之本，挾脊腎募本經之京門穴，

It continues to descend to traverse Rì Yuè (GB-24), which is below Qì Mén (LR-14) of the liver channel; this point (GB-24) is the location where this channel meets with the foot tàiyīn spleen channel and extraordinary channel yángwéi [vessel].

Thereupon, it descends obliquely to traverse the floating rib, arriving at the haunch bone that is located in the lumbar [region]. It descends to Jīng Mén (GB-25) of this channel, the collecting point of the kidneys, which clasps the spine at the base of the floating rib in the lumbus [region].

又下過季脇一寸八分，臍上二分兩旁各七寸半之奇經帶脈穴，又下過帶脈穴下三寸，水道旁五寸五分，本經之五樞穴，亦本經與奇經帶脈相會之處，

It continues to descend to traverse Dài Mài (GB-26), which is 1 cùn 8 fēn below the floating rib, 2 fēn[229] above the umbilicus, and 7 and a half cùn to the side. It continues to descend traversing to Wǔ Shū (GB-27), which is 3 cùn below Dài Mài (GB-26) and 5 cùn 5 fēn to the side of Shuǐ Dào (ST-28); it is also the place where this channel meets with the extraordinary channel dài vessel.

又下過章門下五寸三分，本經之維道穴，亦本經與奇經相會之處，又下過章門下八寸三分之居膠穴，乃本經與奇經陽蹻相會之處，

It continues to descend traversing to Wéi Dào (GB-28) of this channel, which is 5 cùn 3 fēn below Zhāng Mén (LR-13); it is also the place where this channel meets with the extraordinary channel [dài vessel].

It continues to descend traversing to Jū Liáo (GB-29), which is 8 cùn 3 fēn below Zhāng Mén (LR-13); it is the place where this channel meets with the extraordinary channel yángqiāo [vessel].

遂入足太陽膀胱經挾脊之上膠、中膠二穴，下過奇經督脈之長強穴，與前之入髀厭者環跳穴相合，而爲足太陽與本經相會之所，乃下循髀外，行足太陽、足陽明二經之間，歷垂手中指盡處，兩筋之間，本經風市穴，

Thereupon, it enters the two foot tàiyáng bladder channel points that clasp the spine, Shàng Liáo (BL-31) and Zhōng Liáo (BL-33). It descends traversing to Cháng Qiáng (DU-1) of extraordinary channel dū vessel, then at Huán Tiào (GB-30), it joins together with the aforementioned [pathway] that enters the hip joint; it is where this channel and the foot tàiyáng [channel] meet. It descends following the outside of the thigh, travelling in between the two channels of the foot tàiyáng and foot yángmíng and passing through Fēng Shì

---

[229]"2 fēn" is "3 fēn" in the secondary manuscript.

(GB-31), which is where the middle finger rests [on the thigh], in the space of the two sinews.

又歷髀之外，膝上五寸，分肉間陷中之中瀆穴，乃本經膝上之別絡，走歷厥陰肝經之所，乃下膝之外，陽陵泉上三寸，犢鼻外陷中，本經之陽關穴，

It continues along the outside of the thigh to Zhōng Dú (GB-32), which is 5 cùn above the knee, in the depression at the parting of flesh; this is the diverging network-vessel of this channel above the knee, which travels to the foot juéyīn liver channel. It continues to descend on the outside of the thigh to Yáng Guān (GB-33) of this channel, which is 3 cùn above Yáng Líng Quán (GB-34), in the depression on the outside of the knee.

又下膝下一寸，腨外廉陷中，本經之陽陵泉穴，爲本經所入爲合土，又自陽陵泉下於輔骨前，足外踝上七寸，斜屬足太陽、足少陽、足陽明分肉之間，爲本經之陽交穴，乃奇經陽維之郄，

It continues to descend to Yáng Líng Quán (GB-34) of this channel, which is 1 cùn below the knee, in the depression on the outside of the lower leg; the channel enters here as the uniting and earth point.

From Yáng Líng Quán (GB-34), it descends to Yáng Jiāo (GB-35) of this channel, which is in front of the assisting bone, 7 cùn above the outer ankle [bone]; it obliquely adjoins to the parting of flesh in between the foot tàiyáng, foot shàoyáng, and foot yángmíng [channels]; moreover, it is the cleft point of the extraordinary channel yángwéi [vessel].

又歷外踝上六寸，本經之外丘穴，又歷外踝上五寸之光明穴，又爲足少陽膝下之絡，別走足厥陰肝經之所，

It continues to Wài Qiū (GB-36) of this channel at 6 cùn above the outer ankle [bone]. It continues to Guāng Míng (GB-37) at 5 cùn above the outer ankle [bone]; it is the network point of the foot shàoyáng below the knee, it diverges to the foot juéyīn liver channel.

又歷足外踝上四寸，輔骨前，絕骨端三分，去本經在足丘墟穴上七寸，本經之陽輔穴，乃本經所行爲經火，

It continues to Yáng Fǔ (GB-38), which is 4 cùn above the outer ankle [bone], in front of the assisting bone, 3 fēn from the tip of the severed bone, and 7 cùn above Qiū Xū (GB-40) of this channel; the channel flows here as the river and fire point.

又歷足外踝上三寸，動脈中之尋摸骨尖之懸鍾穴，爲足三陽之大絡，按之陽明脈絕，乃取之。

It continues to Xuán Zhōng (GB-39), which is 3 cùn above the outer ankle [bone], on the pulsating vessel, and at the tip of the bone; it is the great network point of the three yáng; by pressing it (GB-39), the yángmíng pulse[230] ceases, that is how to locate it.

遂下行至足，過足外踝下從前陷中，骨縫中，去本經臨泣穴三寸之丘墟穴，爲本經所過爲原，

Thereupon, it descends to arrive at the foot and traverses to Qiū Xū (GB-40), which is in the depression below and in front of the outer ankle [bone], within the bone cleft, and 3 cùn from [Zú] Lín Qì (GB-41) of this channel; the channel traverses here as the source point.

又前行至足小指次指本節後陷中，去本經俠谿穴一寸五分之臨泣穴，爲本經所注爲腧木，又前行過足小指次指本節後一寸，本經之地五會穴，

It continues forwards to arrive at [Zú] Lín Qì (GB-41), which is in the depression behind the base joint of the fourth toe, and 1 cùn 5 fēn from Xiá Xī (GB-43) of this channel; the channel pours here as the stream and wood point. It continues forwards to Dì Wǔ Huì (GB-42) of this channel, which is in the depression 1 cùn behind the base joint of the fourth toe.

又前行足小指次指歧骨間，本節前陷中之俠谿穴，本經所溜爲榮水，乃至足小指次指外側之爪甲如韭葉之竅陰穴，爲本經所出爲井金，而足少陽膽經四十三穴者，至此而終；

It continues forwards to Xiá Xī (GB-43), which is in the depression in front of the base joint, in the space where the little toe and fourth toe diverge; the channel gushes here as the brook and water point. It arrives at [Zú] Qiào Yīn (GB-44), which is located on the outer side of the fourth toe, at one chive leaf's width from the nail corner; the channel emerges here as the well and metal point. The foot shàoyáng gallbladder channel has forty-three points [prior] to arriving at this point, where it terminates.

其支別者，又自足跗面臨泣，別行入足大指，循歧骨出大指，還貫入爪甲，出三毛，以交於足厥陰肝經也。

From [Zú] Lín Qì (GB-41) on the instep of the foot, a branch diverges to enter the big toe, follows where the bones diverge to enter the big toe, where it turns to pierce the nail, re-emerging at the [region of] the three hairs, where it intersects with the foot juéyīn liver channel.

---

[230] I.e., the stomach pulse at ST-42.

Diseases of the Foot Shàoyáng Gallbladder Channel

足少陽膽經病

是動病則爲口苦，以膽汁味苦也。爲善太息，以膽氣不舒也。爲心脇痛不能轉側，以脈循脇裏，出氣街也。甚則面有微塵，體無膏澤，以脈所歷處，少陽氣鬱所爲病。足外反熱，以脈循髀陽，出膝外廉，下外輔骨，抵絕骨，下外踝也，是膽屬少陽，而陽氣上厥使然也。

When there are changes resulting in disease, there will be bitter taste in the mouth, which is because the gallbladder's discharge has a bitter flavour. For frequent sighing, this is because the qì of the gallbladder is constrained. For rib-side pain with inability to turn to the side, this is because the vessel follows the interior of the rib-sides and emerges at Qì Jiē (ST-30). When it is severe, there will be a slightly dusty facial complexion and the lack of oily lustre on the body, this is because when the shàoyáng qì is depressed, it will result in these diseases in the locations where the vessel travels through.

For heat on the outside of the feet, this is because the vessel follows the yáng of the thigh,[231] emerges on the outer ridge of the knee, descends on the outside of the assisting bone to arrive at the severed bone,[232] and descends the outer ankle [bone]; as these [areas] belong to the shàoyáng, this [disease] manifests because of the upwards reversal of the yáng qì.

所生病爲頭痛，以本經行於頭之側也。爲頷腫，以脈循頰車也。爲目銳眥痛，以脈起於目銳眥也。爲缺盆中腫痛，以脈入缺盆，支合缺盆也。爲腋下腫，以脈從缺盆下腋過脇也。爲馬刀俠癭，以頭項腋脇，皆脈所過也。爲汗出，以少陽有火也。

For disease itself engenders, there is headache, which is because the channel travels around the side of the head. There is swelling under the chin, this is because the vessel follows the cheek carriage.[233] For pain of the outer canthus, this is because the vessel commences at the outer canthus. For swelling and pain in Quē Pén (ST-12), this is because the vessel enters at Quē Pén (ST-12), and the branches unite at Quē Pén (ST-12).

For swelling in the armpit, this is because the vessel descends from Quē Pén (ST-12) to the armpit and traverses the rib-side. For sabre and pearl-string lumps,[234] this is because the head, nape, armpit, and rib-side are all places

---

[231] I.e., the outer face of the thigh.
[232] Note: Severed bone is another name for GB-39.
[233] I.e., the joint of the lower jaw, also the name of ST-6.
[234] I.e., scrofula.

where the vessel traverses. For sweating, this is because of the presence of fire in the shàoyáng.

爲振寒瘧，以少陽爲一陽，巨陽之裏，內有三陰，乃爲半表半裏，故爲振寒瘧。爲胸、脇、肋、髀、膝外至脛絕骨皆痛，爲足四指不用。如邪氣盛則疾去其鍼以泄之，如正氣虛則久留其鍼以補之，脈陷下則用艾以灸之。

For shivering due to cold malaria, this is because the shàoyáng is the one yáng[235] and it is the interior of the great yáng;[236] as the three yīn[237] are interior to it, [the shàoyáng] is half-interior and half-exterior, thus there is shivering with cold malaria, pain in the chest, rib-side, side of the chest, thigh, outside of the knee, and the severed bone on the lower leg, as well as inability to move the four digits on the foot.

If the evil qì is exuberant, the needle should be swiftly removed in order to drain it; if the upright qì is vacuous, the needle should be retained for a period of time in order to supplement it; when the vessel is sunken, mount the moxa cone to [warm it].

如人迎之脈大於寸口一倍，則本經爲實，當泄膽經而補肝經。如人迎之脈小於寸口一倍，則本經爲虛，當補膽經而泄肝經。如不實不虛，則直取本經，而不必求之肝經也。

When the rényíng pulse in comparison to the cùnkǒu pulse is one times larger, the principal channel is replete, one ought to drain the gallbladder channel and supplement the liver channel. When the rényíng pulse in comparison to the cùnkǒu pulse is one times smaller, the principal channel is vacuous, one ought to supplement the gallbladder channel and drain the liver channel. When [the principal channel] is neither replete nor vacuous, choose the principal channel, and there is no need to choose the liver channel.

Meeting and Diverging Points
與別經會穴

在頭瞳子髎穴，與手太陽小腸經、手少陽三焦經會。客主人穴，與手少陽三焦經、足陽明胃經會。頷厭穴，與手少陽三焦經、足陽明經會。懸顱穴，與手少陽三焦經、足陽明經會。懸釐穴，與手少陽三焦經、足陽明經會。

---

[235] Note: according to *Sùwèn* Chapter 79, "one yáng" refers to the shàoyáng.
[236] I.e., the tàiyáng according to *Sùwèn* Chapter 31.
[237] I.e., the tàiyīn, shàoyīn, and juéyīn.

On the head: Tóng Zi Liáo (GB-1) meets with the hand tàiyáng small intestine channel and hand shàoyáng sānjiāo channel. Kè Zhǔ Rén (GB-3) meets with the hand shàoyáng sānjiāo channel and foot yángmíng stomach channel.

Hàn Yàn (GB-4) meets with the hand shàoyáng sānjiāo channel and foot yángmíng channel. Xuán Lú (GB-5) meets with hand shàoyáng sānjiāo channel and foot yángmíng channel. Xuán Lí (GB-6) meets with the hand shàoyáng sānjiāo channel and foot yángmíng channel.

曲鬢穴，與足太陽膀胱經會。天衝穴，與足太陽膀胱經會。浮白穴，與足太陽膀胱經會。竅陰穴，與足太陽膀胱經、手少陽三焦經會。完骨穴，與足太陽膀胱經會。

Qū Bìn (GB-7) meets with the foot tàiyáng bladder channel. Tiān Chōng (GB-9) meets with the foot tàiyáng bladder channel. Fú Bái (GB-10) meets with the foot tàiyáng bladder channel. [Tóu] Qiào Yīn (GB-11) meets with the foot tàiyáng bladder channel and hand shàoyáng sānjiāo channel. Wán Gǔ (GB-12) meets with the foot tàiyáng bladder channel.

本神穴，與奇經陽維會。陽白穴，與奇經陽維、手、足陽明大腸胃經會。臨泣穴，與足太陽膀胱、陽　維會。目窗、正營、風池，三穴皆與陽維會。以上在頭本經與別經相會之穴，共十七穴。

Běn Shén (GB-13) meets with the extraordinary channel yángwéi [vessel]. Yáng Bái (GB-14) meets with the extraordinary channel yángwéi [vessel], the hand and foot yángmíng large intestine and stomach channels. [Tóu] Lín Qì (GB-15) meets with the tàiyáng bladder [channel] and yángwéi [vessel]. The three points, Mù Chuāng (GB-16), Zhèng Yíng (GB-17), and Fēng Chí (GB-20), all meet with the yángwéi [vessel]. The above are points of this channel located on the head that meet with other channels, in total, there are seventeen points.

在肩胸腋腹：肩井穴，與手少陽三焦經、足陽明胃經、奇經陽維會。輒筋穴爲膽募，與足太陽會。日月穴，與足太陰脾經、奇經陽維會。帶脈、五樞、維道三穴，皆奇經帶脈會。居髎穴，與奇經陽蹻會。以上肩胸腋腹與別經相會之穴，共七穴。

On the shoulder, chest, armpit, and abdomen: Jiān Jǐng (GB-21) meets with the hand shàoyáng sānjiāo channel, foot yángmíng stomach channel, and the extraordinary channel yángwéi [vessel]. Zhé Jīn (GB-23) is the gallbladder collecting point, it meets with the foot tàiyáng [channel]. Rì Yuè (GB-24) meets with the foot tàiyīn spleen channel and the extraordinary channel yángwéi [vessel]. These three points, Dài Mài (GB-26), Wǔ Shū (GB-27), and Wéi Dào (GB-28), all meet with the extraordinary channel dài vessel. Jū Liáo (GB-29) meets with the extraordinary channel yángqiáo [vessel]. The above are points on the shoulder, chest, armpit, and abdomen that meet with other channels, in total, there are seven points.

在股：環跳穴，與足太陽膀胱經會。中瀆穴，爲本經上別厥陰。以上膝上、股中與別經相會之穴，共二穴。在膝下：陽交穴，與陽維會。光明穴，爲本經下別絡走厥陰。懸鍾穴，爲足三陽之大絡。以上膝下與別經相會之處，共三穴。

On the thigh: Huán Tiào (GB-30) meets with the foot tàiyáng bladder channel. Zhōng Dú (GB-32) is the upper [network-vessel] of this channel that diverges to the juéyīn [channel]. The above are points on the thigh that meet with other channels, in total, there are two points.

Below the knee: Yáng Jiāo (GB-35) meets with the yángwéi [vessel]. Guāng Míng (GB-37) is the lower network-vessel of this channel that diverges to the foot juéyīn [channel]. Xuán Zhōng (GB-39) is the great network point of the three yáng. The above are locations below the knee that meet other channels, in total, there are three points.

足少陽在身之側，足太陽在其後，足陽明在其前，前聯陽明，後聯太陽，中交陽蹻、陽維，所以此經與手足各經所會之穴獨多。共穴四十四，與各經會者二十九穴焉。

While the foot shàoyáng is located on the side of the body, the foot tàiyáng is located on the behind [of the body], and the foot yángmíng is located on the front [of the body]; in front, [the foot shàoyáng] joins with the yángmíng [channel]; behind, it joins with the tàiyáng [channel]; in the middle, it intersects with the yángqiāo and yángwéi [vessels]; therefore, this channel alone has a considerable number of points that meet with other channels of the hand and foot. Of all forty-four points [of this channel], twenty-nine points meet with other channels.

The Sinew Channel of the Foot Shàoyáng
足少陽經筋

足少陽之筋，起於足小指之次指，即第四指之竅陰穴，由俠谿、地五會、臨泣，結於外踝之丘墟，上循脛外廉懸鍾、陽輔、光明、外丘、陽交，結於膝外廉之陽陵泉穴；

The sinew [channel] of the foot shàoyáng commences at the toe next to the little toe, which is namely [Zú] Qiào Yīn (GB-44) on the fourth toe; by way of Xiá Xī (GB-43), Dì Wǔ Huì (GB-42), and [Zú] Lín Qì (GB-41), it knots at Qiū Xū (GB-40) on the outer ankle. It ascends following Xuán Zhōng (GB-39), Yáng Fǔ (GB-38), Guāng Míng (GB-37), Wài Qiū (GB-36), and Yáng Jiāo (GB-35) on the outer ridge of the lower leg, and knots at Yáng Líng Quán (GB-34) on the outside ridge of the knee.

其支者，別起外輔骨，上走於髀，其在前，則結於陽明胃經伏兔之上，其在後，則結於督脈之尻尾上；

A branch diverges from the outer assisting bone,[238] and ascends to the thigh; in the front, it knots above Fú Tù (ST-32) of the foot yángmíng channel; in the rear, it knots above the tail of the coccyx on the dū vessel.

其直者，上乘眇之季脇，上走於腋之前廉，系於膺乳間，上結於缺盆；又其直者，上出於腋，貫於缺盆，出太陽之前，循耳後，上額角，交巔上，下走於頷，上結於頄；又其支者，結於目眥為外維。

The vertical [pathway] ascends over the flank through the floating rib, ascends to go to the front ridge of the armpit, connects with the space between the breasts, and ascends to knot at Quē Pén (ST-12).

Another vertical [pathway] ascends and emerges from the axilla, pierces Quē Pén (ST-12), emerges in front of tàiyáng, follows the behind the ear, ascends the frontal angle, intersects at the vertex, descends to the chin, and ascends to knot at the cheekbone.

Another branch knots at the canthus of the eye as the outer link.[239]

診尺篇謂目痛，赤脈從外走內者少陽病。及其為病，則小指之次指當為轉筋，引於膝外轉筋，其膝不可屈伸，其膕中之筋甚急，前引於髀，後引於尻，即上乘眇之季脇而痛，上引缺盆、膺乳、頸維之筋皆急。

"Chapter on Diagnosing the Cubit"[240] states, "For eye pain... with red vessels that begin from the outside and move interiorly, this is a shàoyáng disease."[241]

When [the sinew channel] is diseased, there will be cramping of the toe next to the little toe, which extends to cramping on the outside of the knee, with inability to bend and extend the knee; the sinews behind the knee will be

---

238 I.e., the fibula.

239 Regarding "link outside," according to the Tàisù, "太陽為目上綱，陽明為目下綱　少陽為目外維。 The tàiyáng is the net above the eye, the yángmíng is the net below the eye, and the shàoyáng is the outer link." In addition, Zhāng Jǐngyuè further notes in the Lèijīng that "凡人能左右盼視者，正以此筋為之伸縮也。 Whenever people can look left and right, it is precisely because of the extension and contraction of this sinew."

240 The cubit (chǐ) here indicates the pulse felt at the elbow at LU-5 (hence, it is named "Cubit Marsh"), which is an ancient method of diagnosis recorded in some chapters of the Nèijīng. Later, this position was redefined to become the proximal wrist pulse.

241 Língshū Chapter 74. Note: the full title of this chapter is "論疾診尺 Discussion of Disease by Diagnosing the Cubit."

extremely tense, extending to the thigh in the front and extending to the coccyx behind; at the floating rib exactly where [the sinew channel] ascends over, it will be painful, which will radiate upwards to Quē Pén (ST-12), the breasts, and the linking sinews of the neck; all of which will be tense.

從左以之於右，其右目必不開，上過右角，並蹻脈而行，左絡於右，故傷左角，其右足不能舉用，爲左所傷，命曰維筋相交。

When [there is a disease in] the left, it will impact the right; as such, one will not be able to open the right eye. [The sinew channel] ascends over the right temple and travels together with the [yáng] qiāo vessel, thus, the left [pathway] networks with the right; therefore, when there is a damage to the left temple, one will not be able to raise the right foot, this is because of damage on the left side; that is namely the decree, "the linking sinews intersect with each other."[242]

First Point of the Gallbladder Channel
Tóng Zi Liáo – Pupil Bone-Hole (GB-1)
膽經第一穴瞳子髎

一名太陽
Alternate name: Tài Yáng

一名前關
Alternate name: Front Pass[243]

穴在目去外眥五分，手太陽小腸經、手少陽三焦經，與本經相會之處。《素》注：灸三壯，鍼三分。

This point is located 5 fēn from the outer canthus. It is the location where this channel meets with the hand tàiyáng small intestine channel and the hand shàoyáng sānjiāo channel. *The Sùzhù* states, "Moxa 3 cones, and needle 3 fēn."

　　注：穴名瞳子髎者，以穴在目銳眥後五分，此穴之內與瞳人相近，故曰瞳子髎。乃手太陽小腸經之支行者，從缺盆循頭之天窗、天容，上頰抵顴髎，上至目銳眥，過瞳子髎者，與本經相會之處。又爲手少陽三焦之又支者，從耳後翳風穴，入耳中過聽宮，歷耳門禾髎，却出至目銳眥瞳子髎，與本經相會之處。本經足少陽原有相火，而手太陽亦爲火經，手三焦亦爲火經，此一穴乃三火聚會之所也。

---

242 From *Língshū* Chapter 10.
243 *Grasping the Wind* names it "Foregate."

Explanation: regarding this point name Tóng Zi Liáo (Pupil Bone-Hole), it is located 5 fēn behind the outer canthus, in addition, the inside of this point is close to the pupil, thus it is called Tóng Zi Liáo (Pupil Bone-Hole). Indeed, from Quē Pén (ST-12), a branch of the hand tàiyáng small intestine channel follows Tiān Chuāng (SI-16) and Tiān Róng (SI-17) on the head, ascends to Quán Liáo (SI-18) on the cheek, ascends to arrive at the outer canthus, traversing Tóng Zi Liáo (GB-1), which is where it meets with the [gallbladder] channel.

Furthermore, regarding another branch of the hand shàoyáng sānjiāo, from Yì Fēng (SJ-17) behind the ear, it enters the ear and traverses Tīng Gōng (SI-19), passing through Ěr Mén (SJ-21) and Hé Liáo (SJ-22),[244] and then re-emerges at Tóng Zi Liáo (Pupil Bone-Hole) at the outer canthus, which is where it meets with the principal [gallbladder] channel. By nature, this channel inherently possesses the ministerial fire,[245] in addition, the hand tàiyáng is a fire channel, and the hand sānjiāo is also a fire channel; thus, this one point is the place where these three entities of fire converge.

瞳子髎之肝病：目癢，翳膜白，青盲無見，遠視昏昏，赤痛淚出，多眵矄，內眥癢，頭痛，喉閉。

Liver diseases of Tóng Zi Liáo: itchy eyes, white membranous eye screens, clear-eye blindness[246] with inability to see, seeing dimly afar, redness and pain [of the eye] with tearing, copious discharge of the eye, itchy inner canthus, headache, and throat impediment.

注：本穴既爲三火聚會之地，而近於目，故目病宜泄此穴，以散三經之火。少陽頭痛，多在頭之側，泄三焦之火，而偏頭痛自息。喉閉亦膽經病也，亦宜泄此火穴。

Explanation: not only is this point where the three entities of fire converge, but it is also nearby the eye; thus, for eye disease, it is appropriate to drain this point in order to disperse the fire of the three channels. Regarding the shàoyáng headache, it is predominantly located on the side of the head, drain the fire of the sānjiāo and the hemilateral headache will cease naturally. Throat impediment is also a gallbladder channel disease, it is appropriate to drain this fire point.

---

[244] Hé Liáo 禾髎 is the name of LI-19, however, it does not align with the pathway described in this context. Meanwhile, Hé Liáo 和髎 (SJ-22, Harmony Bone-Hole) is a homophone with Hé Liáo 禾髎 (LI-19, Grain Bone-Hole); in addition, Hé Liáo 禾髎 is also an alternate name for SJ-22. Therefore, we interpret this point to be SJ-22 instead of LI-19.

[245] I.e., based on the study of five movements and six qì, shàoyáng governs the ministerial fire.

[246] According to the *Practical Dictionary*, clear-eye blindness may be associated with optic atrophy.

Second Point of the Gallbladder Channel
Tīng Huì – Hearing Convergence[247] (GB-2)
膽經第二穴聽會

一名後關

Alternate name: Rear Pass[248]

一名聽河

Alternate name: Hearing River[249]

穴在耳微前陷中，上關穴下一寸，動脈宛宛中，張口得之。《銅人》：鍼三分，留三呼，得氣即泄，不須補。日灸五壯，止三七壯，十日後依前數灸。《明堂》：鍼三分，灸三壯。

This point is located in the depression slightly in front of the ear, 1 cùn below Shàng Guān (GB-3), in the depression of the pulsating vessel, which is located by opening the mouth. *The Tóngrén* states, "Needle 3 fēn,[250] and retain for 3 respirations; obtain qì then promptly drain, one does not need to supplement it. Moxa 5 cones daily, stopping at 21 cones;[251] after 10 days, repeat the aforementioned number[252] of moxa [cones]." *The Míngtáng* states, "Needle 3 fēn, and moxa 3 cones."

注：穴名聽會者，以此穴專主乎聽事，故曰聽會。

Explanation: regarding this point name Tīng Huì (Hearing Convergence), it is because this point specifically governs matters regarding Tīng (Hearing), thus it is called Tīng Huì (Hearing Convergence).

聽會之腎病：耳鳴耳聾。

Kidney disease of Tīng Huì: tinnitus with deafness.

注：耳雖為腎竅，而其部分乃在足少陽之處，少陽之火炎於上，而耳為之鳴，久則聾矣，故宜泄此穴之火。

---

[247] *Grasping the Wind* names it "Auditory Convergence."

[248] *Grasping the Wind* names it "Hind Gate."

[249] *Grasping the Wind* list another alternate name as "聽呵 Hearing Laughter." Note: In extant acupuncture literature, the alternate name of this point is listed as either 聽訶 (Hearing Scolds) or 聽河 (Hearing River); in our brief research, we have not been able to locate the source of the name listed in *Grasping the Wind*.

[250] For "3 fēn," *the Tóngrén* actually says "7 fēn."

[251] For "21 cones," *the Tóngrén* actually states "14 cones."

[252] I.e., start again with 5 cones daily, and slowly increasing up to 21 cones.

Explanation: although the ear is the orifice of the kidneys, yet, this area is surely the location of the foot shàoyáng; when the fire of shàoyáng blazes above, the ears will have ringing;[253] if it remains for an extended period of time, there will be deafness, thus it is appropriate to drain the fire of this point.

聽會之胃病：牙車臼脱，相離一二寸，牙車急不嚼物，齒痛惡寒。

Stomach diseases of Tīng Huì: dislocation of the jaw separated by 1 or 2 cùn,[254] tension of the jaw with inability to chew food, and toothache with aversion to cold.

注：前症雖爲胃經病，而部分在內鉤結之所，正此穴也，宜取此穴。齒痛惡寒，乃中風寒之邪也，宜灸此穴。

Explanation: although the above signs are stomach channel diseases, yet the area is the place where [the branch of this channel] curves and knots on the inside [of the mouth],[255] which is exactly where this point is located; thus, it is appropriate to choose this point. Toothache with aversion to cold is due to evil strike by wind and cold, it is appropriate to moxa this point.

聽會之肝病：狂走瘈瘲，恍惚不樂，中風口喎，手足不隨。

Liver diseases of Tīng Huì: manic walking with tugging and slackening, abstraction with unhappiness, wind stroke with deviated mouth, and paralysis of the hands and feet.

注：前症皆肝火同膽火上炎之極，宜先用鍼泄其火，而後灸以去風。

Explanation: all of the above signs are due to the extreme upwards blazing by the combination of liver fire and gallbladder fire, it is appropriate to utilise needling to drain the fire, and subsequently moxa to eliminate the wind.

---

253 Tinnitus is a conjunction of ears and ringing in Chinese.

254 For "1 or 2 cùn," it was originally "3 cùn" in the primary manuscript. The editors of this manuscript, Zhāng and Zhà, have amended it in accordance with *the Tóngrén*.

255 This likely refers to the branch that extends from GB-1 to, ST-5, SI-18, and then ST-6.

Third Point of the Gallbladder Channel
Kè Zhǔ Rén – Guest and Host-Person[256] (GB-3)
膽經第三穴客主人

一名上關

Alternate name: Upper Pass[257]

穴在耳前骨上，開口有空，動脈宛宛中，張口取之，手、足少陽、陽明之會。
《銅人》：灸七壯，禁鍼。《明堂》：鍼一分，得氣即泄，日灸七壯至二百壯。
《下經》：灸十壯。《素》注：鍼三分，留七呼，灸三壯。《素問》：禁刺深，
深則交脈破爲內漏耳聾，欠而不得欱。一曰：刺上關不得深，下關不得久。

**This point is located above the bone in front of the ear, where a hollow
appears upon opening the mouth, in the depression of the pulsating vessel,
which is located by opening the mouth. It is the meeting of the hand and foot
shàoyáng and yángmíng [channels]. *The Tóngrén* states, "Moxa 7 cones, and
needling is contraindicated."[258] *The Míngtáng* states, "Needle 1 fēn, obtain qì
and then promptly drain, and moxa 7 to 200 cones daily."**

***The Xiàjīng* states, "Moxa 10 cones." *The Sùzhù* states, "Needle 3 fēn, retain for
7 respirations, and moxa 3 cones." *The Sùwèn*[259] states, "Deep needling is
contraindicated, if it is needled deeply, it will break the intersecting network
vessels; as a result, there will be leaking in the interior[260] and deafness; in
addition, when one attempts to yawn, one will not be able to open the mouth
widely." One source states, "Do not pierce Shàng Guān (GB-3) deeply, and do
not retain the [needle in] Xià Guān (ST-7) for a long period."**

注：穴名客主人者，手少陽爲火，而生胃土，足少陽爲木，而尅胃土。土
木有相尅之理，而胃經自下而上會十一穴，有客與主人之義，故曰客主人。

Explanation: regarding the point name Kè Zhǔ Rén (Guest and Host-Person),
as the hand shàoyáng is fire, it engenders stomach-earth; as the foot shàoyáng is
wood, it restrains stomach-earth. There exists the natural order where earth and
wood restrain each other; still, the stomach channel ascends from the below to meet

---

[256] *Grasping the Wind* names it "Guest-Host-Person."

[257] *Grasping the Wind* names it "Upper Gate."

[258] For "needling is contraindicated," *the Tóngrén* actually states "禁不可鍼深 deep needling
is contraindicated."

[259] While the text states this quote comes from *the Sùwèn*, the statement appears to be
loosely based on the commentary from Chapter 52 of *the Sùzhù*.

[260] I.e., internal bleeding.

with the eleven points,[261] which depicts the concept of a Kè (Guest) and Zhǔ Rén (Host-Person),[262] thus it is called Kè Zhǔ Rén (Guest and Host-Person).

手陽明之會於此穴也，乃自左右相交於承漿之後，却循頤後下廉，出人迎，循頰車而上耳前，歷下關過客主人穴，而與本經相會也。

For the hand yángmíng [channel] to meet at this point, after the intersection of the left and right [pathways] at Chéng Jiāng (REN-24), it returns to follow the lower ridge behind the lower cheek, emerges at Rén Yíng (ST-9), following Jiá Chē (ST-6), ascends to the front of the ear, passing through Xià Guān (ST-7) and traversing Kè Zhǔ Rén (Guest Host-Person), where [the hand yángmíng] meets with this channel.

手少陽會於此穴也，乃其支者，從耳後翳風穴入耳中，過聽宮，歷耳門、禾髎，却至目外眥瞳子髎處，而客主人穴，在瞳子髎下之旁，手少陽之脈至瞳子髎者，必過客主人，而與本經合也。

For the hand shàoyáng [channel] to meet at this point, from Yì Fēng (SJ-17) behind the ear, a branch enters into the ear, traverses Tīng Gōng (SI-19), passes through Ěr Mén (SJ-21) and Hé Liáo (SJ-22), returns to arrive at the location of Tóng Zi Liáo (GB-1) at the outer canthus; however, as Kè Zhǔ Rén (Guest Host-Person) is located below and to the side of Tóng Zi Liáo (GB-1), when the vessel of the hand shàoyáng arrives at Tóng Zi Liáo (GB-1), it must have traversed Kè Zhǔ Rén (Guest Host-Person), and that is where [the hand shàoyáng channel] meets with this channel.

客主人之肝病：青盲，瞋目眩眩，瘈瘲沫出，寒熱，痙引骨痛。

---

[261] This line can be interpreted and translated alternatively as "from the below to the above, the stomach channel meets at eleven points [of the gallbladder channel]." As of this moment, we do not know what these "eleven points" are referring to, whether they indicate an array of eleven gallbladder head points as the primary translation, or all the points where the stomach channels meet with the gallbladder channels as the secondary translation. The stomach channel has 8 points on the head while the gallbladder channel has 20 points on head; furthermore, according to Yuè Hánzhēn, the stomach channel has 8 meeting points with the gallbladder channel, while the gallbladder channel has 7 meeting points with the stomach channels; thus, the math does not add up in any case. We have truly stumbled on this riddle, as the Chinese saying goes, we shall need the guidance from brilliant and worthy ones in the future.

[262] From our speculation, the meaning implied by "earth and wood restraining each other" is that earth and wood maintain an uneasy balance between the two of them, as they will always be separated and never engender or transform into each other (which engendering cycle would do). Thus, for this point name, the host indicates the gallbladder wood, whereas the guest indicates the stomach earth; in addition, it describes stomach channel intersections with the gallbladder channel, despite their uneasy relationship in terms of the five phases.

Liver diseases of Kè Zhǔ Rén: clear-eye blindness, squinting the eyes with blurred vision, tugging and slackening with ejection of foam, chills and fever, tetany with pain that radiates into the bones.

注：前症取此穴，乃泄木之旺也。木旺生火，火旺生風，故取此穴，以泄其風。

Explanation: for the above signs, choose this point to drain the effulgence of wood. When wood is effulgent, it will engender fire; when fire is effulgent it will engender wind, thus choose this point in order to drain the wind.

客主人之腎病：耳鳴耳聾。

Kidney disease of Kè Zhǔ Rén: tinnitus and deafness.

注：前症取此穴，乃泄少陽之火也。以手少陽三焦經自耳中出，故取此穴，以泄耳中之火。

Explanation: for the above signs, choose this point to drain the fire of shàoyáng. Because the hand shàoyáng sānjiāo channel emerges from within the ear, thus choose this point in order to drain the fire within the ear.

客主人之胃病：唇吻口強上，口眼偏邪，惡風寒，牙齒齲，口噤，嚼物鳴痛。

Stomach diseases of Kè Zhǔ Rén: stiffness of the lips and mouth, deviation of the mouth and eyes due to evil, aversion to wind and cold, tooth decay, clenched jaw, pain and sounds [in the temporomandibular joint] while chewing things.

注：前症皆胃經病，以足陽明自下來，而會本經於此穴，故灸此穴，以去胃經之風。

Explanation: all of the above signs are stomach channel diseases, this is because the stomach channel comes here from below and meets with this channel at this point, thus moxa this point in order to eliminate the wind in the stomach channel.

Fourth Point of the Gallbladder Channel
Hàn Yàn – Submandibular Fullness[263] (GB-4)
膽經第四穴頷厭

穴在曲周下，顳顬上廉，手、足少陽、陽明之會。《銅人》：灸三壯，鍼七分，留七呼，深刺令人耳聾。

This point is located below the curved periphery,[264] on the upper ridge of the temple region. It is the meeting of the hand and foot shàoyáng, and yángmíng [channels]. *The Tóngrén* **states, "Moxa 3 cones, needle 7 fēn, and retain for 7 respirations; piercing deeply will cause deafness."**

注：此穴有載曲角之下，腦空之上者，《大成》載曲周下。按曲周，《內經》載乃胃煩車之別名。以其穴在耳下曲煩端，動脈環繞一周，故曰曲周。今頷厭穴在額角之端，按之口動，則此穴亦動，乃下與頷相關之所，故曰頷厭。而曰曲周下廉，則漫不相干矣，當以曲角爲正。曲角者，乃額之側頭面盡，有角者是也。

Explanation: it is recorded that this point is below the angle of the temple and above Nǎo Kōng (GB-19); however, it is recorded in *the Dàchéng* that it is below the curved periphery.

Note by [Master Sīlián]: regarding "curved periphery," it is recorded in *the Nèijīng* as an alternate name for Jiá Chē (ST-6).[265] As this point[266] is located below the ear and at the edge of the jaw corner, where the pulsating vessel encircles [the lower jaw] in its periphery, thus [this structure] is called the curved periphery.

Now, Hàn Yàn (Submandibular Fullness) is located at the edge of the frontal eminence; while pressing [this point], if one moves the mouth, the point will also move; as such, [this point] is a location that is associated with the Hàn (Submandibular Region) below; therefore, it is called Hàn Yàn (Submandibular Fullness).

As for the remark that it is "located on the lower ridge of the curved periphery,"[267] it is a liberal and irrelevant [remark]. One should regard [the point location] at the angle of the temple as the orthodoxy. Regarding the angle of the

---

[263] *Grasping the Wind* names it "Forehead Fullness."

[264] While curved periphery most commonly refers to the temporal hairline, in the later passage, Yuè Hánzhēn seems to interpret it as the lower jaw instead.

[265] This likely refers to this line found in *Língshū* Chapter 26 which states "顧痛，刺足陽明曲周動脈，見血，立已；不已，按人迎於經，立已。For cheek pain, pierce the pulsating vessel at the curved periphery on the foot yángmíng [channel], once blood is discharged, [the pain] will immediately cease; if it does not cease, apply pressure to Rén Yíng (ST-9) and it will then cease."

[266] I.e., ST-6.

[267] I.e., the location description by *the Dàchéng*.

temple, it is located on the side of the forehead and at the edge of complexion, where there is an angle.

手三焦少陽之會於此穴也，乃三焦之支行者，從膻中而上缺盆之外，上項過大椎，循天牖上耳後，經翳風、瘈脈、顱顖，直上出耳上角，至角孫，過懸釐，而與本經會於此穴也。

For the hand sānjiāo shàoyáng [channel] to meet at this point, a branch pathway of the sānjiāo [channel] ascends from Dàn Zhōng (REN-17) to the outside of Quē Pén (ST-12), ascends the nape to traverse Dà Zhuī (DU-14), follows Tiān Yǒu (SJ-16) to ascend behind the ear, and passes through Yì Fēng (SJ-17), Chì Mài (SJ-18), and Lú Xìn (SJ-19);[268] thereupon, it ascends vertically to emerge at the angle [of the forehead] above the ear, arrives at Jiǎo Sūn (SJ-20), traverses Xuán Lí (GB-6), and then meets with this channel at this point.

足陽明經之會本經於此穴也，乃胃經左右相交於承漿之後，却循頤後下廉，出大迎，循頰車，上耳前，歷下關，過客主人，循髮際懸釐、頷厭，絡頭維穴者，而與本經會此穴也。此穴在頭維之外，本神之下，絲竹空之上，稍斜懸釐之上。按：手陽明大腸經，歷考諸經，無上行會頷厭之處。

For the foot yángmíng channel to meet with this channel at this point, after the left and right [pathways] of the stomach channel intersect with each other at Chéng Jiāng (REN-24), it returns to follow the lower ridge of the cheek towards the rear, emerges at Dà Yíng (ST-5), follows Jiá Chē (ST-6), ascends in front of the ear, passes through Xià Guān (ST-7), traverses Kè Zhǔ Rén (GB-3), follows Xuán Lí (GB-6) and Hàn Yàn (Submandibular Fullness) on the hairline, networks with Tóu Wéi (ST-8), and then meets with this channel at this point. This point is located outside of Tóu Wéi (ST-8), below Běn Shén (GB-13), above Sī Zhú Kōng (SJ-23), and slightly obliquely above Xuán Lí (GB-6).

Note by [Master Sīlián]: regarding the hand yángmíng large intestine channel, I have investigated various canons, but I could not find a place where its ascending pathway meets with Hàn Yàn (Submandibular Fullness).

頷厭之腎病：耳鳴。

Kidney disease of Hàn Yàn: tinnitus.

注：耳鳴，少陽經有火也，取此穴以泄少陽之火。

Explanation: tinnitus is due to the presence of fire in the shàoyáng channel, choose this point in order to drain the fire of shàoyáng.

---

[268] This is an alternate name for SJ-19.

頷厭之肝病：目無見，目外眥急，偏頭痛，風眩頭痛，驚癇，手捲手腕痛，歷節風汗出。

Liver diseases of Hàn Yàn: blindness, tension at the outer canthus, hemilateral headache, wind dizziness with headache, fright epilepsy, clenched hands with pain of the hand and wrist, and joint-running wind with sweating.

注：前症皆本經有風，及手少陽三焦有風痰所致，宜泄此穴，以去其風痰。但不宜鍼深，灸過三壯耳。

Explanation: all of the above signs are due to the presence of wind in this channel, as well as the presence of wind and phlegm in the hand shàoyáng sānjiāo [channel], it is appropriate to drain this point in order to eliminate the wind and phlegm. However, it is not appropriate to needle deeply, and moxa should not exceed 3 cones.

頷厭之肺病：好嚏。

Lung disease of Hàn Yàn: sneezing.

注：嚏者，肺受風也，而此穴在額角，亦被風之穴，宜灸之。

Explanation: when there is sneezing, the lung has contracted wind; as this point is located on the frontal angle, it is also a point that is affected by wind, thus it is appropriate to moxa it.

Fifth Point of the Gallbladder Channel
Xuán Lú – Suspended Skull (GB-5)
膽經第五穴懸顱

穴在曲角下，顳顬中廉，手、足少陽、足陽明之會。《銅人》：灸三壯，鍼三分，留七呼。《明堂》：鍼三分。《素》注：鍼七分，留七呼，刺深令人耳無所聞。

This point is located below the angle of the temple, on the middle aspect of the temple. It is the meeting of the hand and foot shàoyáng and foot yángmíng [channels]. *The Tóngrén* states, "Moxa 3 cones, needle 3 fēn, and retain for 7 respirations."[269] *The Míngtáng* states, "Needle 3 fēn."[270] *The Sùzhù* states, "Needle 7 fēn, and retain for 7 respirations; piercing deeply will cause the person to have inability to hear."

---

[269] For "7 respirations," *the Tóngrén* actually states "3 respirations."
[270] For "3 fēn," the secondary manuscript states "2 fēn."

注：穴名懸顱者，以其懸於頭顱之側，故曰懸顱。曲角曲周之辨，已詳於前穴頷厭之下矣。手、足少陽、陽明之會於此穴，亦詳於前穴之下。

Explanation: this point is named Xuán Lú (Suspended Skull), because it is [as if it is] Xuán (Suspended) on the side of the Lú (Skull), thus it is called Xuán Lú (Suspended Skull). As for the distinction between the angle of the forehead and the curved periphery, it has already been discussed thoroughly in the previous point, Hàn Yàn (GB-4). The hand and foot shàoyáng and yángmíng [channels] meet at this point, this has also been discussed extensively in the previous point already.

懸顱之肝病：頭偏痛，引目外眥赤。

Liver diseases of Xuán Lú: hemilateral headache that radiates to the outer canthus with redness [of the eyes].

注：前症乃少陽經之火，宜泄此穴。

Explanation: the above sign is due to the fire of the shàoyáng channel, it is appropriate to drain this point.

懸顱之胃病：頭痛，牙齒痛，面膚赤腫。

Stomach diseases of Xuán Lú: headache, toothache, redness and swelling of the facial skin.

注：前症乃胃經病也，以胃土上會此穴而泄之。

Explanation: the above signs are stomach channel diseases, as stomach earth ascends to meet at this point, thus drain it.

懸顱之肺病：熱病煩滿，汗不出，身熱，鼻淵濁下不止，傳爲衄蔑瞑目。

Lung diseases of Xuán Lú: febrile disease with vexation and fullness, absence of sweating, generalised heat [effusion], and incessant deep-source nasal congestion with turbid discharges, which has become a snivelling [nose] with dull vision and closed eyes.

注：前症皆少陽之火及於肝，肝上於肺，而有是症，故泄此穴。

Explanation: all of the above signs are the fire of shàoyáng affecting the liver, when the liver ascends [to interfere] with the lung, there will be these signs, thus drain this point.

Sixth Point of the Gallbladder Channel
Xuán Lí – Suspended Tuft (GB-6)
膽經第六穴懸釐

穴在曲周上，顳顬下，手、足少陽、陽明之會。《銅人》：鍼三分，灸三壯。
《素》注：鍼三分，留七呼。

**This point is located above the curved periphery, below the temple region. It is
the meeting of the hand and foot shàoyáng and yángmíng [channels].** *The
Tóngrén states, "Needle 3 fēn, and moxa 3 cones." The Sùzhù states, "Needle 3
fēn, and retain for 7 respirations."*

注：此穴按圖及各經，僅在懸顱之上，各經皆未明註分寸陷中動脈等的切
其處，止以曲周、曲角、顳顬、腦空四名上、中、下廉記載，

Explanation: regarding this point, according to the illustrations and various
canons, they only [state] that it is above Xuán Lú (GB-5). None of the canons
explains clearly the fēn and cùn [measurement], depression, or pulsating vessel,
where one can palpate. They only record the four terms of curved periphery, angle
of the forehead, temple, and Nǎo Kōng (GB-19), as well as being in their upper,
middle, or lower aspect.

曲周爲頰車，在耳之下取之，而證此穴，已爲不倫，

Since the "curved periphery" is Jiá Chē (ST-6), this point would be located
below the ear; thus, it is incongruent to identify [the location of] this point with [the
curved periphery].

至若顳顬，既稱腦空，在承靈後一寸五分，玉枕骨下取，而證前之額角之
穴，而又不明言其分寸，

As for the "temple," Nǎo Kōng (GB-19) is located 1 cùn 5 fēn behind Chéng
Líng (GB-18) and below the jade pillow bone. When [this account] seeks to identify
the location of this point with the "frontal angle" in front, why does it not provide a
clear description of its fēn and cùn [measurement]?

且在前此之穴，如本經之本神穴，胃經之頭維，三焦之絲竹空，皆確有的
據可指，而何不取此上下左右之穴，證其分寸，

Furthermore, for the points in front of this [point], such as Běn Shén (GB-13)
of this channel, Tóu Wéi (ST-8) of the stomach channel, and Sī Zhú Kōng (SJ-23) of
the sānjiāo [channel], all of them have solid basis [for their locations] that can serve
as landmarks; why does it not utilize these points above, below, left, and right to
locate [Xuán Lú (GB-5)]?

而乃以在下之曲周，在上之腦空，皆遠而難考之穴，證其分寸，而混言以上、中、下廉記此穴，則亦少詳矣。

Instead, it utilises the "curved periphery" below and "Nǎo Kōng (GB-19)" above, both of which are points that are far away and unhelpful to locate [this point], or to identify its fēn and cùn [measurement]. In addition, it mixes in remarks of "upper, middle, or lower aspect" to record this point; yet, once again, it is not described clearly.

幸此穴所治之症，皆可以他穴代之，不然者，鍼學湮沒，日漸失傳，無穴可代，將奈何。

It is fortunate that all of the signs treated by this point can be [treated] by other substituted points; or else, the study of needling would be consigned to oblivion, gradually losing its transmission with each passing day, until there is no point left that can serve as a substitute. At that time, what can one do?

所治之病，皆與前穴同，不贅。面皮赤腫，偏頭痛，煩心不欲食，中焦客熱，熱病汗不出，目銳眥赤痛。

[This point] treats the same diseases as the point prior, it is unnecessary to elaborate. Redness and swelling of the facial skin, hemilateral headache, vexation with no desire to eat, lodged heat in the middle jiāo, febrile disease with absence of sweat, and redness with pain at the outer canthus.

Seventh Point of the Gallbladder Channel
Qū Bìn – Temporal Hairline Curve (GB-7)
膽經第七穴曲鬢

一名曲髮
Alternate name: Hair Curve

穴在耳上髮際，曲隅陷中，鼓頷有空，足少陽、太陽之會。《銅人》：鍼三分，灸七壯。《明堂》：灸三壯。

This point is located on the hairline above the ear, in the depression at the curved corner,[271] where a hollow appears while moving one's jaw.[272] It is the meeting of the foot shàoyáng and tàiyáng [channels]. *The Tóngrén* states, "Needle 3 fēn, moxa 7 cones." *The Míngtáng* states, "moxa 3 cones."

---

[271] I.e., temporal hairline.
[272] Alt. trans. clenching one's teeth.

注：此穴雖在二耳際，乃在耳微前，髮際曲隅陷中，以鼓頷有空證之。耳上髮際，鼓頷則不動，耳微前髮際，鼓頷則有動處，穴名曲鬢，則在耳上微前，不在正耳上矣。

Explanation: although this point is located at the border of the ear, in fact, it is slightly in front of the ear, in the depression at the Qū (Curved) corner, on the hairline, where a hollow appears by moving one's jaw, which will confirm [the location]. Whereas the hairline above the ear does not move when one moves the jaw, the hairline slightly in front of the ear moves when one moves the jaw. Regarding the point name Qū Bìn (Temporal Hairline Curve), it is indicating that it is above and slightly in front of the ear, and not located directly above the ear.[273]

曲鬢之肝病：頷頰腫，引牙車不得開，急痛，口噤不能言，頸項不得回顧，腦兩角痛爲癲風，引目眇。

Liver diseases of Qū Bìn: swelling under the chin and on the cheeks that radiates to the jaw, which makes one unable to open [the mouth], acute pain, clenched jaw with inability to speak, [stiffness] of the neck and nape with inability to look behind, and severe pain at the corners of the brain,[274] which results in epileptic wind and leads to blindness.

注：前症乃本經病也，而泄此穴者，以除少陽部分之風。

Explanation: the above signs are diseases of this channel, thus drain this point in order to eliminate the wind in the division of shàoyáng.

---

[273] Note: In Chinese, qū 曲 is often used as an opposite term to 直 (straight) and 正 (direct) in a two-dimensional space; thus, here, it is saying that since this point is not directly above the ear, it is qū 曲 (crooked). As such, according to Yuè Hánzhēn's interpretation, this point should be understood as "crooked temporal hair," as a point that is around the temporal hair but not directly above the ear; however, as the reader may already be aware, this translation would be easily misunderstood, as there is no equivalent spatial concept of "crooked vs. straight/direct" in English (*the closest terms might be "deviate vs. axial," which may sound rather foreign to most readers*); in addition, we would misinterpret that "crooked" as a modifier for the temporal hair, not for the placement of the point, unless we change the name to something akin of "not directly [above the ear] on the temporal hair" or "crooked [placement] on the temporal hair" – which in terms would render this point name excessively wordy. For that reason, we have kept the original name from the *Grasping the Wind* and conveyed the nuances in this footnote.

[274] I.e., head.

Eighth Point of the Gallbladder Channel
Shuài Gǔ – Valley Lead (GB-8)
膽經第八穴率谷

穴在耳上入髮際寸半陷者宛宛中，嚼而取之，足少陽、太陽之會。《銅人》：鍼三分，灸三壯。《神農經》：治頭風，兩角疼痛，可灸三壯至五壯。小兒急慢驚風，灸三壯，炷如小麥。

This point is located above the ear, in the depression 1 cùn and a half into the hairline, which is located by chewing. It is the meeting of the foot shàoyáng and tàiyáng [channels]. *The Tóngrén* **states, "Needle 3 fēn, and moxa 3 cones."** *The Shénnóng Jīng* **states, "To treat head wind and pain at the two angles [of the head], one can moxa 3 to 5 cones; for chronic fright wind in children, moxa 3 cones, with cones the size of a wheat grain."**

注：此穴在曲鬢之上，有躍然上行之勢，故曰率谷。爲足太陽之會者，乃足太陽自通天穴處，有絡下散於耳上，少陽橫部諸穴，所以養筋脈者，前自耳前曲鬢穴，後至耳後完骨穴，橫布六穴，皆太陽橫下散絡養諸筋之處，故六穴皆有太陽與本經相會之文。

Explanation: as this point is located above Qū Bìn (GB-7), it displays a motion of leaping upwards, thus it is called Shuài Gǔ (Valley Lead).

Regarding the meeting of the foot tàiyáng [channel], from the place of Tōng Tiān (BL-7), the foot tàiyáng [channel] has a network-vessel that spreads out downwards to [the area] above the ear and the various points located in the horizontal area of the shàoyáng [channel]; this is what nourishes the sinew-vessels. From Qū Bìn (GB-7) anterior to the ear in the front, to Wán Gǔ (GB-12) posterior to the ear in the rear, six points spread out horizontally,[275] all of which are the places where the tàiyáng spreads out its network-vessel horizontally and downwards to nourish the various sinews; thus, for these six points, all of them have written accounts of where the tàiyáng [channel] and this channel meet with each other.

率谷之本病：腦兩角痛，頭重，醉後皮膚腫。

Principal diseases of Shuài Gǔ: pain at both angles of the brain, heavy-headedness, and swelling of the skin after intoxication.

注：前症乃少陽經頭側所過部分，此穴正在頭側，宜泄此穴，以去其風與火。

Explanation: the above signs [occur] at the area where the shàoyáng channel traverses on the side of the head, as this point is located exactly on the side of the

---

[275] From GB-7 to GB-12.

head, it is appropriate to drain this point in order to eliminate wind and fire of the [shàoyáng].

率谷之胃病：胃寒，飲食煩滿，嘔吐不止，痰氣膈痛。

Stomach diseases of Shuài Gǔ: stomach cold, vexation and fullness [after intake of] food and drink, incessant retching and vomiting, and phlegm qì occlusion with pain.

注：少陽之木旺，故尅胃土，少陽之火衰，而胃亦寒，嘔吐不止，少陽之氣逆上也，酌其寒熱，而施補泄。痰氣膈痛，泄此穴以舒鬱氣。

Explanation: when the wood of shàoyáng is effulgent, it will restrain stomach earth; when the fire of shàoyáng[276] is debilitated, it will lead to stomach cold; for incessant retching and vomiting, this is counterflow ascent of the qì of shàoyáng; for these, one should deliberate on the cold and heat [condition] and apply supplementation and drainage accordingly. For phlegm qì occlusion with pain, drain this point in order to soothe the depressed qì.

Ninth Point of the Gallbladder Channel
Tiān Chōng – Celestial Surge[277] (GB-9)
膽經第九穴天衝

穴在耳後髮際二寸，耳上如前三分，足少陽、太陽之會。《銅人》：灸七壯。《素》注：鍼三分，灸三壯。

This point is located 2 cùn into the hairline, [in line with] the posterior [border of] the ear, and 3 fēn in front of the apex of the ear. It is the meeting of the foot shàoyáng and tàiyáng [channels]. *The Tóngrén* states, "Moxa 7 cones." *The Sùzhù* states, "Needle 3 fēn, and moxa 3 cones."[278]

注：此穴去率谷而又高矣，有衝上之義，故曰天衝。

Explanation: after departing from Shuài Gǔ (GB-8), this point reaches even higher, which has the image of Chōng (Surging) upwards, thus it is named Tiān Chōng (Celestial Surge).

天衝之本病：癲疾，風痙頭痛，善驚恐。

Principal diseases of Tiān Chōng: epileptic disease, wind tetany with headache, and susceptibility to fright and fear.

---

[276] I.e., the ministerial fire.
[277] *Grasping the Wind* names it "Celestial Hub."
[278] For "3 cones," *the Sùzhù* actually states "5 cones."

注：前症皆少陽本經病也，泄此穴以去風火症也。但不宜多灸耳，三壯足矣。

Explanation: all of the above signs are diseases of the shàoyáng principal channel, drain this point in order to eliminate the wind and fire signs. Nevertheless, it is not appropriate to moxa excessively, 3 cones should be sufficient.

天衝之胃病：牙齦腫。

Stomach disease of Tiān Chōng: swollen gums.

注：此雖胃經病，而少陽之火亦能致之，故泄此穴。

Explanation: although this [sign] is a stomach channel disease, the fire of shàoyáng can also cause it, thus drain this point.

Tenth Point of the Gallbladder Channel
Fú Bái – Floating White (GB-10)
膽經第十穴浮白

穴在耳後入髮際一寸，足太陽、少陽之會。《銅人》：鍼三[279]分，灸七壯。《明堂》：灸三壯。

This point is located 1 cùn into the hairline, behind the ear. It is the meeting of the foot tàiyáng and shàoyáng [channels]. *The Tóngrén* states, "Needle 3 fēn, and moxa 7 cones." *The Míngtáng* states, "Moxa 3 cones."

注：此穴在天衝之下，斜曲在後，乃降而不遽降，有浮之象焉，故曰浮白。

Explanation: this point is located below Tiān Chōng (GB-9), in a slope and down the curve to the behind; while it does descend [from the previous point], it does not descend abruptly; thus, it has an image of Fú (floating), therefore it is called Fú Bái (Floating White).

浮白之本病：耳聾耳鳴，嘈嘈無所聞，頸項瘦瘤癰腫，不能言，肩背不舉，發寒熱，喉痺。

Principal diseases of Fú Bái: deafness and tinnitus, tumult [in the ears] with inability to hear, goitre and swollen welling-abscess in the neck and nape, inability to speak, inability to raise the shoulder and upper-back, chills and fever, and throat impediment.

---

[279] For "3 fēn," *the Tóngrén* actually says "5 fēn."

注：前症皆本經正病，以此穴近耳，故耳病取此。瘻瘤皆少陽之鬱，泄此穴以散少陽之鬱。肩背皆少陽部分，故取上穴，以散其鬱。寒熱亦本經病，宜灸此穴，以退其寒熱。喉痺亦少陽之火也，泄上穴以散其火。

Explanation: all of the above signs are precisely the diseases of the principal channel; in addition, as this point is nearby the ear, thus for ear disease, choose this point. All goitres are due to depression of shàoyáng, drain this point in order to disperse the depression in shàoyáng. The shoulder and upper-back are both shàoyáng areas, thus choose this point above in order to disperse the depression.

Chills and fever are also diseases of the principal channel, it is appropriate to moxa this point in order to abate the chills and fever. Throat impediment is also due to the fire of shàoyáng, drain this point above in order to disperse the fire.

浮白之肺病：胸滿不得息，胸痛，咳逆痰沫。

Lung diseases of Fú Bái: fullness in the chest with inability to catch the breath, chest pain, and cough and counterflow with foamy phlegm.

注：前症則爲肺病，而少陽之脈下胸過脇者，有鬱焉致之，故泄此穴，以散之。

Explanation: the above signs are actually lung diseases, as the vessel of the shàoyáng descends to the chest to traverse the rib-sides, when there is depression [in these areas], these [signs] will be the result, thus drain this point in order to disperse it.

Eleventh Point of the Gallbladder Channel
[Tóu] Qiào Yīn – [Head] Yīn Orifice (GB-11)
膽經第十一穴竅陰

一名枕骨
Alternate name: Pillow Bone[280]

穴在完骨上，枕骨下，動搖有空，足太陽、手少陽、足少陽相會之地。《銅人》：鍼三分，灸七壯。《甲乙》：鍼四分，灸五壯。《素》注：鍼三分，灸三壯。

This point is located above the completion bone,[281] below the pillow bone, where a hollow appears while shaking the head. It is the place where the foot

---

[280] According to the *Practical Dictionary*, it is the occipital bone.
[281] According to the *Practical Dictionary*, it is the mastoid process of the temporal bone, and also the name of GB-12.

tàiyáng, hand shàoyáng, and foot shàoyáng [channels] meet with one another. *The Tóngrén* states, "Needle 3 fēn, and moxa 7 cones." *The Jiǎyǐ* states, "Needle 4 fēn, and moxa 5 cones." *The Sùzhù* states, "Needle 3 fēn, and moxa 3 cones."

注：以此穴有空，可按而得，故曰竅，下浮白而在於陰，故曰竅陰。

Explanation: as this point is in a hollow, which can be located by palpating, thus it is called Qiào (Orifice); as it is below Fú Bái (GB-10), therefore it is located in the Yīn (Yīn), thus it is called [Tóu] Qiào Yīn ([Head] Yīn Orifice).

竅陰之本病：目痛，頭項頷痛，引耳嘈嘈無所聞，喉痺口苦，四肢轉筋，手足煩熱，汗不出。

Principal diseases of [Tóu] Qiào Yīn: eye pain, pain of the head, nape, and chin, which causes noisy tumult in the ears with the inability to hear, throat impediment with bitter taste in the mouth, cramping of the four limbs, heat vexation in the hands and feet, and absence of sweating.

注：前症皆少陽本經病，以其近耳，故取此穴，以泄少陽之火。喉痺口苦，四肢轉筋，皆少陽本病，亦宜泄此穴。手足煩熱，此少陽之熱，忌汗下者，宜取此穴以解之。

Explanation: all of the above signs are shàoyáng principal channel diseases, as this [point] is nearby the ear, thus choose this point in order to drain the fire of shàoyáng. For throat impediment with bitter taste in the mouth, cramping of the four limbs, these are both shàoyáng principal diseases, it is appropriate to drain this point. For heat vexation in the hands and feet, this is the heat of shàoyáng, when it is contraindicated to sweat or precipitate, it is appropriate to choose this point in order to resolve it.

竅陰之心病：舌本出血，舌強，脅痛咳逆，癰疽發屬。

Heart diseases of [Tóu] Qiào Yīn: bleeding from the root of the tongue, stiff tongue, pain of the rib-sides with cough and counterflow, and eruption of both welling- and flat abscesses.

注：舌竅乎心，舌本則肝經所歷之處，泄膽火者，泄肝火也。咳逆乃胃病也，舌強，脅痛而咳逆，則少陽有逆上之火矣，故泄此穴，以散上逆之火。癰疽皆心病，而發屬則有風症，泄此穴以去少陽之風。

Explanation: the tongue is the orifice of the heart, yet, the root of the tongue is the place where the liver channel passes through; by draining gallbladder fire, it will also drain liver fire. Cough and counterflow is a stomach disease; however, a stiff tongue with rib-side pain and cough and counterflow, this is counterflow ascent of shàoyáng fire, it is appropriate to drain this point in order to disperse the counterflow ascent of fire.

Both welling- and flat-abscess are heart diseases, when they erupt there will be wind signs, drain this point in order to eliminate the wind of shàoyáng.

Twelfth Point of the Gallbladder Channel
Wán Gǔ – Completion Bone (GB-12)
膽經第十二穴完骨

穴在耳後入髮際四分，足少陽、太陽之會。《銅人》：鍼三分，灸七壯。《素》注：鍼六分，留七呼，灸三壯。《明堂》：鍼二分，灸以年爲壯。

This point is 4 fēn into the hairline, behind the ear. It is the meeting of the foot shàoyáng and tàiyáng [channels]. *The Tóngrén* **states, "Needle 3 fēn,**[282] **and moxa 7 cones."** *The Sùzhù* **states, "Needle 6 fēn,**[283] **retain for 7 respirations, and moxa 3 cones."** *The Míngtáng* **states, "Needle 2 fēn, and moxa the number of cones according to one's age."**

注：耳後高起之骨，爲完骨，入髮際四分，正當此骨之上，故名以誌之。

Explanation: the Gǔ (Bone) that rises up behind the ear is the Wán Gǔ (Completion Bone); as [this point] is 4 fēn into the hairline, it is directly above this Gǔ (Bone), thus its name serves as the landmark.

完骨之本病：足痿失履不收，牙車急，煩腫頭面腫，頸項痛，頭風耳後痛，喉痺。

Principal diseases of Wán Gǔ: wilting of the legs with inability to walk, tension of the tooth carriage, swelling of the cheek with swelling of the head and face, pain of the neck and nape, head wind with pain behind the ear, and throat impediment.

注：前症皆少陽本病，頭側、頸項、耳後皆少陽部分，故取此穴，以泄少陽之風與火。肺經有火，而喉亦爲之痺，故取此穴，以泄膽火。

Explanation: all of the above signs are shàoyáng principal diseases; as the side of the head, neck, nape,[284] and behind the ear are all areas of shàoyáng, thus choose this point in order to drain the wind and fire of shàoyáng. When there is a presence of fire in the lung, it will lead to the throat becoming impeded, thus choose this point in order to drain the gallbladder fire.

完骨之心病：煩心，小便赤黃，癲疾。

---

[282] For "3 fēn," *the Tóngrén* actually states "5 fēn."

[283] For "6 fēn," *the Sùzhù* actually states "3 fēn."

[284] "頸項 neck and nape" is originally "頭項 head and nape" in the manuscript. The editors of this manuscript, Zhāng and Zhà, have amended it according to the previous paragraph.

Heart diseases of Wán Gǔ: vexation of the heart, red and yellow urine, and epileptic disease.

注：前症雖心症，而少陽上行之火亦能助之，故取此穴，以降少陽之火。

Explanation: although the above signs are heart signs, when the fire of shàoyáng ascends, it will exacerbate [the heart fire], thus choose this point in order to descend the fire of shàoyáng.

完骨之胃病：齒齲，口眼喎斜。

Stomach diseases of Wán Gǔ: tooth decay, and deviated eyes and mouth.

注：此雖胃病，而少陽部分多在面側，故取此穴，以泄其風與火。

Explanation: although these are stomach diseases, as the area of shàoyáng is predominantly located on the side of the face, thus choose this point in order to drain the wind and fire.

Thirteenth Point of the Gallbladder Channel
Běn Shén – Root Spirit (GB-13)
膽經第十三穴本神

穴在足太陽經曲差穴旁一寸五分，直耳上，入髮際四分，足少陽、陽維之會。
《銅人》：鍼三分，灸七壯。

This point is located 1 cùn 5 fēn to the side of Qū Chà (BL-4) of the foot tàiyáng channel, directly above the ear, and 4 fēn into the hairline. It is the meeting of the foot shàoyáng [channel] and yángwéi [vessel]. *The Tóngrén states, "Needle 3 fēn, and moxa 7 cones."*

注：惟木有本，此穴乃本經自完骨外折回，上至於額之上，與督之神庭橫直，先取神庭爲中，後旁一寸五分，爲太陽之曲差，又再旁取一寸五分，爲此穴，三穴橫列而稍向後，故曰本神，言膽經之神所在也。其與陽維會也，乃陽維自風池而上行，至於此穴而會之也。

Explanation: only wood is that which has Běn (Roots); regarding this point, this channel returns[285] from outside of Wán Gǔ (GB-12), ascends to arrive at the top

---

[285] "折回 return" is originally "折四 turn, four" in the manuscript. We suspect this to be a typographical error in this manuscript, as it is difficult to comprehend the meaning of the original wording; if any, we could only speculate that it means that this is saying that Wán Gǔ (GB-12) is located at the fourth fold of the gallbladder channel on the head. Nevertheless, it is more possible that "四 four" is a typographical error for "回 return," as the two characters are similar in writing and commonly misrecognized, especially if 回 is written in its variant form 囬.

of the forehead, on a horizontal line with Shén Tíng (DU-24) of the dū [vessel]. First locate Shén Tíng (DU-24) on the midline; next, at 1 cùn 5 fēn to the side, it is Qū Chà (BL-4) of the tàiyáng [channel]; a further 1 cùn 5 fēn from [Qū Chà (BL-4)], it is this point; these three points line up horizontally and move slightly towards the rear, thus [this point] is called Běn Shén (Root Spirit), as this is referring to where the Shén (Spirit) of the gallbladder is located.

Regarding its meeting with the yángwéi [vessel], the yángwéi [vessel] ascends from Fēng Chí (GB-20) and arrives at this point to meet with [the gallbladder channel].

本神之本經病：驚癇吐涎沫，癲癇吐涎沫，偏風頭項強急痛，目眩，胸脇相引不得轉側。

Principal channel diseases of Běn Shén: fright epilepsy with ejection of foamy drool, epilepsy with ejection of foamy drool, hemilateral wind with stiffness and tension and pain of the head and nape, dizzy vision, [pain] that radiates between the chest and rib-sides[286] with inability to turn to the sides.

注：前症皆少陽經風、火、痰三邪所致之症也，俱泄此穴。

Explanation: all of the above signs are caused by the three evils, which are namely wind, fire, or phlegm, in the shàoyáng channel; for all cases, drain this point.

Fourteenth Point of the Gallbladder Channel
Yáng Bái – Shàoyáng White[287] (GB-14)
膽經第十四穴陽白

穴在眉上一寸，直瞳子，手、足陽明、少陽、陽維五脈之會。《素》注：鍼三分。《銅人》：鍼二分，灸三壯。

This point is located 1 cùn above the eyebrow, in line with the pupil. It is the meeting of the five vessels, the hand and foot yángmíng and shàoyáng [channels], as well as the yángwéi [vessel]. *The Sùzhù* states, "Needle 3 fēn." *The Tóngrén* states, "Needle 2 fēn, and moxa 3 cones."

注：陽者，少陽也。此穴上不入髮，下不入眉，乃在眉髮之間，髮眉皆黑，而此在其白處，故曰陽白。

---

286 "脇 Rib-sides" was absent in the manuscript and supplemented in accordance with *the Collated Explanations of the Zhēnjiǔ Dàchéng*.
287 *Grasping the Wind* names it "Yáng White."

Explanation: Yáng (Yáng) is referring to the shàoyáng. To the above, this point does not enter the hairline; to the below, this point does not enter the eyebrow; as such, it is in the space between the eyebrow and the hair[line]. Whereas both the hair and eyebrow are black, this [point] is located at the Bái (White) place, thus it is called Yáng Bái (Shàoyáng White).

陽維之會本經於此穴也，自風池而上行也。胃經之會此穴也，乃自交承漿而後，循頤下廉出大迎，循頰車，上耳前，歷下關，過本經客主人，循髮行本經懸顱、懸釐，經頭維會於督之神庭，而過此穴也。

For the yángwéi [vessel] to meet this channel at this point, it ascends from Fēng Chí (GB-20). For the stomach channel to meet at this point, after intersecting at Chéng Jiāng (REN-24), it follows the lower ridge of the cheek to emerge at Dà Yíng (ST-5), follows Jiá Chē (ST-6) to ascend to in front and above the ear, passes through Xià Guān (ST-7), traverses Kè Zhǔ Rén (GB-3) of this channel, follows Xuán Lú (GB-5) and Xuán Lí (GB-6) of this channel on the hairline, passes Tóu Wéi (ST-8) to meet with Shén Tíng (DU-24) of the dū [vessel], and further traverses to this point.

手陽明無會於此穴者。手少陽之會於此穴也，乃支行者，從膻中而上出缺盆，上過大椎，循天牖上耳後，循翳風、瘈脈、顱顖，直上出耳上角，至角孫，過懸顱、頷厭，乃過陽白者而會於此穴也。

The hand yángmíng does not meet with this point. For the hand shàoyáng to meet at this point, a branch ascends from Dàn Zhōng (REN-17) to emerge from [the outside of] Quē Pén (ST-12), ascends traversing Dà Zhuī (DU-14), follows Tiān Yǒu (SJ-16) to ascend behind the ear, follows Yì Fēng (SJ-17), Chì Mài (SJ-18), and Lú Xìn (SJ-19), ascends vertically to emerge at the corner [of the forehead] above the ear, arrives at Jiǎo Sūn (SJ-20), traverses Xuán Lú (GB-5) and Hàn Yàn (GB-4), thereupon traversing Yáng Bái (GB-14) and meeting with this point.

陽白之本病：瞳子癢痛，目上視，遠視眈眈，昏夜無見，目痛目眵。

Principal diseases of Yáng Bái: pain and itchiness in the pupils, upward gazing eyes, seeing dimly afar, poor vision at twilight and night, and eye pain with discharge.

注：前症皆少陽經本病，此穴緊在目上，故取之以治目病，而泄下行之火。

Explanation: all of the above signs are principal diseases of the shàoyáng channel, this point is located very close to the top of the eye, thus choose it in order to treat eye diseases and drain the descending fire.[288]

陽白之肺病：背膝寒慄，重衣不得溫。

Lung diseases of Yáng Bái: cold in the interstices of the upper back with shivering, and inability to get warm despite [wearing] additional clothing.

注：此肺部受風寒也，以陽維會於此穴，陽維管一身之陽，宜灸此穴，以溫諸陽。

Explanation: these [signs] are due to the contraction of wind and cold in the lung area; as the yángwéi [vessel] meets at this point,[289] and as the yángwéi [vessel] officiates the yáng of the whole body, it is appropriate to moxa this point in order to warm all the yáng.

Fifteenth Point of the Gallbladder Channel
[Tóu] Lín Qì – [Head] Overlooking Tears (GB-15)
膽經第十五穴臨泣

穴在上直入髮際五分陷中，令患人正坐正睛取穴，足太陽、足少陽、陽維之會。《銅人》：鍼三分，留七呼。

This point is located in the depression 5 fēn directly into the hairline; have the patient sitting upright and looking straight in front to locate this point. It is the meeting of the foot tàiyáng and foot shàoyáng [channels], as well as the yángwéi [vessel]. *The Tóngrén* states, "Needle 3 fēn, and retain for 7 respirations."

注：膽經有二臨泣，一在目之上，一在足之上，此爲上臨泣，以此穴正在睛上，故曰臨泣。陽維自後風池前上行，會本經於此穴，太陽自睛明上行者過此穴，故爲三經之會。

---

288 Note: Based on the orientation of the gallbladder channel, in case of eye disease caused by gallbladder fire, the fire would descend from GB-14 to enter the eye.

289 For "此肺部受風寒也，以陽維會於此穴 these [signs] are due to the contraction of wind and cold in the lung area; as the yángwéi [vessel] meets at this point…" the primary manuscript has, "此肺部受風也，寒以陽維會於此穴 these [signs] are due to the contraction of wind in the lung area, after which, the cold [evil] follows the yángwéi [vessel] to reach this point…" The editors of this manuscript, Zhāng and Zhà, have amended it according to the secondary manuscript.

Explanation: the gallbladder channel has two Lín Qì (Overlooking Tears) [points]: one is located above the eye, and the other is located on the foot. This one is the upper Lín Qì (Overlooking Tears), as this point is located directly above the eyeball, thus it is called Lín Qì (Overlooking Tears).

From Fēng Chí (GB-20) in the rear, the yángwéi [vessel] moves to the front and ascends to meet with this channel at this point; from Jīng Míng (BL-1), the ascending pathway of the tàiyáng [channel] traverses this point; thus, it said that [this point] is the meeting of the three channels.

臨泣之本經病：目眩，目生白翳，目淚，大風自目外眥痛，卒中風不識人，驚癇反視，枕骨合顱痛。

Principal channel diseases of [Tóu] Lín Qì: dizzy vision, generation of white eye screens, tearing, great wind with pain at the outer canthus, sudden wind stroke with inability to recognise people, fright epilepsy with the eyes rolled back, and pain at the pillow bone and skull union.[290]

注：前症皆本經正病，穴在目上，故治諸目病。驚癇、中風，皆本經正病，故取此穴，以治風癇之症。枕骨合顱，皆本經之脈回折處，故責此穴。

Explanation: all of the above signs are principal diseases of this channel, as this point is above the eye, thus it treats various eye diseases. For fright epilepsy and wind stroke, both of these are principal diseases of this channel, thus choose this point in order to treat the signs of wind epilepsy. Both the pillow bone and skull union are bends where the vessel of this channel turns around, thus seek this point.

臨泣之肺病：惡寒鼻塞。

Lung disease of [Tóu] Lín Qì: aversion to cold with nasal congestion.

注：前症乃肺受風也，以此穴近鼻之上，亦責之。

Explanation: the above sign is due to the lung contracting wind, as this point is near the top of the nose, one can also seek it.

---

[290] 枕骨 pillow bone and 合顱 skull union are alternate names for GB-11 and DU-17, respectively.

Sixteenth Point of the Gallbladder Channel
Mù Chuāng – Eye Window (GB-16)
膽經第十六穴目窗

穴在臨泣後一寸半，足少陽、陽維之會。《銅人》：鍼三分，灸五壯，三度刺，目大明。

This point is located 1 cùn and a half behind [Tóu] Lín Qì (GB-15). It is the meeting of the foot shàoyáng [channel] and yángwéi [vessel]. *The Tóngrén* states, "Needle 3 fēn, and moxa 5 cones; pierce it 3 times and the vision will brighten."

注：穴名目窗者，以此穴正在目之上，刺之目明，如目之有窗者然，故曰目窗。

Explanation: this point is named Mù Chuāng (Eye Window) because this point is directly above the Mù (Eye); by piercing it, the Mù (Eyes) will brighten, it is as though the Mù (Eye) has a Chuāng (Window), thus it is called Mù Chuāng (Eye Window).

目窗之本病：目赤痛，忽頭旋，目䀮䀮視不明，頭面浮腫，頭痛寒熱，汗不出惡寒。

Principal diseases of Mù Chuāng: redness and pain of the eye, sudden spinning of the head, blurred vision with dim vision, puffy swelling of the head and face, headache with chills and fever, and absence of sweating with aversion to cold.

注：目症乃本經病也，宜責此穴。頭面浮腫，又頭之側浮腫，乃本經受風而然，故宜責此穴。寒熱者，少陽經症，汗不出，宜灸此穴。

Explanation: eye diseases are indeed diseases of this channel, it is appropriate to seek this point. Regarding puffy swelling of the head and face, as well as puffy swelling on the side of the head, these are caused by this channel contracting wind, thus it is appropriate to seek this point. For chills and fever, that is a shàoyáng channel sign; for absence of sweating, it is appropriate to moxa this point.

Seventeenth Point of the Gallbladder Channel
Zhèng Yíng – Upright Construction (GB-17)
膽經第十七穴正營

穴在目窗後一寸半，足少陽、陽維之會。《銅人》：鍼三分，灸五壯。

This point is located 1 cùn and a half behind Mù Chuāng (GB-16). It is the meeting of the foot shàoyáng [channel] and yángwéi [vessel]. *The Tóngrén* **states, "Needle 3 fēn, and moxa 5 cones."**

注：臨泣與太陽經五處穴、督經上星穴橫直，目窗與太陽經承光穴、督經顖會穴橫直，正營與太陽通天穴、督經前頂穴橫直，正當頭頂之偏，故曰正營。其與陽維會，已見前穴。

Explanation: [Tóu] Lín Qì (GB-15) is in a horizontal line with Wǔ Chù (BL-5) of the tàiyáng channel and Shàng Xīng (DU-23) of the dū channel. Mù Chuāng (GB-16) is in a horizontal line with Chéng Guāng (BL-6) of the tàiyáng channel and Xìn Huì (DU-22) of the dū channel. Zhèng Yíng (Upright Construction) is in a horizontal line with Tōng Tiān (BL-7) of the tàiyáng [channel] and Qián Dǐng (DU-21) of the dū channel; as such, it is situated Zhèng (Exactly)[291] to the side of the vertex, thus it is called Zhèng Yíng (Upright Construction). Regarding its meeting with the yángwéi [vessel], it is already presented in the previous point.

正營之本病：目眩瞑，頭頂偏痛。

Principal diseases of Zhèng Yíng: dizzy dim vision and unilateral vertex headache.

注：目疾乃本經正病，頭頂偏痛，乃本穴部分，故取之。

Explanation: eye disease are surely the principal diseases of this channel; unilateral vertex headache in the area of this point, thus choose it.

正營之胃病：牙齒痛，唇吻急強，齒齲痛。

Stomach diseases of Zhèng Yíng: toothache, tension and stiffness of the lips, and tooth decay and pain.

注：前症乃胃病，而取此穴者，散少陽之火也。

Explanation: the above signs are indeed stomach signs, yet choose this point to disperse the fire of shàoyáng.

---

[291] As an adjective, the character zhèng 正 can mean "upright, right, principal, orthodox… etc.;" however, according to the context, the character should be read as an adverb instead as "just, precisely, exactly… etc." This nevertheless leads to the issue of how we can render the point name with an adverb and an unexplained character yíng 營 (construction, camp, circuit… etc.); as such, due to the lack of information, we have kept the point name rendered by *Grasping the Wind*, even though it may not completely fit the context here. Further Note: based on pure speculations, as DU-20 is often depicted as the north star of the human body, the yíng 營 is likely a verb (circulate, garrison) used to describe the points surrounding it, like the stars circulating and stationing around the north star.

Eighteenth Point of the Gallbladder Channel
Chéng Líng – Divine Support[292] (GB-18)
膽經第十八穴承靈

穴在正營後一寸五分，足少陽、陽維之會。灸三壯，禁鍼。

This point is located 1 cùn 5 fēn behind Zhèng Yíng (GB-17). It is the meeting of the foot shàoyáng [channel] and yángwéi [vessel]. Moxa 3 cones, needling is contraindicated.

注：此穴與足太陽絡却、督經百會穴橫直，靈指百會而言，有君象焉，此穴與之橫直，有承君之象，故曰承靈。陽維之會，解見前穴。

Explanation: this point is in a horizontal line with Luò Què (BL-8) of the foot tàiyáng [channel] and Bǎi Huì (DU-20) of the dū channel. Líng (Divine) is referring to Bǎi Huì (DU-20), which has the image of an emperor; as this point is in line with it, it has the image of Chéng (Supporting) the emperor, thus, it is called Chéng Líng (Divine Support). Regarding the meeting with the yángwéi [vessel], see the explanation in the previous point.

承靈之本病：腦風頭痛，惡風寒。

Principal diseases of Chéng Líng: brain wind with headache, and aversion to wind and cold.

注：腦風頭痛、惡風寒，本經傷風病也，宜灸此穴。

Explanation: for brain wind with headache, aversion to wind and cold, these are diseases of wind damage to this channel, it is appropriate to moxa this point.

承靈之肺病：衄鼽鼻窒，喘息不利。

Lung diseases of Chéng Líng: snivelling and nosebleed with nasal congestion, and panting with inhibited [breathing].

注：此雖肺症，此穴在頂，風寒中之，亦能致此症，宜灸此穴。

Explanation: although these are lung signs, this point is located on the vertex; when wind or cold strikes it, it could result in these signs, it is appropriate to moxa this point.

---

[292] *Grasping the Wind* names it "Spirit Support."

Nineteenth Point of the Gallbladder Channel
Năo Kōng – Brain Hollow (GB-19)
膽經第十九穴腦空

一名顳顬
Alternate name: Temple Region

穴在承靈後一寸五分，挾玉枕下陷中，足少陽、陽維之會。《素》注：鍼四分。
《銅人》：鍼五分，得氣即泄，灸三壯。

This point is located 1 cùn 5 fēn behind Chéng Líng (GB-18), in the depression that clasps the jade [pillow] bone.[293] It is the meeting of the foot shàoyáng [channel] and yángwéi [vessel]. *The Sùzhù* states, "Needle 4 fēn." *The Tóngrén* states, "Needle 5 fēn, obtain qì then promptly drain, and moxa 3 cones."

　　注：此穴雖與太陽經玉枕穴、督經後頂穴橫直，然至此，則頭之形削而
下，故此穴在玉枕骨下有陷中者是，以指搯之甚痛者是也。陽維之會，解見前。

　　Explanation: this point is in a horizontal line with Yù Zhěn (BL-9) of the tàiyáng channel and Hòu Dǐng (DU-19) of the dū channel. Upon arriving here, the shape of the head descends sharply; namely, this point is located in the middle of the depression below the jade pillow bone, where it is severely painful upon pinching it with one's fingers. Regarding the meeting with the yángwéi [vessel], see the previous explanation.

腦空之本病：頸項强不得回顧，頭重痛不可忍，目瞑心悸，發即爲癲風，引目
眇，鼻痛。

Principal diseases of Năo Kōng: stiffness in the neck and nape with inability to look behind, unbearable heaviness and pain in the head, dim vision with heart palpitations that manifests with epileptic wind, which also leads to blindness and pain in the nose.

　　注：前症皆少陽之在頭，中風邪之甚者，故取此穴治之。

　　Explanation: all of the above signs are severe [conditions] due to strike by wind evil at the shàoyáng [channel] on the head, thus choose this point in order to treat these [signs].

腦空之肺病：勞疾羸瘦，體熱。

Lung diseases of Năo Kōng: taxation disease with marked weakness and emaciation, and generalised heat.

---

[293] Yù Zhěn 玉枕 (Jade Pillow) is also the name of BL-9.

注：此肺症也，取此穴者，以散上逆之火耳。

Explanation: these are lung signs, choose this point in order to disperse the counterflow ascent of fire.

Twentieth Point of the Gallbladder Channel
Fēng Chí – Wind Pool (GB-20)
膽經第二十穴風池

穴在耳後顬顬後，腦空下，髮際陷中，按之引於耳中，手少陽、陽維之會。
《素》注：鍼四分。《明堂》：鍼三分。《銅人》：鍼七分，留七呼。《甲
乙》：鍼三分。患大風者，先補後泄。少可患者，以經取之。留五呼，泄七吸，
灸不及鍼，日七壯至百壯。《千金》:治癭氣，灸百壯。

This point is located at the rear of the temple region behind the ear, below Năo Kōng (GB-19), in the depression at the hairline; upon pressing it, [a sensation] will radiate into the ear. It is the meeting of the hand shàoyáng and yángwéi [vessel]. *The Sùzhù* **states, "Needle 4 fēn."** *The Míngtáng* **states, "Needle 3 fēn."**

The Tóngrén **states, "Needle 7 fēn, and retain for 7 respirations."** *The Jiǎyǐ* **states, "Needle 3 fēn. For a patient suffering from great wind,[294] initially supplement then subsequently drain. For a patient who is slightly relieved [after treatment], choose [the point] according to which channel [the condition occurs in]. Retain for 5 respirations, drain for 7 respirations; moxa is inferior to needling [it], moxa 7 to 100 cones."** *The Qiānjīn* **states, "To treat goitre qì, moxa 100 cones."**

注：風之中人，多在身之後，則頭之上，頭之後，皆其所也。然風每中於
身之虛處，如督經之中行在頭者有風府，亦督經之虛處也。膽經之風池，亦膽經之
虛處也。陽維脈自下而上者，入於此穴之中，而始上行於少陽在首腦空以上諸穴
也。

Explanation: when a person is struck by Fēng (Wind), it predominantly [strikes] the rear of the body; consequently, both the top of the head and the rear of the head are such locations. Fēng (Wind) always strikes the vacuous spaces of the body, for example, on the midline of the head, there is Fēng Fǔ (Wind Mansion, DU-16) of the dū channel, which is also a vacuous place on the dū channel; furthermore,

---

294 *The Practical Dictionary* states that "great wind" is leprosy and is "a transmissible disease that is characterised by localised numbing and subsequent appearance of red patches which swell and rupture without suppuration and that may spread to other parts of the body."

Fēng Chí (Wind Pool) of the gallbladder channel is also a vacuous place on the gallbladder channel.

The yángwéi vessel ascends from below to enter into this point; this is where it begins to ascend to the various head points of the shàoyáng [channel] above Nǎo Kōng (GB-19).

傷寒有中風一症，少汗而服桂枝不效者，或鍼或灸此穴，服桂枝則無不效矣。

There is one pattern of Fēng (Wind) strike in cold damage, when there is little sweating and the prescription of Guìzhī [Tāng][295] turns out ineffective. One may needle or moxa this point; afterwards, one should again prescribe Guìzhī [Tāng], and without exception, it will always be effective.[296]

風池之本病：洒淅寒熱，傷寒溫病汗不出，目眩，苦偏正頭痛，瘧癧，頸項如拔，痛不得回顧，目淚出涕，耳塞目不明，腰脊俱痛，腰傴僂引項無力不收，大風中風氣塞，涎上不語昏危，欠氣多，癭氣。

Principal diseases of Fēng Chí: chills and fever as though after a soaking, cold damage and warm disease with absence of sweating, dizzy vision, suffering from hemilateral or medial headache, intervallic malaria, [sensation] that resembles dislocation of the neck and nape and pain with inability to look behind, tearing and snivelling, blocked ear with dim vision, pain of both the lumbus and spine, stooped low back with [pain] that radiates to the nape and with lack of strength and loss of use [in the low back], great wind with wind stroke and qì blockage, [excessive] ascent of drool with inability to speak and critical clouding, frequent yawning, and goitre qì.

注：少陽經所主者，多爲風病，多爲目病，爲寒熱病，爲筋病。而風池一穴，尤爲本經最要之穴，以在頭爲虛處，後風之來易傷之，而又爲離首入項之第一穴。本經在首之二十穴，至此而盡，故所治病爲多。至癭氣、欠氣多，亦責此穴者，皆本經鬱而不暢之症，故灸之也。

Explanation: what the shàoyáng channel governs is predominantly wind diseases, predominantly eye diseases, chills and fever diseases, and sinew diseases. As for this one point, Fēng Chí (GB-20), it is the point of the utmost importance on this channel, as it is located at a vacuous place on the head, where it is easily damaged by wind that comes from the behind; in addition, after departing from the head, it is also the first point to enter the nape.

---

[295] I.e., Guìzhī Tāng 桂枝湯 (Cinnamon Twig Decoction).
[296] This seems to allude to Line 24 of *Shānghán Lùn*.

For the twenty points of this channel on the head, they terminate upon arriving here, thus, it is the reason why it treats many diseases.[297] For goitre qì and frequent yawning, also seek this point, as these are signs of depression leading to inhibition of this channel, thus moxa it.

風池之肺病：鼻鼽衄。

Lung disease of Fēng Chí: snivelling with nosebleed.

注：此陽明經病也，責此穴者，泄少陽之風與火，使不上逆也。

Explanation: this is a yángmíng channel disease, seek this point to drain the wind and fire of shàoyáng, so that the ascending counterflow can be prevented.

Twenty-First Point of the Gallbladder Channel
Jiān Jǐng – Shoulder Well (GB-21)
膽經第二十一穴肩井

一名膊井
Alternate name: Shoulder Well[298]

穴在肩上陷中，缺盆上，大骨前一寸半，以三指按取，當中指下陷中，手、足少陽、足陽明、陽維之會，連入五臟，刺五分，灸五壯，先補後泄。《千金》：凡產難，鍼兩肩井一寸，泄之，須臾即生。又云：治卒忤，灸百壯。又云：臂重不舉，灸隨年壯至百壯，刺五分補之。

This point is located in the depression on top of the shoulder, above Quē Pén (ST-12), 1 cùn and a half in front of the great bone;[299] when using three fingers to locate it, it is exactly in the depression under the middle finger. It is the meeting of the hand and foot shàoyáng, the foot yángmíng [channels], and the yángwéi [vessel]. It links up with the five zàng-viscera, pierce 5 fēn, and moxa 5 cones; initially supplement and then subsequently drain.

The Qiānjīn states, "For all difficult childbirth, needle both Jiān Jǐng (GB-21) with 1 cùn [depth], drain it, in an instant [the woman] will give birth." It also states, "To treat sudden hostility, moxa 100 cones." It further states, "For

---

[297] In the secondary manuscript, there are five extra characters of "較首上諸穴 in contrast to various points on the head above."

[298] Note: While both Bó Jǐng 膊井 (the alternate name) and Jiān Jǐng 肩井 (the main name) are translated as "shoulder well," Jiān 肩 specifically refers to the shoulder, whereas Bó 膊 is more ambiguous and can be defined as limb, upper arm, or shoulder.

[299] I.e., the scapula.

heaviness of the arm with inability to raise it, moxa cones according to one's age, [gradually increasing] up to 100 cones, and pierce 5 fēn to supplement it."

注：此穴在肩之上，其下內五臟，其深不測，如井然，故曰肩井。

Explanation: this point is located on top of the Jiān (Shoulder); underneath it, it enters into the five zàng-viscera, with an unfathomable depth that resembles a Jǐng (Well), thus it is called Jiān Jǐng (Shoulder Well).

手少陽、陽明之會本經於此穴也，以手少陽脈上臂，歷清冷淵、消濼，行手太陽之裏，手陽明之外，上肩循臂之臑，上肩過肩髎，將至頰，過天髎穴，出足少陽之後，過肩井而與本經相會也。足陽明之會本經於此穴也，以足陽明之支別者，從水突、氣舍，入缺盆，肩井緊在缺盆之上，故此穴有胃經與本經在此穴有相會之處。

For both the hand shàoyáng and yángmíng to meet with this channel at this point, the hand shàoyáng vessel ascends the arm, passes through Qīng Lěng Yuān (SJ-11) and Xiāo Luò (SJ-12), [ascending] inside of the hand tàiyáng [channel] and outside of the hand yángmíng [channel], ascends the shoulder by following the upper arm, and ascends the shoulder by traversing Jiān Liáo (SJ-14); prior to arriving at the cheek, it traverses Tiān Liáo (SJ-15), emerges behind the foot shàoyáng [channel] to traverse Jiān Jǐng (GB-21), where it meets with this channel.

For the yángmíng [vessel] to meet with this channel at this point, a diverging branch of the foot yángmíng [channel] follows Shuǐ Tū (ST-10) and Qì Shè (ST-11) to enter Quē Pén (ST-12); as Jiān Jǐng (GB-21) is nearby the top of Quē Pén (ST-12), this point serves as a location where the stomach channel meets with this channel, here at this point.

陽維之會本經於此穴也，以陽維之脈，自下而上，循脅肋斜上，肘上會手陽明、手、足太陽於臂臑之後，遂過肩前，與手少陽會於肩前之臑會、天髎，却會手、足少陽、足陽明於肩井也。但忌鍼深，以內過五臟也，若鍼深悶倒，急補足三里。

For the yángwéi [vessel] to meet with this channel at this point, the vessel of the yángwéi ascends from below, follows the rib-sides to ascend obliquely, and meets with the hand yángmíng, hand and foot tàiyáng [channels] above the elbow and behind Bì Nào (LI-14); thereupon, it traverses in front of the shoulder to meet with the hand shàoyáng [channel] at Nào Huì (SJ-13) and Tiān Liáo (SJ-15), and it returns to meet with the hand and foot shàoyáng, and foot yángmíng [channels] at Jiān Jǐng (GB-21).

Nonetheless, deep needling should be avoided, as it passes through the five zàng-viscera inside; if it is needled deeply, there will be oppression [in the chest] and collapse; in that case, urgently supplement Zú Sān Lǐ (ST-36).

肩井之本病：中風氣塞，涎上不語，氣逆，頭項痛，臂痛，手不能向頭，五勞七傷。

Principal diseases of Jiān Jǐng: wind strike with qì blockage, inability to speak due to ejection of saliva, qì counterflow, pain in the head and nape, arm pain, inability to move the hand towards the head, five taxations and seven damages.

注：前症皆本經中風之症，宜取此穴，以通其滯，而去其邪。五勞七傷，取此穴者，乃暢其滯氣也。必先補而後泄。

Explanation: all of the above signs are signs of wind strike at this channel, it is appropriate to choose this point in order to free the stagnation and eliminate the evil. For five taxations and seven damages, choose this point to soothe the qì stagnation. One must initially supplement and then subsequently drain.

肩井之婦人病：婦人難產，墮胎後手足厥逆，鍼此穴立愈。

Women's diseases of Jiān Jǐng: difficult childbirth in women, reverse flow of the hands and feet after a miscarriage; needle this point and there will be immediate recovery.

注：此穴雖爲手、足少陽並足陽明、陽維之會，而各經之入缺盆者，無不相及之，故治產難也。

Explanation: although this point is [only said to be] the meeting place of the hand and foot shàoyáng, the foot yángmíng, and the yángwéi [vessels], yet, as other channel [pathways] enter Quē Pén (ST-12), without exception, all of them reach [this point], thus it treats difficult childbirth.

Twenty-Second Point of the Gallbladder Channel
Yuān Yè – Armpit Abyss (GB-22)
膽經第二十二穴淵液

一名泉液
Alternate name: Spring Humour[300]

穴在腋下三寸宛宛中，舉臂取之。《銅人》：禁灸。《明堂》：鍼三分。

---

[300] Note: "泉 spring" in this instance means a fountain or source of water. On the other hand, "液 humour" means thick body fluid.

This point is located in the depression 3 cùn below the armpit, lift the arm to locate it. *The Tóngrén* **states, "Moxa is contraindicated."** *The Míngtáng* **states, "Needle 3 fēn."**

注：此穴在腋下，有淵深之意，故曰淵液。禁灸者，以此經氣多而血少，恐助其火也。

Explanation: as this point is located below the Yè (Armpit), it has the meaning of a deep Yuān (Abyss),[301] thus it is called Yuān Yè (Armpit Abyss). Regarding the contraindication of moxa, it is because this channel has copious qì and scant blood, thus there is a fear that [moxa] will exacerbate the fire.

淵液之本病：寒熱，馬刀瘍，胸滿無力，臂不舉。

Principal diseases of Yuān Yè: chills and fever, sabre lumps and sores, fullness in the chest with lack of strength, and inability to raise the shoulder.

注：前症皆邪中本經之正病，但多宜於補之以藥，不宜助之以火，鍼泄其氣可也，斷不可出血。不宜灸，令人生腫蝕。馬刀瘍，內潰者死，寒熱者生。

Explanation: all of the above signs are principal diseases of evil striking this channel; however, [for these diseases], while it is more appropriate to supplement with herbs, it is not appropriate to exacerbate it with fire;[302] one can needle to drain the qì, but one absolutely must not perform bloodletting. It is inappropriate to moxa, as this will cause the swelling and erosion [of the armpit]. Regarding sabre lumps and sores, if they rupture internally, the person will die; if there are chills and fever, the person will live.

Twenty-Third Point of the Gallbladder Channel
Zhé Jīn – Sinew Seat[303] (GB-23)
膽經第二十三穴輒筋

一名神光
Alternate name: Spirit Light

---

301 For "淵深 deep abyss," the scribal manuscript has two rare characters, "浮漫," here instead, both of which with unclear definition (river soaked?). The editors of this manuscript, Zhāng and Zhà, have changed it to "淵深 deep abyss" in accordance with the secondary manuscript.

302 I.e., fire needling or moxibustion.

303 This seat refers to those of an ancient chariot, according to *Grasping the Wind*, "the rib cage is said to resemble the sides of a chariot in the area above the way."

一名膽募

Alternate name: Gallbladder Collecting Point

穴在腋下三寸，復前一寸三肋端，橫直蔽骨旁七寸五分，平直兩乳，側臥屈上足取之，膽之募，足太陽、少陽之會。《銅人》：灸三壯，鍼六分。《素》注：鍼七[304]分。

This point is located 3 cùn below the armpit, 1 cùn towards the front [of the body] in the third intercostal, 7 cùn 5 fēn in a horizontal line to the side of the sheltered bone, and in line with the two nipples; to be located while lying on the side and bending the top leg. It is the collecting point of the gallbladder. It is the meeting of the foot tàiyáng and shàoyáng [channels]. *The Tóngrén states,* **"Moxa 3 cones, and needle 6 fēn."** *The Sùzhù states, "Needle 7 fēn."*

注：足少陽所主骨筋，而本經之筋上行者，前結於伏兔，後結於尻。其直者，上乘䏚季脇，上走腋前廉，系於膺乳，結於缺盆。此穴乃本經上脇之筋所行處，故曰輒筋。

Explanation: the foot shàoyáng is that which governs the bones[305] and Jīn (Sinews); as for the ascending pathway of the Jīn (Sinew) [channel] of this channel, it knots at Fú Tù (ST-32) in the front, and it knots at the coccyx in the rear. The vertical [pathway] ascends over the flank, free rib, and rib-side, ascends and travels to the front aspect of the armpit, connects with the breast, and knots at Quē Pén (ST-12). As this point is in the location where this channel ascends over the Jīn (Sinews) of the rib-side, thus it is called Zhé Jīn (Sinew Seat).

輒筋之本病：太息善悲，嘔吐宿汁，吞酸。

Principal diseases of Zhé Jīn: sighing with tendency to sorrow, retching and vomiting of lodged fluids, and acid regurgitation.

注：前症乃少陽之氣滯所有之症，取此穴以舒少陽之鬱氣。

Explanation: all of the above signs are signs caused by the stagnation of shàoyáng qì, choose this point in order to soothe the depressed qì of shàoyáng.

輒筋之肺病：胸中暴滿不得臥。

Lung disease of Zhé Jīn: sudden fullness in the chest with inability to lie down.

注：少陽之氣，上逆於胸中，而有是症，宜泄此穴，以舒少陽之逆。

---

304 For "7 fēn," *the Sùzhù* actually states "6 fēn."

305 Note: According to *Língshū* Chapter 10, "膽足少陽之脈... 是主骨所生病者 the vessel of gallbladder shàoyáng... it is that which governs the engendered diseases of bones."

Explanation: when there is counterflow ascent of the qì of shàoyáng into the chest, this sign will occur; it is appropriate to drain this point in order to soothe the counterflow of shàoyáng.

甄筋之脾病：小腹熱，欲走，多唾，言語不正，四肢不收。

Spleen diseases of Zhé Jīn: heat in the lower abdomen, desire to walk, copious spittle, incoherent speech, and loss of use of the four limbs.

注：肝腎之氣逆於下，木旺尅土之義也，宜取此穴以泄木之旺。

Explanation: when there is counterflow qì of the liver and kidney in the below, this is the meaning of "effulgent wood will restrain earth;" thus, it is appropriate to choose this point in order to drain the effulgence of wood.

Twenty-Fourth Point of the Gallbladder Channel
Rì Yuè – Sun and Moon (GB-24)

膽經第二十四穴日月

一名神光

Alternate name: Spirit Light

穴在肝經期門穴下五分，足太陰、少陽、陽維三經所會之處，鍼七分，灸五壯。
《千金》：嘔吐宿汁，吞酸，灸神光百壯。

This point is located 5 fēn below Qì Mén (LR-14) of the liver channel. It is the place where the three channels, foot tàiyīn, shàoyáng, and yángwéi [vessel] meet. Needle 7 fēn, moxa 5 cones. *The Qiānjīn* states, "For retching and vomiting with lodged fluids and acid regurgitation, moxa 100 cones on Shén Guāng (GB-24)."

注：此穴在肝經期門之下，人身南面而立，此穴正在東西，猶日月之出没於東西也，別無所取義焉。

Explanation: this point is below Qì Mén (LR-14) of the liver channel. [By orientation], the human body stands erected facing the south,[306] and this point is located exactly in the east and west, as though the rising and setting of Rì Yuè (Sun and Moon) in the east and west. Besides this, there is no other meaning [of this name].

---

[306] This is reminiscent of *Sùwèn* Chapter 6, which states, "聖人南面而立 by facing the south, the sage stands erected."

本經淵液之穴，直在腋下三寸，至輒筋則平前一寸，橫直蔽骨前七寸五分，至此穴則又斜下在期門下五分，上為肝經之期門，下一寸五分為脾經之腹哀，而此穴在其中，故足太陰會本經於此穴。

The point Yuān Yè (GB-22) of this channel is 3 cùn directly below the armpit. [The pathway subsequently] arrives at Zhé Jīn (GB-23), which is 1 cùn in front, in a horizontal line with the concealed bone that is 7 cùn 5 fēn in front. [The pathway then] arrives at this point, which is 5 fēn obliquely below Qī Mén (LR-14). In the above, it is Qī Mén (LR-14) of the liver channel; 1 cùn 5 fēn below, it is Fù Āi (SP-16) of the spleen channel; thus, this point is in the middle between them, therefore, the foot tàiyīn [vessel] meets with this channel at this point.

陽維循膝外廉上髀厭，抵小腹側，會足少陽於居髎穴，循脇肋斜上而行，故會本經於此穴。

The yángwéi [vessel] follows the outer aspect of the knee to ascend to the hip bone, arrives at the side of the lower abdomen, meets with Jū Liáo (GB-29) of the foot shàoyáng [channel], and follows the rib-side to ascend obliquely; thus, [the yángwéi vessel] meets with this channel at this point.

日月之本病：太息善悲，腹熱欲走，多唾，言語不正，四肢不收。

Principal diseases of Rì Yuè: sighing with tendency to sorrow, heat in the abdomen with desire to walk, copious spittle, incoherent speech, and loss of use of the four limbs.

注：前症皆本經鬱滯所致，故泄此穴。

Explanation: all of the above signs are a result of depression and stagnation in this channel, thus drain this point.

Twenty-Fifth Point of the Gallbladder Channel
Jīng Mén – Capital Gate (GB-25)
膽經第二十五穴京門

一名氣腧
Alternate name: Qì Transport Point

一名氣府
Alternate name: Qì Mansion

穴在監骨下腰中季肋本挾脊，腎之募。《銅人》：灸三壯，鍼三分，留七呼。

This point is located below the haunch bone, on the lumbus, where the base of the free rib clasps the spine. It is the collecting point of the kidneys. *The Tóngrén* **states, "Moxa 3 cones, needle 3 fēn, and retain for 7 respirations."**

注：前穴居脾經腹哀之上，此穴又折而斜下，至季肋之本，斜過肝經上行章門穴之上，斜下而至於季肋本，此穴應與足太陽之脈下行者相會，乃眇之所，人身至虛之處，

Explanation: the previous point (GB-24) is situated above Fù Āi (SP-16) of the spleen channel. As for this point, [the pathway] turns to descend obliquely towards the base of the free rib. It obliquely traverses above Zhāng Mén (LR-13) on the ascending pathway of the liver channel, and descends obliquely to arrive at the base of the free rib. This point should meet with the descending pathway of the foot tàiyáng vessel at the flank,[307] which is the most vacuous location in the entire human body.

曰氣府，曰氣腧，以本經少血而多氣耳。其曰腎募者，此穴部分，乃在內爲腎所繫處，而膽經過之，與腎有相通者，故曰腎募也。

It is called Qì Fǔ (Qì Mansion) and Qì Shù (Qì Transport Point) because this channel has scant blood and copious qì. It is also called the collecting point of the kidneys because the area of this point is where the kidneys fasten themselves on the inside; as such, the gallbladder channel traverses it and has a [pathway] that communicates with the kidneys; therefore, it is the kidney collecting point.

其取義於京門者，以此穴在後，爲身最虛之處，猶門焉。京者，大也。

For the meaning of Jīng Mén (Capital Gate), it is because this point is located in the rear, at the location where the body is most vacuous, it is like the image of a Mén (Gate). Regarding Jīng (Capital), this is because it is a large [area].

京門之本病：肩背寒痙，肩胛內廉痛，寒熱，腹脹引背不得息，髀樞引痛。

Principal diseases of Jīng Mén: cold tetany of the shoulder and upper back, pain of the inside ridge of the scapula, chills and fever, abdominal distension that radiates to the upper back with inability to catch the breath, and pain that radiates to the thigh pivot.

注：前症皆本經上下中風寒所致，故取此穴，以去上下之風寒。

Explanation: all of the above signs are a result of a wind or cold strike at this channel, either in the above or below, thus choose this point in order to eliminate the wind or cold that is either in the above or below.

---

[307] This is the soft area below the free ribs.

京門之腎病：腰痛不能俯仰久立，水道不利，溺黃，小腹急腫。

Kidney diseases of Jīng Mén: lumbar pain with inability to bend forwards and backwards and [inability to] stand for long periods, inhibited water pathways, yellow urine, urgency and swelling of the lower abdomen.

注：此穴近腎，膽氣逆於腎，故有俯仰不得之症，水道不利，皆氣滯之所致也。溺黃，乃熱也；小腹急脹，亦氣滯也。均泄此穴，以泄少陽之氣於腎。

Explanation: as this point is nearby the kidneys, the gallbladder qì counterflow can reach the kidneys, thus there is the sign of inability to bend forwards and backwards, as well as inhibited water pathways; both of these are a result of qì stagnation. Yellow urine is due to heat; for urgency and distension of the lower abdomen, there is also qì stagnation; without exception, drain this point in order to drain the [counterflow] qì of shàoyáng that is reaching the kidneys.

京門之大小腸病：腸鳴，小腸痛，腸鳴洞泄。

Large intestine and small intestine diseases of Jīng Mén: rumbling intestines, pain in the small intestine, and rumbling intestines with throughflux diarrhoea.

注：前症皆膽氣有餘，干於二腸，故泄此穴。

Explanation: all of the above signs are due to superabundance of gallbladder qì that is interfering with both of the intestines, thus drain this point.

Twenty-Sixth Point of the Gallbladder Channel
Dài Mài – Dài Vessel [Point] (GB-26)

膽經第二十六穴帶脈

穴在季肋下一寸八分陷中，臍上二分，兩旁各七寸半，足少陽、帶脈二經相會之處。《銅人》：鍼六分，灸五壯。《明堂》：灸七壯。

This point is located in the depression 1 cùn 8 fēn below the floating rib, 2 fēn above the umbilicus, and 7 and a half cùn on each side [of the abdomen]. This is the location where the two channels, the foot shàoyáng [channel] and dài vessel, meet with each other. *The Tóngrén* **states, "Needle 6 fēn, and moxa 5 cones."** *The Míngtáng* **states, "Moxa 7 cones."**

注：帶脈橫束乎腰，凡十二經上下往來，皆爲帶脈束之。上之帶脈，中之五樞，下之維道，上下三穴，皆帶脈所橫治之處。

Explanation: the Dài Mài (Dài Vessel) binds the waist horizontally. For all [pathways] of the twelve channels that come and go between the above and below, they are all bound by the Dài Mài (Dài Vessel). With Dài Mài (Dài Vessel [Point]) in the above, Wǔ Shū (GB-27) in the middle, and Wéi Dào (GB-28) in the below, all of these three points from the above to the below are the locations governed by the horizontal [pathway] of Dài Mài (Dài Vessel).

其經起於季脇，足厥陰之章門穴，圍身一周，如束帶然，總束諸脈，使不妄行，如人束帶而前垂，故名帶脈。

The channel commences under the rib-side at the floating rib, at Zhāng Mén (LR-13) of the foot juéyīn [channel]. It encircles the body in a [horizontal] circuit, as though one is bound with a Dài (Sash).[308] It binds all of the vessels together, so that they do not shift freely. As it resembles a person's bound Dài (Sash) that is hanging down in front, thus it is named the Dài Mài (Dài Vessel).

婦人惡露，隨帶脈而下，故謂之帶下。十二經與奇經七經，皆上下周流，惟帶脈橫束乎腰，而衝任二脈，循腹脇挾臍旁，傳流於氣衝，属於帶脈，絡於督脈。衝、任、督三經，同起而異行，一原而三歧，皆絡帶脈。

For lochia [diseases] in women, as it follows the Dài Mài (Dài Vessel) to discharge, thus it is called "the Dài (Sash) discharge."[309] Whereas all of the twelve channels and the [other] seven channels of extraordinary vessels ascend and descend in their circuits of flow, the dài vessel is the only one that binds the waist horizontally. As for the two vessels of the chōng and rèn, they follow the abdomen and rib-side while clasping the umbilicus, to spread at Qì Chōng (ST-30), adjoin to the Dài Mài (Dài Vessel), and network to the dū vessel. For the three channels of the chōng, rèn, and dū, they commence together but [diverge into] different pathways, with one origin but three forks; yet, they all network with the Dài Mài (Dài Vessel).

因諸經往來上下，遺熱於帶脈之間，客熱鬱抑，白物滿溢，隨溺而下，綿綿不絕，是爲白帶，凡有此病者，每按此穴，莫不應手酸痛，令灸之，無有不愈。若更灸百會尤佳，所謂下有病上取之，是之謂也。

Because all of the channels come and go between the above and below [at the dài vessel], they bequeath heat in the space of the dài vessel; when this lodged

---

[308] Note: *The Practical Dictionary* translates dài mài 帶脈 as the "girdling vessel;" in addition, another common translation is "belt vessel." Of the two choices, "belt" is fitting, but dài 帶 is wider in width and often worn purely for decorative purpose rather than the functional purpose of securing one's clothing; on the other hand, "girdling" or "girdle" depicts the width properly, yet it is worn as an undergarment for form-shaping purpose, which is not what dài 帶 is worn for. So, we have elected "waist sash," or "sash" in short, as our translation choice, because we believe that it is closer to the appearance and function of dài 帶.

[309] I.e., vaginal discharge.

heat is depressed or repressed, white substances will fill and overflow, discharging along with the urine continuously and unceasingly; this is known as "white Dài (Sash)."[310] In general, for those with this disease, whenever this point is pressed, there will always be ache and pain in response to the hand [pressure], without exception, moxa it, and there will be none who do not recover. Furthermore, it is particularly brilliant to also moxa Bǎi Huì (DU-20); this is exactly what is meant by the saying, "when there is disease below, choose a [point] above."[311]

帶脈之本病：腰腹縱，溶溶如囊水之狀，婦人小腹痛，裏急後重，瘈瘲，月事不調，赤白帶下。又腎着病，腰痛冷如冰，身重，腰如帶五千錢，不渴，小便利，勞汗出，衣裏冷濕而得，久則變爲水也，宜灸此穴。

Principal diseases of Dài Mài: slackening of the abdomen and lumbus with dissolution [of the lumbus] that resembles the appearance of a pouch of water, lower abdominal pain in women, internal urgency and heaviness in the rectum, tugging and slackening, irregular menstruation, red and white vaginal discharge.

Also, in kidney fixity disease,[312] there is lumbar pain that is as cold as ice, generalised heaviness, [heavy sensation in] the lumbus as though one is carrying 5,000 coins, and absence of thirst with uninhibited urination; upon taxation, there is sweating, which makes the clothing cold and damp inside; as a result, one contracts [this disease]. After an extended period of time, it will transform into water [diseases], it is appropriate to moxa this point.

注：悉見前。

Explanation: all [explanations] can be found in previous [points].

Twenty-Seventh Point of the Gallbladder Channel
Wǔ Shū – Pivot of the Five [Zàng-Viscera][313] (GB-27)
膽經第二十七穴五樞

穴在帶脈下三寸，水道旁五寸五分，足少陽、帶脈之會。《銅人》：鍼一寸，灸五壯。《明堂》：灸三壯。

---

[310] I.e., white vaginal discharge.
[311] This likely is a paraphrase to this statement from *Sùwèn* Chapter 70, "病在下，取之上。When the disease is located below, choose the above."
[312] This following paragraph is a paraphrase of *Jīnguì Yàolüè* Line 11.16.
[313] *Grasping the Wind* names it "Fifth Pivot."

This point is located 3 cùn[314] **below Dài Mài (GB-26) and 5 cùn 5 fēn to the side of Shuǐ Dào (ST-28). It is the meeting of the foot shàoyáng [channel] and the dài vessel.** *The Tóngrén* **states, "Needle 1 cùn, and moxa 5 cones."** *The Míngtáng* **states, "Moxa 3 cones."**

注：少陽爲樞，帶脈下三寸，正當腰際，乃一身曲折之所，故曰五樞，言五臟之樞也。

Explanation: the shàoyáng is the Shū (Pivot); [as this point is] located 3 cùn below Dài Mài (GB-26), it is exactly on the waist, the place where the whole body can bend and twist, thus it is called Wǔ Shū (Pivot of the Five [Zàng-Viscera]), which is indicating it as the Shū (Pivot) of the Wǔ (Five) zàng-viscera.

五樞之本病：男子寒疝，陰卵上入小腹痛，婦人赤白帶下，裏急，瘦瘕，痃癖。

Principal diseases of Wǔ Shū: cold mounting in males, retraction of the testicles into the lower abdomen with pain, red and white vaginal discharge in women, internal urgency, tugging and slackening, strings and aggregations.

注：疝責肝經，肝膽相爲表裏，此穴在腰脇之間，正受寒之所，宜灸之。此穴去帶脈不遠，故亦治帶下之病。瘦瘕亦本經正病，故亦取之。痃癖之在下者，下焦肝膽之氣寒而滯，而積因之而生，故灸此穴。

Explanation: for mounting diseases, blame the liver; yet, as the liver and gallbladder are an exterior and interior [pair], and as this point is located between the lumbus and rib-side, it is exactly the place that contracts cold; thus, it is appropriate to moxa this point. Because this point is not far from Dài Mài (GB-26), it can also be used to treat diseases of vaginal discharge.

Tugging and slackening are also principal diseases of this channel, thus choose this [point]. For strings and aggregations that are located below, when qì of the liver and gallbladder in the lower jiāo becomes stagnated due to cold, it will subsequently lead to accumulations and the engenderment [of these diseases], thus moxa this point.

---

[314] "3 cùn" is originally '3 fēn.' The editors of this manuscript, Zhāng and Zhà, have amended it according to the secondary manuscript and the *Zhēnjiǔ Dàchéng*.

Twenty-Eighth Point of the Gallbladder Channel
Wéi Dào – Yángwéi Path[315] (GB-28)
膽經第二十八穴維道

一名外樞
Alternate name: Outer Pivot

穴在肝經章門穴下五寸三分，足少陽、帶脈之會。《銅人》：鍼八分，留六呼，灸三壯。

This point is located 5 cùn 3 fēn below Zhāng Mén (LR-13) of the liver channel. It is the meeting of the foot shàoyáng [channel] and dài vessel. *The Tóngrén* states, "Needle 8 fēn, retain for 6 respirations,[316] and moxa 3 cones."

注：帶脈之橫束諸經也，上下凡三穴，而此穴乃其最下穴也，又向裏折斜而下。陽維自循膝外廉，上髀厭，抵少腹側，會本經於居髎之後，上循脅肋斜上，此正其自下斜上之處，故曰維道。

Explanation: the horizontality of the dài vessel binds all other channels together. In total, there are three [dài vessel] points from the above and to the below, and this point is the lowest point. It further turns obliquely inwards and then descends. The yángwéi [vessel] follows the outer aspect of the knee, ascends the hip joint, and reaches the side of the lower abdomen. After it meets with this channel at Jū Liáo (GB-29), it follows the rib-side above to ascend obliquely. As this [point] is located exactly at the place where the [yángwéi vessel] begins to ascend obliquely from the below, thus it is called Wéi Dào (Yángwéi Path).

維道之本病：嘔逆不止，水腫，三焦不調，不嗜食。

Principal diseases of Wéi Dào: incessant vomiting counterflow, water swelling, failure of the sānjiāo to regulate, and no pleasure in eating.

注：嘔逆乃少陽經正病也，泄此穴以降少陽之逆氣。水腫、三焦不調、不嗜食，乃帶脈病也，可灸此穴，以散腰中之水氣。

Explanation: vomiting counterflow is surely a principal disease of the shàoyáng channel, drain this point in order to descend the counterflow qì of shàoyáng. Regarding water swelling, failure of the sānjiāo to regulate, and no pleasure in eating, these are diseases of the dài vessel, one can moxa this point in order to disperse the water qì within the waist.

---

[315] *Grasping the Wind* names it "Linking Path."
[316] "Retain for 6 respirations" is absent in *the Tóngrén*.

Twenty-Ninth Point of the Gallbladder Channel
Jū Liáo – Sitting Bone-Hole[317] (GB-29)
膽經第二十九穴居髎

穴在肝經章門穴下八寸三分，監骨上陷中，足少陽、陽蹻之會。《銅人》：鍼八分，留六呼，灸三壯。

This point is located 8 cùn 3 fēn below Zhāng Mén (LR-13) of the liver channel, in the depression above the haunch bone. It is the meeting of the foot shàoyáng [channel] and yángqiāo [vessel]. *The Tóngrén* **states, "Needle 8 fēn, retain for 6 respirations,[318] and moxa 3 cones."**

注：居者，坐也。人坐則此穴而在腹與肢折曲之處，故曰居髎。陽蹻之脈，自附陽爲郄之後，直上循股外廉，上循脇，此穴正在上股上循脇之所，故曰足少陽、陽蹻之會。

Explanation: regarding Jū (Sitting), it means sitting. When a person sits, this point is situated at the location where the abdomen and [lower] limbs bend and twist, thus it is called Jū Liáo (Sitting Bone-Hole).

From its cleft point at Fù Yáng (BL-59), the vessel of the yángqiāo ascends vertically following the outside of the thigh, and ascends following the rib-side; this point is located exactly at the place on the upper thigh where [the yángqiāo vessel] ascends to follow the rib-side, thus it is said to be the meeting of the foot shàoyáng [channel] and yángqiāo [vessel].

居髎之本病：腰引小腹痛，肩引胸臂攣急，手臂不得舉以至肩。

Principal diseases of Jū Liáo: pain that radiates from the lumbus to the lower abdomen, hypertonicity of the shoulder that radiates to the chest and arm,[319] and inability to lift the arm to reach the shoulder.

注：此穴正腰股相連之處，有氣滯則相引痛，取此穴以泄之。肩引胸臂等病，而取此穴者，身之側正少陽部分也，上有病取之下，所以取此穴，以散上之風邪。

Explanation: this point is in the exact location where the lumbus and thigh link together; when there is qì stagnation, there will be pain that radiates between them,[320] choose this point in order to drain it. Regarding diseases such as shoulder

---

[317] *Grasping the Wind* names it "Squatting Bone-Hole."
[318] "Retain for 6 respirations" is absent in *the Tóngrén.*
[319] "Chest" is originally "lumbus." The editors of this manuscript, Zhāng and Zhà, have amended it according to the secondary manuscript and the *Zhēnjiǔ Dàchéng.*
[320] I.e., the lumbus and thigh.

[hypertonicity] that radiates to the chest and arm, this point is chosen because the side of the body is exactly the area of the shàoyáng. "When there is a disease above, choose [a point] below."[321] That is the reason why this point is chosen, so that the wind evil above can be dispersed.

Thirtieth Point of the Gallbladder Channel
Huán Tiào – Ring Leaping[322] (GB-30)
膽經第三十穴環跳

穴在髀樞中，側臥伸下足，屈上足，以右手摸穴，左搖撼取之，足少陽、太陽之會。《銅人》：灸五十壯。《素》注：鍼一寸，留二呼，灸三壯。《指微》：已刺不可搖，恐傷鍼。

This point is located on the thigh pivot. [Have the patient] lie on the side, with the bottom leg extended while the top leg bent;[323] use the right hand to palpate for the point, which is located by shaking [the top leg] with the left [hand]. It is the meeting of the foot shàoyáng and tàiyáng [channels]. *The Tóngrén states, "Moxa 50 cones." The Sùzhù states, "Needle 1 cùn, retain for 2 respirations,[324] and moxa 3 cones." The Zhǐwēi states, "While being needled, one must not move, as there is a risk of needle injury."*

注：此穴乃上下二骨錯扣之處，屈上足，以手按其兩骨錯扣之處搖撼，則穴之空開。徐徐下鍼，先語患人，即痛亦不可少動其股，蓋股已伸，則骨之錯扣者，必掩閉其穴，而鍼傷於內，至要之禁也。

Explanation: this point is at the location where the two bones from the above and below interlock. [Have the patient] bend the top leg, use the [right] hand to press the place where the two bones interlock while shaking [the top leg with left hand], and the hollow of this point will appear. Insert the needle steadily and slowly. Prior [to needling], inform the patient that they must not move the thigh the slightest even if there is pain. If the [top] thigh were extended, then the interlocking bones would certainly shut and close this point; as a result, there will be internal needle injury. This caution is of the utmost importance.

---

[321] This likely is a paraphrase to this statement from *Sùwèn* Chapter 70, "病在上，取之下。 When the disease is located above, choose the below."

[322] *Grasping the Wind* names it "Jumping Round."

[323] E.g., While lying on the right side, straighten the right leg (i.e., the bottom leg) that is contacting the bed, bend the left leg (i.e., the top leg) slightly, and touch the bed with the left foot if needed, so that one can maintain balance with this posture. Vice versa for lying on the left side.

[324] For "2 respirations" the *Sùzhù* actually states "20 respirations."

曰環跳者，骨縫錯扣之處，上如環以扣其骨，股之能屈伸往來者，以環故也，跳則走動之象，此為少陽入股之第一穴，足太陽之支別行背者，自第二行附分而下至秩邊者，橫入此穴中，故與本經會於此穴也。

For it to be called Huán Tiào (Ring Leaping), at the juncture where the bones interlock, the upper part resembles a Huán (Ring) so that it is able to fasten the [thigh] bone. The thigh is able to bend and stretch, moving back and forth, it is all because of this Huán (Ring). Tiào (Leaping) depicts an image of the feet moving, as this is the first point of the shàoyáng [channel] when it enters the thigh.

A branch of the foot tàiyáng diverges to travel the upper back, descends from Fù Fēn (BL-36) on the second [vertical] pathway [of foot tàiyáng] to arrive at Zhì Biān (BL-54), horizontally enters this point, thus [the foot tàiyáng] and this channel meet at this point.

環跳之本病：冷風濕痹不仁，風疹遍身，半身不遂，腰胯痛寒，膝不得轉側伸縮。

Principal diseases of Huán Tiào: cold, wind, and damp impediment with insensitivity, wind papules over the whole body, hemiplegia, lumbar and hip pain, inability of the knees to turn to the sides, extend, or flex.[325]

注：冷風寒濕之傷人下部，未有不先中此穴者，故一切腿膝艱難痛苦之病，皆取此穴。又環跳穴痛，恐生附骨疽。

Explanation: when cold-wind and cold-damp damage the lower part of the body, it is unprecedented that they do not strike this point first, thus for all difficult and agonising diseases of the leg and knee, always choose this point. Moreover, when there is pain at Huán Tiào (GB-30), I am afraid that there may be the engenderment of bone-clinging flat-abscess.[326]

---

[325] "膝不得轉側伸縮 inability of the knees to turn to the sides, extend, or flex" is originally "膝不得轉側不仁 inability of the knees to turn to the sides with insensitivity." The editors of this manuscript, Zhāng and Zhà, have amended it according to the secondary manuscript and the *Zhēnjiǔ Dàchéng*.

[326] According to *the Practical Dictionary*, bone-clinging flat-abscess "is a headless flat-abscess located on a bony and sinewy part of the body… it takes the form of a bread swelling with a head, and without any change in skin colour. After rupturing, there is a persistent dribbling discharge of pus from the opening, which does not heal easily, any pieces of dead bone must be remove before healing is possible."

Thirty-First Point of the Gallbladder Channel
Fēng Shì – Wind Market (GB-31)
膽經第三十一穴風市

穴在膝外上廉兩筋中，以手着腿，中指盡處是穴。鍼五分，灸五壯。

This point is located in the middle between the two sinews, on the upper ridge outside of the knee; with the hand touching the legs, this point is located at the tip of the middle finger. Needle 5 fēn, and moxa 5 cones.

注：陽蹻之脈，以附陽爲郄之後，直上循股外廉而上行者，正與少陽之循髀樞下行者往來相遇，陽蹻爲病，動苦腰背痛，又爲癲癎僵臥羊鳴，惡風，偏枯瘴痺，身體强硬等症。

Explanation: after its cleft point, Fù Yáng (BL-59), the vessel of the yángqiāo ascends vertically on the outer ridge of the thigh. It just so happens that this ascending pathway [of the yángqiāo vessel] encounters the incoming shàoyáng pathway that descends following the hip joint.

When the yángqiāo [vessel] is diseased, there will be diseases such as discomfort in movement and pain in the lumbus and upper back; in addition, there may be signs such as epilepsy, lying motionless and making sounds like the bleating of goats, aversion to wind, hemilateral withering with paralysis and impediment, stiffness and rigidity of the whole body.

而少陽之所主病，亦與此類，皆風病也。風之所中，在下體入此穴者多，故曰風市，言風往來之所也。

Moreover, regarding the diseases governed by the shàoyáng, they are also the likes of these, as they are all Fēng (Wind) diseases. Regarding the places where the Fēng (Wind) strikes, in the lower region of the body, [wind] predominantly enters at this point, thus it is called Fēng Shì (Wind Market), this is speaking of the place where Fēng (Wind) comes and goes.

風市之本病：中風腿膝無力，脚氣，渾身搔癢，麻痺，癘風瘡。

Principal diseases of Fēng Shì: wind strike with lack of strength in the leg and knee, leg qì, itchiness all over the body, paralysis, and pestilential wind with sores.

注：風之中腿膝也，多在股膝之側，此穴在風往來之所，取此穴而灸之甚效。

Explanation: when the wind strikes the leg and knee, it predominantly [strikes] the side of the thigh and knee; this point is the place where the wind comes and goes, choose this point and moxa it; it is extremely effective!

Thirty-Second Point of the Gallbladder Channel
Zhōng Dú – Middle River[327] (GB-32)
膽經第三十二穴中瀆

穴在髀外膝上五寸，分肉間陷中，足少陽絡別走厥陰。《銅人》：灸五壯，鍼五分，留七呼。

This point is located 5 cùn above the knee on the outside of the thigh, in the depression at the parting of flesh. It is the foot shàoyáng network point that diverges to the foot juéyīn. *The Tóngrén* states, "Moxa 5 cones, needle 5 fēn, and retain for 7 respirations."

注：瀆者，行水之名，足太陽在其後，足陽明在其前，故曰中瀆。膝下有足少陽之絡，曰光明，去外踝五寸，別走厥陰，此膝下之絡也。此絡乃膝之上，別走厥陰者，下絡管膝下而絡於厥陰，上絡管膝上而絡於厥陰。

Explanation: regarding Dú (River), it is the name of where water flows; as the foot tàiyáng [channel] is located behind it, and the foot yángmíng [channel] is located in front of it, thus it is called Zhōng Dú (Middle River).

There is a network point of the foot shàoyáng [channel] below the knee, it is called Guāng Míng (GB-37), which is located 5 cùn from the outer ankle [bone]; it diverges to the foot juéyīn, serving as the network point below the knee. This network point[328] is above the knee, it [also] diverges to the foot juéyīn [channel]. While the network point below manages [the limb] below the knee and networks with the juéyīn, this network point above manages [the limb] above the knee and also networks with the juéyīn [channel].

中瀆之本病：寒氣客於分肉間，攻痛上下，筋痹不仁。

Principal diseases of Zhōng Dú: cold qì that is lodged in the parting of flesh, pain that attacks the above and below, and sinew impediment with insensitivity.

---

[327] *Grasping the Wind* names it "Central River."
[328] I.e., GB-32.

注：股之能動者，筋主之也，而風之傷筋也，多在股之外，此穴與上穴，皆其所也，故取此穴灸之，以溫其寒。

Explanation: regarding the ability of the thigh to move, the sinews govern it; yet when wind damages the sinews, it predominantly occurs on the outside of the thigh. Both this point and the previous point are locations where [wind damages the sinews], thus choose this point and moxa it in order to warm the cold.

Thirty-Third Point of the Gallbladder Channel
Yáng Guān – Yáng Pass[329] (GB-33)
膽經第三十三穴陽關

一名陽陵
Alternate name: Yáng Mound

穴在陽陵泉上三寸，犢鼻外陷中。《銅人》：鍼五分，禁灸。

This point is located 3 cùn above Yáng Líng Quán (GB-34), in the depression outside of the Dú Bí (ST-35). *The Tóngrén* **states, "Needle 5 fēn, and moxa is contraindicated."**

注：此穴在膝之外，上下兩骨之間，上下之脈過之，下交於上，上交於下，如關然。以爲足少陽之所統也，故曰陽關。

Explanation: as this point is located outside of the knee, between the bones above and below, where the vessels above and below traverse through; this is where the lower [pathways] intersect with the above and where the upper [pathways] intersect with the below, as such, it resembles a Guān (Pass).[330] As it is controlled by the foot shàoyáng, thus it is called Yáng Guān (Yáng Pass).

陽關之本病：風痺不仁，膝痛不可屈伸。

Principal diseases of Yáng Guān: wind impediment with insensitivity, knee pain with inability to bend and stretch.

注：膝之所以能屈伸者，正在此穴之氣血通暢故也。如風寒客之，則上下之氣血爲風寒所滯，而屈伸不能矣，故取此穴，鍼以通其滯氣。禁灸者，此穴之皮薄肉少，恐內傷筋也。

---

[329] *Grasping the Wind* names it "Yáng Joint."

[330] Note: this "關 Pass" should be understood as a fortified gate guarded by military presence, which is typically located at a choke point created by natural landscape and/or artificial fortifications.

Explanation: what enables the knee to bend and stretch, it is precisely because the qì and blood flow freely and smoothly at this point. If wind and cold lodge here, the qì and blood from above and below will become stagnant here; as a result, one will no longer be able to bend and stretch; thus, choose this point and needle it in order to free the stagnated qì. Regarding the contraindication of moxa, this is because the skin is thin and the flesh is thin at this point, there is fear that [moxa] will damage the sinews inside.

Thirty-Fourth Point of the Gallbladder Channel
Yáng Líng Quán – Yáng Mound Spring (GB-34)
膽經第三十四穴陽陵泉

穴在膝下一寸，骱外廉陷中，蹲坐取之，足少陽所入爲合土。《銅人》：鍼六分，留十呼，得氣即泄，又宜久留鍼，日灸七壯至七七壯。《素》注：灸三壯。《明堂》：灸一壯。

This point is located 1 cùn below the knee, in the depression on the outer ridge of the shin, to be located by squatting. The foot shàoyáng enters here, as the uniting and earth point. *The Tóngrén* states, "Needle 6 fēn, retain for 10 respirations,[331] obtain qì and then promptly drain; it is also appropriate to retain the needle for a long period, or to moxa 7 to 49 cones daily." *The Sùzhù* states, "Moxa 3 cones." *The Míngtáng*[332] states, "Moxa 1 cone."

注：穴之稱陵也，以僅在膝之下，膝有高陵之象焉，故曰陵。陽者，以本經而得名也。泉者，乃本經之脈至此下注，有泉之象焉。如本經自下而上昇，又爲所入爲合土，脈自土中出，又有泉象。《難經》曰：筋會陽陵泉。疏曰：筋病治此。

Explanation: this point is named Líng (Mound) because it is nearby the base of the knee; as the knee has an image of a high Líng (Mound), thus [this point] is called Líng (Mound). Regarding Yáng (Yáng), it is named as such because of the channel [it is on]. Regarding Quán (Spring), this is surely because upon arriving here, the vessel of this channel pours into the below, which has the image of a Quán (Spring).

As this channel ascends from the below to enter here as the uniting and earth point, the vessel emerges from earth [at this location], which again has the image of a Quán (Spring). *The Nànjīng* states, "The sinews meet at Yáng Líng Quán

---

[331] "Retain for 10 respirations" is absent in *the Tóngrén*.

[332] "明堂 *The Míngtáng*" is "明下 *the Míngxià*" in both the secondary manuscript and *the Zhēnjiǔ Dàchéng*.

(Yáng Mound Spring)."[333] [*The Nànjīng*] *Shū* states, "For sinew diseases, choose this point."

陽陵泉之本病：膝伸不得屈，髀樞膝骨冷痹，內外廉不仁，偏風半身不遂，腳冷無血色，足筋攣，頭面腫，苦嗌中介然。

Principal diseases of Yáng Líng Quán: the knee can extend but not bend, cold impediment at the thigh pivot and knee bone with insensitivity on both the inside and outside, hemilateral wind with hemiplegia, cold leg with absence of the colour of blood,[334] hypertonicity of the sinews in the leg, swelling of the head and face, and immoveable discomfort in the throat.

注：凡腿腳病，皆筋中風寒濕爲之也，取此穴無不效者，乃筋會此穴故也。若頭腫又爲嗌中介然，亦責之何也？頭腫必在頭之側腫，爲少陽盤折之處，乃風中於上也，上有病取之下，以散其風也。嗌中介然，乃肝病也，肝之經上入頏顙之所爲也。責此穴者，乃上裏有病，散之下表也。

Explanation: in general, all diseases of the legs and feet manifest when the sinews are struck by wind, cold, or damp; it is unheard of that it would not work by choosing this point, because the sinews meet at this point.

As for swelling of the head and immoveable discomfort in the throat, for what reason should one seek this [point]? This swelling of the head must be swelling located on the side of the head, at the location where the shàoyáng [channel] turns and winds; [the swelling] is caused by wind strike at the above; when there is a disease above, choose [a point] below in order to disperse the wind. Regarding the immoveable discomfort in the throat, this is surely a liver disease because the liver channel ascends to enter the nasopharynx [region]. This point is sought because when the interior [partner] is diseased above, disperse it from below with its exterior [partner].

Thirty-Fifth Point of the Gallbladder Channel
Yáng Jiāo – Yáng Intersection (GB-35)
膽經第三十五穴陽交

一名別陽
Alternate name: Divergent Yáng

一名足窌
Alternate name: Leg Bone-Hole

---

[333] From *Nànjīng* Difficulty 45.
[334] I.e., absence of a healthy skin colour.

穴在足外踝上七寸，斜屬三陽分肉之間，陽維之郄。《銅人》：鍼六分，留六呼，灸三壯。

This point is located 7 cùn above the outer ankle [bone], it obliquely adjoins to the space at the parting of flesh in between the three yáng [channels]. It is the cleft point of the yángwéi [vessel]. *The Tóngrén* **states, "Needle 6 fēn, retain for 6 respirations,[335] and moxa 3 cones."**

注：陽維自下來者，以此穴爲郄，而遇少陽過之，此穴兩陽相遇，故曰陽交。

Explanation: from the below, the yángwéi [vessel] arrives at this point, which serves as its cleft point; thereupon, it encounters the shàoyáng [channel] that is traversing through [this point]. As this point is where the two Yáng (Yáng) [vessels] encounter each other,[336] thus it is called Yáng Jiāo (Yáng Intersection).

陽交之本病：胸滿腫膝痛，足不收，寒厥驚狂，喉痹面腫，寒痹膝胻不收。

Principal diseases of Yáng Jiāo: fullness and swelling in the chest with knee pain, loss of use of the legs, cold reversal with fright mania, throat impediment with swollen face, cold impediment of the knee and lower leg with loss of use.

注：足膝痛，足不收，膝胻不收，寒厥驚狂，皆本經受風寒之邪所致，故宜泄此穴，以去本經之風寒，兼灸以溫之。至驚狂喉痹之病，則本經之火有餘也，取此穴以泄上逆之火。胸滿腫，乃肝氣上逆也，泄膽所以泄肝也。

Explanation: regarding pain in the legs and knees, loss of use of the legs, loss of use of the knees and lower legs, cold reversal with fright mania, all of these are a result of this channel contracting wind and cold evil, thus it is appropriate to drain this point in order to eliminate the wind and cold in this channel, and concurrently moxa in order to warm it.

When there is a disease of fright mania with throat impediment, this is because of the superabundance of fire in the channel, choose this point in order to drain the counterflow ascent of fire. Fullness and swelling in the chest are due to counterflow ascent of liver qì, drain the gallbladder so as to drain the liver.

---

[335] For "retain for 6 respirations," *the Tóngrén* actually states "retain for 7 respirations.".
[336] I.e., the yángwéi vessel and shàoyáng channel.

Thirty-Sixth Point of the Gallbladder Channel
Wài Qiū – Outer Hill (GB-36)
膽經第三十六穴外丘

穴在外踝上六寸，少陽所生。《銅人》：鍼三分，灸三壯。

This point is located 6 cùn above the outer ankle [bone]. It is where the shàoyáng engenders.[337] ***The Tóngrén* states, "Needle 3 fēn, and moxa 3 cones."**

注：陽交之下於此穴稍高，乃向後稍，自外踝而上六寸，而稍斜向後，得其肉之稍高處是穴，故曰外丘，對厥陰之在外處稍高爲丘。

Explanation: this point (GB-36) is below Yáng Jiāo (GB-35), as the latter (GB-35) is slightly higher and slightly behind it (GB-36). Ascend 6 cùn from the outer ankle [bone] and turn slightly backwards, where the flesh is slightly elevated by palpation, that is the point; thus, it is called Wài Qiū (Outer Hill), which is in accordance with its location on the Wài (Outside) of the juéyīn and its slightly elevated [flesh] as the Qiū (Hill).

外丘之本病：癲疾瘻痺，頭項痛，惡風寒，猘犬咬傷毒不出，發寒熱，速以三壯艾，可灸所咬處及足少陽絡光明穴，兼灸此穴。

Principal diseases of Wài Qiū: epileptic disease with wilting and impediment, pain in the head and nape, and aversion to wind and cold; for rabid dog bite with undischarged toxin as well as chills and fever, swiftly moxa 3 cones; one

---

[337] This strange phrase, literally, "少陽所生 this is where/what the shàoyáng engenders," appears at this point and at GB-38. For GB-38, this phrase most certainly indicates that it is the child point of the gallbladder channel, as wood engenders fire; thus, it is the child point where the gallbladder wood channel engenders the fire phase; however, it proves problematic here, as this point is not a fire point. One possible explanation could be drawn from Dr. Wei-Chieh Young's contemporary analysis of the Master Tung points, where he proposes that assignments of the five phases should not be confined to certain selected points but should be applied to wider regions; as such, for points that fall between two phases, they are endowed with the affinity of the two adjacent phases. Thus, for GB-36, as it falls between an earth point and a fire point, it has affinity to both fire and earth phases. So, in this case, it can also serve as a child point to engender the fire phase. Another possibility is that GB-36 could also have been a fire point at certain time periods in history or by certain acupuncture lineages, and *the Míngtáng* simply preserves this alternate opinion before GB-38 became the commonly accepted fire point by the time of *Língshū* (i.e., when the five transport points were assigned) and *Nànjīng* (i.e., when five phases were assigned to the five transport points). Such idea may be possible, as most of its indications seem to be replete signs that require draining. Nevertheless, this still awaits more investigation and lies outside the scope of this translation. Alternatively, 少陽所生 can also be interpreted as "it is engendered by the shàoyáng;" however, it is equally questionable as it would not provide any information besides stating that it is also a point of the foot shàoyáng channel.

can moxa the location of the bite and the foot shàoyáng network point Guāng Míng (GB-37), in addition to this point.

注：前症皆本經中風之症，故取此穴。猘犬傷，亦灸此穴者，治風毒之外入者也。

Explanation: all of the above signs are signs of wind strike at this channel, thus choose this point. When there is bite from a rabid dog, moxa this point as it will treat the wind toxin that has entered from the exterior.

外丘之肺病：胸脹滿，膚痛，小兒龜胸。

Lung diseases of Wài Qiū: distension and fullness in the chest, skin pain, and pigeon chest in children.

注：前症皆肝氣之逆於胸也，泄此穴，以降肝上逆之氣於其表經。

Explanation: all of the above signs are due to counterflow of liver qì in the chest, drain this point in order to descend the ascending counterflow of liver qì in its exterior [pair] channel.

Thirty-Seventh Point of the Gallbladder Channel
Guāng Míng – Bright Light (GB-37)
膽經第三十七穴光明

穴在外踝上五寸，足少陽之絡別走厥陰。《銅人》：鍼六分，留七呼，灸五壯。《明堂》：灸七壯。

This point is located 5 cùn above the outer ankle [bone]. It is the network point of the foot shàoyáng that diverges to the foot juéyīn [channel]. *The Tóngrén* **states, "Needle 6 fēn, retain for 7 respirations, and moxa 5 cones."** *The Míngtáng*[338] **states, "Moxa 7 cones."**

注：光明之義，無所發明，豈陽有絡以通於陰，以氣相通，有光明之可見耶？難以強解，尚侯高明。虛則痿躄，坐不能起，補之。實則足跗熱，膝痛，身體不仁，善嚙煩，泄之。

Explanation: regarding the meaning of Guāng Míng (Bright Light), I can offer no elucidation. Could it be that the yáng [channel] has a network-vessel that communicates with the yīn [channel] and that they communicate with each other via qì, so that one is able to perceive Guāng Míng (Bright Light)? As it is difficult to

---

[338] "明堂 *The Míngtáng*" is "明下 *the Míngxià*" in both the secondary manuscript and *the Zhēnjiǔ Dàchéng*.

have a compelling explanation, I will leave it for future people of brilliance and knowledge [to explain].

When [the network-vessel] is vacuous, there will be crippling wilt and inability to get up from sitting, supplement it; when it is replete, there will be heat on the instep, knee pain, insensitivity of the body, and tendency to gnaw the cheeks, drain it.

光明之本病：淫瀯，脛痠胻痛，不能久立，熱病汗不出，卒狂。

Principal diseases of Guāng Míng: pain and weakness, aches and pain in the lower leg, inability to stand for long periods, febrile disease with absence of sweating, and sudden mania.

注：脛胻之症，皆本經正症，爲風寒之邪所致而生，宜補而灸之。熱病汗不出而卒狂，宜泄少陽之火，故取此絡穴以泄之，乃實症也。

Explanation: for signs of the lower legs, in all cases, they are principal signs of this channel, and they are engendered from [the contraction of] cold and wind evils, it is appropriate to supplement and moxa it. For febrile disease with absence of sweating and sudden mania, it is appropriate to drain the fire of shàoyáng, thus choose this network point and drain it, as these are surely replete signs.

Thirty-Eighth Point of the Gallbladder Channel
Yáng Fǔ – Yáng Assistance (GB-38)
膽經第三十八穴陽輔

一名分肉
Alternate name: Parting of the Flesh

穴在足外踝上四寸，輔骨之前，絕骨之端三分，去足上丘墟穴七寸，足少陽所行爲經火，膽經實則泄之。《素》注：鍼三分。又曰：鍼七分，留十呼。《銅人》：灸三壯，鍼五分，留七呼。

This point is located 4 cùn above the outer ankle [bone], in front of the assisting bone,[339] 3 fēn from the tip of the severed bone,[340] and 7 cùn above Qiū Xū (GB-40) on the foot. The foot shàoyáng flows here, as the river and fire point; when the gallbladder channel is replete, drain it. *The Sùzhù* states, "Needle 3 fēn." It also states, "Needle 7 fēn, and retain for 10 respirations." *The Tóngrén* states, "Moxa 3 cones, needle 5 fēn, and retain for 7 respirations."

---

[339] I.e., the fibula.

[340] Note: Jué Gǔ 絕骨 (severed bone) is also the name for GB-39.

注：此穴乃少陽之經穴爲火，乃本經所生。曰陽輔者，乃陽極盛之稱，木旺極則生火之義也。

Explanation: this point is the river and fire point of the shàoyáng [channel], it is surely where this channel engenders.[341] Regarding the name of Yáng Fǔ (Yáng Assistance), it is indicative of the utmost exuberance of Yáng (Yáng) as well as the concept that fire will be engendered from the utmost effulgence of wood.

陽輔之本病：腰溶溶如坐水中，膝下浮腫，筋攣，百節疼痛，實無所知，諸節盡痛無常處，喉痺，腋下腫瘻，馬刀挾癭，膝胻疼痛，風痺不仁，厥逆善太息。心脇痛，面塵頭角頷痛，目銳眥痛，缺盆中腫痛，胸中脇肋、髀膝外至絕骨外踝前痛，善潔面青，汗出振寒瘧。

Principal diseases of Yáng Fǔ: dissolution of the lumbus that appears as though one has been sitting in water, puffy swelling below the knees, hypertonicity of the sinews, pain and aching in the one hundred joints yet without knowing the precise location, severe pain in all joints without a fixed location, throat impediment, armpit swelling and wilting, sabre and pearl-string lumps,[342] aching pain in the knees and lower legs, wind impediment with insensitivity, and reverse flow with frequent sighing; pain of the heart and rib-sides, dusty facial complexion with pain at the corners of the head and chin, pain at the outer canthus, pain and swelling at Quē Pén (ST-12), chest, rib-sides, and costal region, pain from the hip and outer knee to the severed bone and the front of the outer ankle [bone], tendency towards cleanliness with green-blue face, sweating with shivering and cold malaria.

注：以上各症，少陽之症可謂備矣，而皆責此一穴者，以少陽本經爲木，而中有相火，此穴乃爲經火之穴，故少陽經風邪、寒邪、火邪、一切有餘之症，皆取此穴者，以泄本經之有餘也，所謂盛則泄其子也。

Explanation: for the various signs above, one may say that they fully account for all signs of the shàoyáng; yet, one ought to always seek this single point, because the shàoyáng channel is wood and possesses the ministerial fire within it; in addition, as this point is indeed [the channel's] river and fire point, thus for [signs of] wind evil, cold evil, fire evils, as well as all signs of superabundance in the shàoyáng channel, this point is always chosen in order to drain the superabundance of this channel, which is known as, "when there is exuberance, drain the child."[343]

---

[341] I.e., it is the child point where the wood channel engenders the fire phase. See also footnote 337 in GB-36.

[342] I.e., scrofula.

[343] From *Nànjīng* Difficulty 69.

Thirty-Ninth Point of the Gallbladder Channel
Xuán Zhōng – Suspended Goblet[344] (GB-39)
膽經第三十九穴懸鍾

一名絕骨
Alternate name: Severed Bone

穴在足外踝上三寸動脈中，尋摸尖骨者是，足三陽之大絡，按之陽明脈絕，乃取之。《銅人》：鍼六分，留七呼，灸五壯。《指微》：斜入鍼二寸許，灸五壯或七壯。

This point is located on the pulsating vessel 3 cùn above the outer ankle [bone], where a sharp and bony object can be palpated. It is the great network point of the three leg yáng; by pressing it (GB-39), the yángmíng pulse ceases, that is how to locate it. *The Tóngrén* states, "Needle 6 fēn, retain for 7 respirations, and moxa 5 cones." *The Zhǐwēi* states, "Insert the needle obliquely with slightly more than 2 cùn [in depth], and moxa 5 or 7 cones."

注：穴名懸鍾者，以其上懸肉開分如鍾形，穴在其內，故曰懸鍾。《難經》云：髓會絕骨。髓病治此。袁氏曰：足能健步，以髓會絕骨也。足三陽從上下者，由頭而至於足，至此穴皆有絡以相通，故曰三陽之大絡。

Explanation: this point is named Xuán Zhōng (Suspended Goblet) because the flesh Xuán (Suspended) above divides up to resemble the shape of a Zhōng (Goblet);[345] as this point is located inside of this [goblet], thus it is called Xuán Zhōng (Suspended Goblet).

The Nànjīng states, "The marrow meets at Jué Gǔ (Severed Bone)." [*The Nànjīng Shū* states], "For marrow diseases, treat this point."[346] Mister Yuán[347] said,

---

[344] *Grasping the Wind* names it "Suspended Bell." Note: The homophonic characters zhōng 鍾 (goblet) and zhōng 鐘 (bell) look very similar and are often used interchangeably in modern times, either by intention or by mistake; in addition, simplified Chinese simply combine them two into one single character of 钟 zhōng, which further adds to the confusion; nonetheless, they carry different meanings according *the Shuōwén Jiězì* 説文解字 (*Explaining Graphs and Analysing Characters*, 2nd century CE). For that reason, we are changing the name to goblet instead of bell, so that it can better reflect its original meaning.

[345] Note: this likely refers to the ancient Chinese goblet, which is commonly called "bronze tripod wine vessel." The flesh above this point resembles the main body of such a goblet, while the flesh that splits to the front and back resemble two legs of the goblet.

[346] "*The Nànjīng Shū* states" has been supplemented to clarify the reference, as the following quote is not found in the *Nànjīng* itself. The same convention is applied to the other Eight Meeting Points.

[347] This is Yuán Kūnhòu 袁坤厚, author of *Nànjīng Běnzhǐ* 難經本旨 (*the Original Purport of the Nànjīng*, c. 14th century CE), which is no longer extant.

"what enables one to be able to walk briskly in strides, it is because the marrow meets at Jué Gǔ (Severed Bone)." As the three leg yáng [channels] descend from the above, from the head[348] towards the feet, when they arrive at this point, there is a network-vessel that communicates all of them with one another, thus it is said to be the great network point of the three yáng.

惟有絡以相通，故按此穴，則足上跗陽之脈絕，乃其紀也。如不絕，再於上下求之，其動脈甚細，須細求之方得。此處皮肉甚薄，故宜斜入，不宜正下。鍼斜入二寸，所以管三陽之大絡也。

It is only because that [this point] has a network-vessel which communicates [with the other channels], that upon applying pressure to this point, the [yángmíng] pulse on the foot instep will Jué (Cease), that is why [its name] was recorded as such. Suppose that [the pulse] does not Jué (Cease), again, search the above and below;[349] as the pulsating vessel is extremely fine, one must search carefully in order to locate [this point]. At this location, the skin and flesh are extremely thin, thus it is appropriate to needle it obliquely, it is not appropriate to needle it perpendicularly. It is needled obliquely to a depth of 2 cùn, so that it can manage the great network-vessel of the three yáng.

懸鍾之本病：腳氣膝胻痛，筋氣痛，足不收，喉痹，頸項強，陰急，中風手足不遂，憂恚。

Principal diseases of Xuán Zhōng: leg qì with pain in the knee and lower leg, sinew and qì pain,[350] loss of use of the legs, throat impediment, stiffness of the neck and nape, tension in the genitals, wind stroke with paralysis of the limbs, anxiety and rage.

注：前症皆因風火濕寒之邪，中於本經，而有是症，宜於此穴泄之。

Explanation: all of the above signs are caused by evils of wind, fire, damp, and cold; when the channel is [struck by these evils], there will be these signs, it is appropriate to drain this point.

懸鍾之胃病：心腹脹滿，胃中熱，不嗜食，泄注，心中咳逆。

Stomach diseases of Xuán Zhōng: distension and fullness in the heart [region] and abdomen, heat in the stomach, no pleasure in eating, outpour diarrhoea, coughing and counterflow in the heart [region].

---

[348] "由頭 from the head" is originally "將胸 from the chest." The editors of this manuscript, Zhāng and Zhà, have changed it in accordance with the secondary manuscript.

[349] I.e., to find the place where it causes the pulse to cease.

[350] "筋氣痛 Sinew and qì pain" is "骨筋攣痛 pain and hypertonicity of the sinews and bones" in the *Zhēnjiǔ Dàchéng*.

注：胃病而亦責此穴者，以本經至此穴，而與足陽明胃經有相通之處，故胃經病亦泄此穴。

Explanation: [for these] stomach diseases, this point is also chosen because when this channel arrives at this point, it is in a location where it communicates with the foot yángmíng stomach channel; thus, for stomach diseases, [one can] also drain this point.

懸鍾之肺病：鼻衄，腸痔瘀血，鼻乾逆氣，煩滿狂易，虛勞寒損。

Lung diseases of Xuán Zhōng: nosebleed, haemorrhoids with blood stasis, dry nose with counterflow qì, vexation and fullness with mania, and vacuity taxation with cold detriment.

注：前症雖肺病也，而少陽之相火與肝之火逆於肺中，亦能致是症，故泄膽經之火以降之。虛勞寒損，宜補此絡穴以足三陽之氣。

Explanation: although the above signs are lung diseases, when there is a counterflow of [both] the shàoyáng ministerial fire and liver fire into the lung, it will also cause these signs; thus drain the fire of the gallbladder channel in order to descend it. Regarding vacuity taxation with cold detriment, it is appropriate to supplement this network point in order to replenish the qì of the three leg yáng [channels].

懸鍾之太陽病：腦疽，二便閉澀。

Tàiyáng diseases of Xuán Zhōng: flat-abscess of the brain, blocked and rough urination and defecation.

注：腦疽乃太陽病也，以此穴而有絡通太陽，故責此穴，以泄太陽之火於下。二便乃膀胱病也，以本穴有絡通太陽，故並取之，以降太陽之滯氣，而大、小便不滯矣。

Explanation: flat-abscess of the brain is indeed a tàiyáng disease, as this point has a network-vessel that communicates with the tàiyáng, thus seek this point in order to drain the fire of the tàiyáng from the below. [Blocked and rough] urination and defecation are surely bladder diseases, as this point has a network-vessel that communicates with the tàiyáng [channel], thus also choose this [point] in order to descend the stagnant qì of the tàiyáng [channel], so that the stool and urine will no longer be stagnant.

Fortieth Point of the Gallbladder Channel
Qiū Xū – Hill Village[351] (GB-40)
膽經第四十穴丘墟

穴在足外踝下，從前陷中骨縫中，去臨泣三寸。又挾谿穴中量上外踝前五寸，足
少陽所過爲原，膽虛實皆拔之。《銅人》：灸三壯。《素》注：鍼五分，留七呼。
《神農經》云：治肋下痛不得息，小腹腎痛，脚腕痛，可灸七壯。

**This point is located below the outer ankle [bone], in the depression in front
[of the ankle bone], in the bone juncture, and 3 cùn from [Zú] Lín Qì (GB-41).
Alternatively, it is 5 cùn above Xiá Xī (GB-43) and in front of the outer ankle
[bone]. The foot shàoyáng traverses here, as the source point. Whether the
gallbladder is vacuous or replete, it will eliminate [the disease].** *The Tóngrén*
states, "Moxa 3 cones." *The Sùzhù* **states, "Needle 5 fēn, and retain for 7
respirations."** *The Shénnóng Jīng* **states, "To treat pain under the rib-sides with
inability to catch the breath, lower abdominal and kidney pain, pain of the
leg[352] and ankle,[353] one can moxa 7 cones."**

注：穴名丘墟者，以在外踝前，外踝之骨大而圓，有丘象焉，其穴在前，
有墟象焉，故曰丘墟。乃膽經入足之始穴，如自竅陰上行，則又爲離足之絡穴，虛
實皆拔之。凡治膽經病，任鍼井、滎、腧、經、合各穴，於原穴一穴，應補則同
補，泄則同泄焉。

Explanation: this point is named Qiū Xū (Hill Village), as it is located in front
of the outer ankle [bone]; the bone of the outer ankle is large and round, which has
the image of a Qiū (Hill); as this point is located in front [of it], it has the image of Xū
(Village), thus it is called Qiū Xū (Hill Village). Indeed, this is where the points of the
gallbladder channel begin to enter the foot. By ascending from [Zú] Qiào Yīn (GB-
44), there is also the network point that departs from the foot; therefore, whether
there is a vacuous or replete [condition], it will always eliminate [the disease].

Whenever one treats diseases of the gallbladder channel, no matter what
one needles, the well point, the brook point, the stream point, the river point, or the
uniting point, one ought to supplement this one point of source point[354]
concurrently when one supplements, and drains [this source point] concurrently
when one drains.

---

351 *Grasping the Wind* names it "Hill Ruins."
352 For "脚 leg," the secondary manuscript has "脚氣 leg qì."
353 Lit. "wrist," which is at times used for ankle as well.
354 For "於原穴一穴 as for the one point of source point," the secondary manuscript has, "原
穴一穴鍼 needle the one point of source point."

丘墟之本病：久瘧振寒，腋下腫，痿厥坐不能起，髀樞中痛，腿胻痛轉筋，卒疝，小腹堅，寒熱頸腫，腰痛太息，胸肋滿痛不得息。

Principal diseases of Qiū Xū: chronic malaria with shivering and chills, swelling of the armpit, wilting reversal with inability to get up from sitting, pain at the thigh pivot,[355] pain and cramping of the leg and calf, sudden mounting, hardness of the lower abdomen, chills and fever with swelling of the neck, lumbar pain with great respiration, fullness and pain of the chest and rib-sides with inability to catch the breath.

注：前症皆少陽經本症也，熱應泄，寒應補，皆取此穴，或降其氣，通其滯。

Explanation: all of the above signs are principal signs of the shàoyáng channel; for heat, one ought to drain; for cold, one ought to supplement. In both cases, one should choose this point to either descend the qì or free the stagnation.

Forty-First Point of the Gallbladder Channel
[Zú] Lín Qì – [Foot] Overlooking Tears (GB-41)
膽經第四十一穴臨泣

穴在足小指次指本節後陷中，去俠谿一寸五分，足少陽所注爲腧木。《甲乙》：鍼二分，留五呼，灸三壯。《千金》：頸漏，腋下馬刀，灸百壯。

This point is located in the depression behind the base joint of the fourth toe, 1 cùn 5 fēn from Xiá Xī (GB-43). The foot shàoyáng pours here, as the stream and wood point. *The Jiǎyǐ* states, "Needle 2 fēn, retain for 5 respirations, and moxa 3 cones." *The Qiānjīn* states, "For neck fistulae, sabre lumps under the armpit, moxa 100 cones."

注：少陽經有二臨泣，在額上者，下臨目之泣也，在足上者，目之臨泣在下也，此穴乃少陽之支別者，別行入大指，循歧骨內，出大指端，還貫入爪甲，出三毛，以交於足厥陰肝經也。

Explanation: the shàoyáng channel has two Lín Qì (Overlooking Tears) [points]; for the one that is located on the head above (GB-15), it descends to Lín (Overlook) the Qì (Tears) of eyes; for the one that is located on the foot (GB-41), it is Lín Qì (Overlooking Tears, GB-15) of the eyes in the below.

At this point, a diverging branch of the shàoyáng [channel] diverges to enter the big toe, follows the inside of where the bones diverge, emerges at the tip of the

---

355 I.e., the greater trochanter.

large toe, where it turns to pierce and enter the nail, re-emerging at [the region of] the three hairs, in order to intersect with the foot juéyīn liver channel.

臨泣之本病：胸中痛，缺盆中及腋下馬刀瘍瘻，善嚙煩，天牖穴中滿，淫濼胻痠，目眩，枕骨合顱痛，洒淅振寒，心痛，周痺痛無常處，瘩瘧日發，婦人月事不利，季脇支滿，乳癰。

Principal diseases of [Zú] Lín Qì: pain in the chest, sabre lumps with open sores and fistulae in the supraclavicular fossa and armpit, tendency to gnaw on the cheeks, fullness at Tiān Yǒu (SJ-16), pain and weakness with aching lower leg, dizzy vision, pain at the pillow bone and skull union, shivering with cold as though after a soaking, heart pain, generalised impediment and pain without a fixed location, intervallic malaria with daily occurrence, inhibited menstruation in women, propping fullness in the free ribs, and mammary welling-abscess.

注：前症皆本經之正症，或爲火逆於上，或被風寒之邪客於上，本穴爲腧木，乃助少陽之火者，故取此穴，而泄其氣於下。

Explanation: all of the above signs are principal signs of this channel, possibly because of counterflow fire above, or possibly because of lodged evil of wind cold above; as this point is the stream and wood point, it is surely what exacerbates the fire of shàoyáng, thus choose this point and drain the qì from below.

臨泣之肺病：厥逆氣喘，不能行。

Lung diseases of [Zú] Lín Qì: reverse flow with panting, and inability to walk.

注：氣喘雖爲肺病，而厥逆、四肢寒，乃筋病也，故責膽經之腧木而泄之。此穴在八法，與奇經帶脈相通，與外關主客相應。

Explanation: although panting is a lung disease, yet, reverse flow and cold sensation in the four limbs are sinew diseases, thus seek the stream and wood point of the gallbladder channel and drain it. Among the eight confluence points, this point communicates with the dài vessel of the eight extraordinary channels; furthermore, it corresponds with Wài Guān (SJ-5) as the host and guest.

Forty-Second Point of the Gallbladder Channel
Dì Wǔ Huì – Earth Fivefold Meeting[356] (GB-42)
膽經第四十二穴地五會

穴在足小指次指本節後陷中，去俠谿一寸，《銅人》：鍼一分，禁灸。

This point is located in the depression behind the base joint of the fourth toe, 1 cùn from Xiá Xī (GB-43). *The Tóngrén* states, "Needle 1 fēn,[357] and moxa is contraindicated."

注：少陽之穴，在足者有五穴，而肝經之太衝穴，有絡橫連地五會，如木之有根在地。此穴乃肝經相會之地也，故曰地五會。

Explanation: for points of the shàoyáng [channel], there are Wǔ (Five) points located on the foot; in addition, Tài Chōng (LR-3) of the liver channel has a network-vessel that horizontally links it with Dì Wǔ Huì (Earth Fivefold Meeting), as though a tree planting its roots in the Dì (Earth). As this point is the Huì (Meeting) place with the liver channel, thus is it called Dì Wǔ Huì (Earth Fivefold Meeting).

地五會之本病：腋痛，足外無膏澤。

Principal diseases of Dì Wǔ Huì: armpit pain, lack of oily lustre on the outside of the feet.

注：腋痛乃本經之氣上逆也，泄之在下。足外無膏澤，乃本經血少也，宜補之。

Explanation: armpit pain is due to counterflow ascent of the qì of this channel, drain it from that which is located below. For the lack of oily lustre on the outside of the feet, this is because the principal channel has scant blood, it is appropriate to supplement it.

地五會之胃病：乳癰。

Stomach disease of Dì Wǔ Huì: mammary welling-abscess.

注：乳病雖陽明經症，而胸脇亦肝膽之火所致之處，泄其下以散少陽之火。

Explanation: although mammary welling-abscess is a yángmíng channel sign, yet the chest and rib-sides are also locations that are affected by the fire of liver and gallbladder, drain it below in order to disperse the fire of shàoyáng.

---

[356] *Grasping the Wind* names it "Earth Fivefold Convergence."
[357] For "1 fēn," *the Tóngrén* actually states "2 fēn."

地五會之肺病：內損脫血。

Lung disease of Dì Wǔ Huì: internal injury with blood desertion.

注：此雖爲肺症，肝膽上炎，則有是症，宜泄此穴，以降少陽之火。

Explanation: although this is a lung sign, when the liver and gallbladder blaze upwards, there will be this sign, it is appropriate to drain this point in order to descend the fire of shàoyáng.

Forty-Third Point of the Gallbladder Channel
Xiá Xī – Clasped Ravine[358] (GB-43)
膽經第四十三穴俠谿

穴在足小指次指歧骨間，本節前陷中，足少陽所溜爲滎水，膽實則泄之。《素》注：鍼三分，留三呼，灸三壯。

This point is located in the space where the bones of the little toe and fourth toe diverge, in the depression in front of the base joint. The foot shàoyáng gushes here, as the brook and water point. When the gallbladder is replete, drain it. *The Sùzhù* states, "Needle 3 fēn, retain for 3 respirations, and moxa 3 cones."

注：穴在二指歧骨之間，故曰俠，所溜爲滎水，故曰谿。

Explanation: this point is located in the space where the two toes diverge, thus it is called Xiá (Clasped); since it gushes as the brook and water point, it is thus called Xī (Ravine).

俠谿之本病：胸中痛不可轉側，痛無常處，耳聾，目外眥赤，目眩，煩頷腫，胸脇支滿，寒熱，傷寒之熱病汗不出。

Principal diseases of Xiá Xī: pain in the chest with inability to turn to the side, pain without a fixed location, deafness, redness in the outer canthus of the eye, dizzy vision, swelling of the cheek and under the chin, propping fullness of the chest and rib-sides, chills and fevers,[359] and febrile disease of cold damage with absence of sweating.

---

[358] *Grasping the Wind* names it "Pinched Ravine."

[359] "Chills and fever" is originally absent in the manuscript. The editors of this manuscript, Zhāng and Zhà, have amended it according to the *Zhēnjiǔ Dàchéng* and explanation in the subsequent paragraph.

注：以上皆少陽本經正病，宜泄其水穴，所以生木，子盛則泄其母之義。
寒熱，傷寒汗不出，乃傳入少陽經之傷寒也，宜補此水穴，以出其少陽之汗。

Explanation: as all the above are principal diseases of the shàoyáng channel, it is appropriate to drain the water point, so that wood can be engendered; this is the meaning of "when the child is exuberant, drain its mother."[360] Regarding chills and fever, cold damage with absence of sweating, this is due to the transmission of cold damage into the shàoyáng channel, it is appropriate to supplement the water point in order to discharge the sweat of shàoyáng.

Forty-Fourth Point of the Gallbladder Channel
[Zú] Qiào Yīn – [Foot] Yīn Opening[361] (GB-44)
膽經第四十四穴竅陰

穴在足小指次指外側，去爪甲角如韭葉，足少陽所出爲井金。《素》注：鍼一
分，留一呼。《甲乙》：留三呼，灸三壯。

This point is located on the outer side of the fourth toe,[362] at one chive leaf's width from the nail corner. The foot shàoyáng emerges here, as the well and metal point. *The Sùzhù states, "Needle 1 fēn, and retain for 1 respiration." The Jiǎyǐ states, "Retain for 3 respirations, and moxa 3 cones."*

注：膽經有二竅陰，一在頭上，一在足下。少陽木也，木之井穴，如木之
根生於地也，故曰陰，必有竅焉，以爲生木之本，故曰竅陰。井亦竅也，陽不離乎
陰，以見陰陽相須之義。

Explanation: the gallbladder channel has two Qiào Yīn (Yīn Opening) [points]; one is located above on the head (GB-11), while the other is located below on the foot (GB-44). As the [leg] shàoyáng is of the wood [phase], this well point of wood resemble the roots of wood that are engendered within the soil, thus it is called Yīn (Yīn); [within the soil], there must [also] be a Qiào [Opening], so that it may serve as the foundation where wood is engendered; therefore, it is called [Zú] Qiào Yīn ([Foot] Yīn Opening). In addition, a well is also a Qiào (Opening). As yáng cannot depart from within Yīn (Yīn), from this, one can observe the meaning of the mutual reliance of Yīn (Yīn) and yáng.

---

[360] This seems to allude to the concept of "母能令子虛 [treating] the mother can make the child vacuous" found in *Nànjīng* Difficulty 75.

[361] *Grasping the Wind* names it "Portal Yīn."

[362] Lit. the toe next to the little toe.

竅陰之本病：脇痛，咳逆不得息，轉筋，肘不得舉，卒聾，目痛小眥痛，頭痛心煩，手足煩熱，汗不出，魘夢。

Principal diseases of [Zú] Qiào Yīn: rib-side pain, cough and counterflow with inability to catch the breath, cramps, inability to raise the elbow, sudden deafness, pain of the eye and outer canthus, headache with heart vexation, heat vexation in the hands and feet, absence of sweating, and nightmares.

注：脇也、筋也、肋也、耳也、目小眥也，皆少陽之經上行部分，上有邪，宜泄之下也。頭痛必偏頭痛，而後可責之。少陽之傷寒，汗不出者，方可責之此穴。肝藏魂者也，肝有邪而夢爲之魘，宜補此穴，以逐肝之邪，補膽所以補肝也。

Explanation: the rib-sides, sinews, costal region, ears, and outer canthus, these are all areas where the channel of shàoyáng travels through; when there is evil above, it is appropriate to drain it below. This headache must be a hemilateral headache, then one can seek this [point].

In cold damage of shàoyáng, one can only seek this point for those with absence of sweating. As the liver stores the ethereal soul, when there is evil in the liver, the dreams will become nightmares; it is appropriate to supplement this point in order to expel the evil of the liver, because by supplementing the gallbladder, one is able to supplement the liver.

竅陰之肺病：喉痺舌強，口乾。

Lung diseases of [Zú] Qiào Yīn: throat impediment with stiff tongue, and dry mouth.

注：喉雖爲肺竅，舌雖爲心竅，口雖爲脾竅，膽之經上通頏顙，少陽之火助之而喉痺也，口乾也，舌強也。皆相火逆也，故從井泄之。

Explanation: although the throat is the lung's orifice, although the tongue is the heart's orifice, although the mouth is the spleen's orifice, the channel of the gallbladder [also] ascends to communicate with the nasopharynx region. As the fire of shàoyáng exacerbates [this region], there will be throat impediment, dry mouth, and stiff tongue; these are all due to counterflow of ministerial fire, thus utilise the well point to drain it.

Extra Points Associated with the Foot Shàoyáng Gallbladder Channel
足少陽膽經奇穴

Fish's Tail (UEX-HN 16)
Yú Wěi – 魚尾

在目眥外頭，兼睛明、太陽，治目症。

This point is located on the outer canthus; along with the points Jīng Míng (BL-1) and Tài Yáng (EX-HN 5), they treat eye diseases.

Yáng Wéi [Point] (UEX-HN 22)
Yáng Wéi – 陽維

在耳後，引耳令前，弦筋上是穴。《千金》云：耳風聾雷鳴，灸陽維十五壯。

This point is behind the ear; pull the ear forwards, this point is located above the string-like sinew. *The Qiānjīn* states "For wind deafness with thunderous [ringing], moxa 15 cones on Yáng Wéi (UEX-HN 22)."

On the Yáng (EX-HN 2)
Dāng Yáng- 當陽

當瞳子，直入髮際內一寸，去臨泣五分是穴。主治頭風眩暈，疼痛，延久不愈，灸三壯。

This point is in a straight line with the pupil, 1 cùn into the hairline, and 5 fēn from [Tóu] Lín Qì (GB-15). To govern the treatment of head wind, dizziness, and headache, that are persistent and failing to recover, moxa 3 cones.

Temple Region (UEX-HN 15)
Niè Rú – 顳顬

《千金翼》云：顳顬在眉眼尾中間，上下有來去絡脈是，鍼灸之所主治，疸氣溫病。

The Qiānjīn Yì states, "Niè Rú (UEX-HN 15) is located in the middle between the eyebrow and the outer corner of the eye, where there is a network-vessel that comes and goes, whether above or below. By needling and moxa, [this point] governs the treatment of jaundice qì and warm diseases.

Point Above the Ear[363] (UEN-HN 19)
Ěr Shàng Xué – 耳上穴

《千金翼》云：治癭氣，灸風池及耳上髮際，各百壯。《千金》作兩耳後髮際。

The Qiānjīn Yì states, "To treat goitre qì, moxa Fēng Chí (GB-20) and Ěr Shàng [Xué] (UEN-HN 19) on the hairline, 100 cones at each [point]." *The Qiānjīn* states, "It is behind both ears on the hairline."

Rib-side Hall (UEX-CA 25)
Xié Tang – 脇堂

在腋下骨間陷中，舉腋取之。主治胸脇氣滿，噎噫喘逆，目黃，遠視晾晾，可灸五壯。

This point is located in the depression between the bones under the armpit; raise the arm to find it. To govern the treatment of fullness of qì in the chest and rib-sides, belching with panting counterflow, yellowing of the eyes, and seeing dimly afar, one can moxa 5 cones.

Rear Armpit Point (UEX-CA 21)
Hòu Yè Xià Xué – 後腋下穴

《千金》云：治頸漏，灸背後兩邊腋下後紋頭，隨年壯。

The Qiānjīn states, "To treat fistulae of the neck, moxa at the top of the crease of the armpit on the upper back on both sides, with [the number of] cones according to one's age."

---

363 This point is commonly listed as Ěr Shàng Fǎ Jì 耳上髮際 (Point Above the Ear on the Hairline).

Armpit Point (UEX-CA 19)
Yè Xià Xué – 腋下穴

《千金翼》云：噦噫，膈中氣閉塞，灸腋下聚毛附肋宛宛中五十壯，神良。

The Qiānjīn Yì states, "[To treat] belching and blockage of qì in the chest, moxa 50 cones in the depression in the armpit, where the hair gathers nearby the rib; it is miraculously effective."

Wind Marketplace[364]
Fēng Shì – 風市

在膝上七寸外側兩筋間。又取法，令正身平直，直垂兩手着腿，當中指頭盡處陷中是穴。鍼五分，灸三五壯。

This point is located in between the two sinews, 7 cùn above the knee on the outer face [of the thigh]. In addition, for the method to locate it, have the person stand upright, with their [arms] hanging straight and hands touching the legs; this point is located in the depression, at tip of the middle finger. Needle 5 fēn, moxa 15 cones.

《千金》云：病輕者，不可減百壯，重者五六百壯。主治腰腿痠痛，足頸麻頑，腳氣，起坐艱難，先泄後補，風病先補後泄，此風痺冷痛之要穴。

The Qiānjīn states, "For mild diseases, one should not moxa less than 100 cones; for serious diseases, [moxa] 500 to 600 cones. To govern the treatment of aching pain in the lumbus and leg, stubborn numbness of the legs and neck, leg qì, and difficulty getting up from sitting, initially drain then subsequently supplement; for wind diseases, initially supplement then subsequently drain. This is an essential point for [the treatment of] wind impediment and cold pain."

《神農經》云：治偏風半身不遂，兩脚疼痛，灸二十一壯。

The Shénnóng Jīng states, "To treat hemilateral wind with hemiplegia, and aching pain in both legs, moxa 21 cones."

---

[364] This point has the same Chinese name and very similar location as GB-31; we are not sure why Yuè Hánzhēn separates the two points. Nevertheless, in order to differentiate the two points, we have named this Wind Marketplace.

The Ankle [Point] (UEX-LE 17)
Zú Huái – 足踝

《千金》云：小舌，灸左足踝上七壯。又云：灸足兩踝上三壯。又治齒痛，灸外踝上高骨前交脈上七壯。又治轉筋，十指攣拘，灸足外踝骨上七壯。

The Qiānjīn states, "For the small tongue,[365] moxa 7 cones above the left ankle [bone]." It also states, "Moxa 3 cones on both ankle [bones]." In addition, "To treat toothache, moxa 7 cones on the intersecting vessels in front of the elevated bone above the outer ankle [bone]." Furthermore, "To treat cramps and hypertonicity of the ten digits,[366] moxa 7 cones on the outer ankle bone."

Tip of the Outer Ankle [Bone] (EX-LE 9)
Wài Huái Jiān – 外踝尖

在外踝尖上是穴，主治外轉筋，可灸七壯，或刺出血。

This point[367] is located on the tip of the outer ankle [bone]; to govern the treatment of cramping on the outside,[368] one can moxa 7 cones, or pierce to let blood.

---

[365] It is a lump underneath the tongue, which looks like a little or secondary tongue; based on the original context in the *Qiānjīn*, this condition specifically occurs in children.

[366] Note: though it does not specify, we speculate it to mean "ten toes" given its location.

[367] "是穴 This point" is originally "三寸 3 cùn." The editors of this manuscript, Zhāng and Zhà, have amended it according to the *Zhēnjiǔ Dàchéng*.

[368] Note: Based on *the Zhēnjiǔ Dàchéng*, this likely means the cramping that occurs on the lateral aspect of the leg.

The Foot Juéyīn Liver Channel & Points

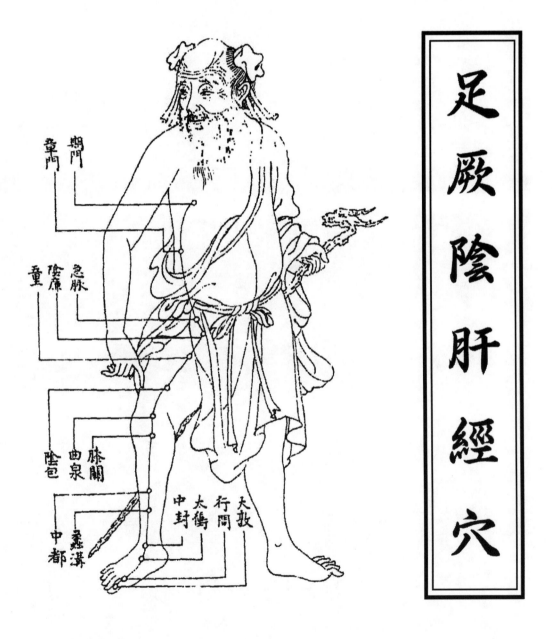

The Foot Juéyīn Liver Channel & Points
足厥陰肝經

Overview of the Foot Juéyīn Liver Channel
足厥陰肝經總論

思蓮子曰：肝之經爲足厥陰，多血少氣。起於足大指橫紋外側之大敦井木穴，循足跗上廉，歷大指縫中之動脈應手行間榮火穴，大指本節後二寸之動脈太衝腧土穴，抵內踝前一寸，筋裏宛宛中之中封經金穴，

Master Sīlián says, the channel of the liver is the foot juéyīn, it has copious blood and scant qì.

It commences at Dà Dūn (LR-1), the well and wood point, on the outside of the transverse crease of the big toe. It follows the upper surface of the foot, passing through Xíng Jiān (LR-2), the brook and fire point, within the seam of the big toe, where the pulsating vessel resonates with the hand. It continues to Tài Chōng (LR-3), the stream and earth point, which is at the pulsating vessel 2 cùn behind the base joint of the big toe. It arrives at Zhōng Fēng (LR-4), the river and metal point, at 1 cùn in front of the inner ankle [bone], in the depression inside of the sinew.

自中封上內踝三寸，過脾經之三陰交穴，經本經內踝上五寸之蠡溝肝絡，別走少陽穴，內踝上七寸骭骨之中都穴，復上一寸，交出足太陰脾經之後，上膕內廉，至犢鼻下二寸之膝關穴，又過曲膝近橫紋，膝股內側，輔骨下，大筋上，小筋下陷中曲泉，肝經所入爲合水穴。

From Zhōng Fēng (LR-4), it ascends 3 cùn above the inner ankle [bone], traverses Sān Yīn Jiāo (SP-6) of the spleen channel, and passes Lí Gōu (LR-5), which is 5 cùn above the inner ankle [bone]; it is the network point of the liver, which diverges to go to the foot shàoyáng points. [It ascends to] Zhōng Dū (LR-6), which is 7 cùn above the inner ankle [bone] and on the shin bone. It then ascends 1 further cùn, where it intersects with and emerges behind the foot tàiyīn spleen channel. It ascends the inner ridge of the back of the knee to Xī Guān (LR-7), which is 2 cùn below Dú Bí (ST-35). It continues and traverses Qū Quán (LR-8), where the liver channel enters as the uniting and water point, nearby the transverse crease at the knee bend, on the inside of the knee and

thigh, below the assisting bone, above the large sinew, and in the depression below the small sinew.

循股內膝上四寸，股內兩筋間，蹻足內側必有槽中之陰包穴，又上過氣衝下三寸，陰股動脈之五里穴，又過去氣衝二寸羊矢下，動脈應手之陰廉穴，遂當脾經衝門，穴在橫骨兩端腹中，去腹中行各四寸半，動脈應手之所，又上至府舍，穴在脾經腹結下二寸，去腹中行各四寸半之處，合足太陰脾經、陰維脈並本經三脈，入腹絡脾肝，結心肺，從脇上至肩，太陰郄、三陰陽明之別處也，

It follows the inner thigh ascending to Yīn Bāo (LR-9), which is 4 cùn above the knee, in the space between the two sinews, where there must be a groove on the inner [thigh] when the leg is curled. It ascends to traverse Wǔ Lǐ (LR-10), which is 3 cùn below Qì Chōng (ST-3), at the pulsating vessel on the yīn of the thigh. It traverses to Yīn Lián (LR-11), which is 2 cùn from Qì Chōng (ST-30) and below the goat faeces,[369] where the pulsating vessel resonates with the hand. It continues to arrive at Chōng Mén (SP-12) of the spleen channel, this point is located on the abdomen at both ends of the pubic bone, 4 and a half cùn on each side of the abdominal midline, where the hand resonates with the pulsating vessel. It continues to ascend to arrive at Fǔ Shè (SP-13), this point is located 2 cùn below Fù Jié (SP-14) of the spleen channel, at the location that is 4 and half cùn on each side of the abdominal midline; here, the three vessels unite, the foot tàiyīn spleen channel, yīnwéi vessel, and this channel [of the liver], they enter the abdomen, network the spleen and liver, bind with the heart and lung, and ascend to reach the shoulder from the rib-side; in addition, it is the tàiyīn cleft point as well as the place where the three yīn and yángmíng [channels] diverge to.

又自府舍入陰毛中，左右相交，環繞陰器，抵小腹而上會任脈之曲骨穴，毛際陷中，動脈應手之所，又上過任脈臍下四寸，膀胱募之中極穴，又上任脈臍下三寸，小腸募之關元穴，乃上循旁至脾經腹哀下三寸五分，大橫穴之外，直季脇肋端，當臍上二寸，兩旁各六寸之章門穴，為脾之募，乃足少陰、厥陰相會之所，

It continues from Fǔ Shè (SP-13) to enter the pubic hair region, where the left and right [pathways] intersect and encircle the yīn organs. Upon reaching the lower abdomen, it ascends to meet with Qū Gǔ (REN-2) of the rèn vessel, which is in the depression at the pubic hair region, at the place where the pulsating vessel resonates with the hand.

It continues to ascend and traverse Zhōng Jí (REN-3) of the rèn vessel, the collecting point of the bladder, which is 4 cùn below the umbilicus. It continues to ascend Guān Yuán (REN-4) of the rèn vessel, the collecting point of the small intestine, which is 3 cùn below the umbilicus. Thereupon, it moves

---

[369] I.e., anterior superior iliac crest. It is also designated as an extra point Yáng Shǐ (UEX-LE-1).

to the sides to reach Zhāng Mén (LR-13), the collecting point of the spleen, which is 3 cùn 5 fēn below Fù Āi (SP-16) of the spleen channel, outside of Dà Héng (SP-15), directly [below] the edge of the floating rib, at precisely 2 cùn above the umbilicus and 6 cùn on each side [of the midline]; moreover, it is the location where the foot shàoyīn and juéyīn [channels] meet with each other.

又上行至直乳二肋端，胃經不容穴，去中行三寸，旁一寸五分，爲肝之募期門穴，與足太陰脾經、陰維二脈相會之地，挾胃屬肝，下膽經日月穴之所，在期門下五分，乃足太陰脾經、足少陽膽經、陰維三脈相會於此處，而下絡於膽也；

It continues and ascends to Qī Mén (LR-14), the collecting point of the liver, which is in the second intercostal space directly [below] the breast, 1 cùn 5 fēn to the side of Bù Róng (ST-19) of the stomach channel that is 3 cùn from the midline; it is the place where the two vessels of the foot tàiyīn spleen channel and yīnwéi [vessel] meet with each other, where it clasps the stomach and adjoins to the liver. Below, it is the location of Rì Yuè (GB-24) of the gallbladder channel, which is located 5 fēn below Qī Mén (LR-14); in addition, after the three vessels meet at this location, the foot tàiyīn spleen channel, foot shàoyáng gallbladder channel, and yīnwéi [vessel], they descend to network with the gallbladder.

其直行者，又上至期門，上貫膈，行脾經食竇穴之外，穴在脾經天谿穴下一寸六分，去胸中行各六寸，脾經大包穴之裏，穴在膽經淵腋穴下三寸，布胸肋中，出九肋間，爲脾大絡，又上肺經之雲門穴，膽經之淵腋穴之間，

Its vertical pathway ascends to arrive at Qī Mén (LR-14), it further ascends to pierce the diaphragm, travels outside of Shí Dòu (SP-17) of the spleen channel, which is located 1 cùn 6 fēn below Tiān Xī (SP-18) of the spleen channel, 6 cùn on each side of the chest midline; [this pathway travels] inside of Dà Bāo (SP-21) of the spleen channel, which is located 3 cùn below Yuān Yè (GB-22) of the gallbladder channel, it spreads at the intercostals, emerging at the ninth intercostal, as the great network of the spleen. It continues and ascends in the space between Yún Mén (LU-2) of the lung channel and Yuān Yè (GB-22) of the gallbladder channel.

上行至頸人迎穴之外，系頸大脈動脈應手，挾結喉旁一寸五分之所，循喉嚨之後，上入頏顙，行胃經大迎穴、四白穴、膽經陽白穴之外，陽白穴在眉上一寸，直瞳子，內連目系，上出額，行膽經臨泣穴之裏，臨泣穴在眉上，直入髮際五分陷中，又上頂，會於督之百會穴焉；

It ascends to reach the neck outside of Rén Yíng (ST-9), which links with where the large pulsating vessel on the neck resonates with the hand, clasping at 1 cùn 5 fēn to the side of the laryngeal prominence. It follows behind the throat, ascends to enter the nasopharynx [region]. It travels outside of Dà Yíng (ST-5) and Sì Bái (ST-2) of the stomach channel, as well as Yáng Bái (GB-14) of the gallbladder channel; Yáng Bái (GB-14) is located 1 cùn above the eyebrow, in line with the pupil. It continues inwards to link with the eye connector, ascends to emerge at the forehead, travels inside of [Tóu] Lín Qì (GB-15) of the gallbladder channel; [Tóu] Lín Qì (GB-15) is located above the eyebrow, in the depression 5 fēn behind the border of the hairline. It continues and ascends to the vertex, where it meets with Bǎi Huì (DU-20) of the dū [vessel].

其支者，從期門屬肝處，別貫膈，行脾經食竇之外，本經之裏，上注肺，下行至中焦，挾中脘之分，以交於手太陰肺經，而又爲周身之始。《內經》云：厥陰爲闔，闔折則氣絶而喜悲，取之厥陰，視有餘不足，而補泄之焉。

A branch from Qī Mén (LR-14) adjoins to the location of the liver, diverges to pierce the diaphragm, travels outside of Shí Dòu (SP-17) of the spleen channel, at the inside of the principal channel; it ascends to pour into the lung, descends to reach the middle jiāo, clasps the division of Zhōng Wǎn (REN-12), where it intersects with the hand tàiyīn lung channel; as such, it marks the beginning of the circulation around the whole body. *The Nèijīng* states, "Juéyīn closes; when the closing breaks, the qì will exhaust; as a result, one will be susceptible to sorrow, choose the juéyīn [channel]; inspect whether it is superabundant or insufficient, then supplement or drain it accordingly."[370]

Diseases of the Foot Juéyīn Liver Channel
足厥陰肝經病

是動病則爲腰痛不可俯仰，以肝與腎通，則膂筋之脈通於肝也。爲丈夫㿗疝，以睾丸屬肝也。爲婦人少腹腫，以肝脈上抵小腹也。

When there are changes, it will result in diseases such as pain of the lumbus with inability to bend forwards and backwards, this is because as the liver communicates with the kidneys, the vessels of paravertebral sinews likewise communicate with the liver. For slumping mounting in men, this is because the testicles adjoin to the liver. For swelling of the lower abdomen in women, this is because the liver vessel ascends to arrive at the lower abdomen.

爲嗌乾，以肝脈上循喉嚨也。爲面塵脱色，以膽病面塵脱色，肝爲膽之裏，所主病同也。

For dry pharynx, this is because the liver vessel ascends following the throat. For dusty facial complexion with loss of colour,[371] this is because dusty facial

---

370 From *Língshū* Chapter 5.
371 I.e., the loss of a healthy complexion colour.

complexion with loss of colour is a gallbladder disease; as the liver is the interior [pair] of the gallbladder, hence it governs this same disease.

所生病爲胸滿，以脈上貫膈也。爲嘔逆，以脈挾胃也。爲飧泄，以脈抵小腹也。爲狐疝，以脈過陰器，上睾結莖也。爲遺溺，爲閉癃，皆以肝脈上睾結莖也。

For disease itself engenders, there is fullness in the chest, as this vessel ascends to pierce the diaphragm. For vomiting counterflow, this is because the vessel clasps the stomach. For swill diarrhoea, this is because the vessel arrives at the lower abdomen. For fox-like mounting, this is because the vessel traverses the yīn organs, ascends to the testicles, and binds at the penis. For enuresis and dribbling urinary block, both are because the liver vessel ascends to the testicles and binds at the penis.

如寸口較人迎之脈大者一倍，則肝脈爲實，當泄，而膽經爲虛，當補。如寸口較人迎之脈小者一倍，則肝經爲虛，當補，而膽經爲實，當泄也。

When the cùnkǒu pulse in comparison to the rényíng pulse is one times larger, the liver vessel is replete, one ought to drain it; moreover, the gallbladder channel is vacuous, one ought to supplement it. When the cùnkǒu in comparison to the rényíng is one times smaller, the liver vessel is vacuous, one ought to supplement it; moreover, the gallbladder channel is replete, one ought to drain it.

Sinew Channel of the Foot Juéyīn
足厥陰經筋

足厥陰之筋，起於大指之上大敦穴，上結於內踝之前中封，上循於脛，上結於內輔骨之曲泉，以上循陰股之陰包等穴，結於陰器，以絡諸筋。

The sinew [channel] of the foot juéyīn commences at Dà Dūn (LR-1) on the top of the big toe, and it ascends to knot at Zhōng Fēng (LR-4) in front of the inner ankle [bone]. It ascends following the shin, and further ascends to knot at Qū Quán (LR-8) on the inside of the assisting bone. It ascends to Yīn Bāo (LR-9) following the yīn of the thigh, knots at the yīn organs,[372] and networks with the various sinews.

其病當爲足大指內踝之前痛，爲內輔骨痛，爲陰股痛或轉筋，爲陰器不用。若傷於內，則陰器不起。若傷於寒，則陰器縮入。若傷於熱，則陰器縱挺不收。治在行其水，以清陰器。

---

[372] I.e., the external genitals.

Its diseases are pain of the big toe [that radiates to] the front of the inner ankle [bone], pain at the inside of the assisting bone, pain or cramping along the inside of the thigh, and inability to use the yīn organs. If there is damage internally, there will be ineffectiveness of the yīn organ.[373] If there is damage by cold, the yīn organs will retract. If there is damage by heat, the yīn organ will have persistent erection and inability to retract. The treatment is to move water in order to clear [the heat in] the yīn organs.

First Point of the Liver Channel
Dà Dūn – Great Mound[374] (LR-1)
肝經第一穴大敦

穴在足大指端，去爪甲如韭葉，及三毛中。指上有毛處，上有橫紋，名曰三毛聚，此穴乃在外側隱隱陷中。內側爲隱白，乃脾之井。此穴乃肝之井，足厥陰脈所出爲井木。《銅人》：鍼三分，留十呼，灸三壯。《千金》：大便難，灸四壯。又治五淋，灸三十壯。又失溺不禁，灸七壯，小兒灸一壯。又溺血，灸隨年壯。

This point is located on the tip of the big toe, at one chive leaf's width from the nail corner, at the [region of] the three hairs.[375] There is a location with hairs on the [big] toe, above the [transverse] crease, and it is called the "gathering of the three hairs."[376] This point is located in the slight depression on the outside; on the inside, there is Yǐn Bái (SP-1), which is the well point of the spleen. This point is the well point of the liver, the foot juéyīn vessel emerges here, as the well and wood point.

---

[373] I.e., impotence.

[374] *Grasping the Wind* names it "Great Pile." Based on the explanation given, Yuè Hánzhēn seems to have interpreted the character dūn 敦 (honest, sincere) as its homophone, dūn 墩 (earth mound); therefore, we have changed the name to "Great Mound" accordingly. As this would result in same English name as Dà Líng 大陵 (PC-7, "Great Mound"), the difference between líng 陵 and dūn 墩 is that, líng 陵 tends to depict a naturally occurring hill or a burial mound in rare occasions; whereas for dūn 墩, it is usually a mound created by human effort, usually serving as a foundation or a pillar to support something else.

[375] According to the *Practical Dictionary,* it is the "region just proximal to the base of the nail of the great toe, at which a number of hairs are often found growing."

[376] See also the extra point at the end of this chapter, Sān Máo Jù Zhōng 三毛聚中 (Within the Gathering of Three Hairs, UEX-LE 29). Side Note: From historical sources, this point is sometimes referred to as "聚毛 gathering of hair" or "三毛 three hairs;" here, it seems that Yuè Hánzhēn combines these two historical names together for this alternate point locations of LR-1 (note: some early writings indicate that this point is located within the hair region such as *Língshū* Chapter 2).

The Tóngrén states, "Needle 3 fēn, retain for 10 respirations,[377] and moxa 3 cones." *The Qiānjīn* states, "For difficult defecation, moxa 4 cones. In addition, to treat the five stranguries, moxa 30 cones. Also, [to treat] unrestrained enuresis, moxa 7 cones; in children, moxa 1 cone. [To treat] bloody urine, moxa cones according to the patient's age."

注：木之根在下，須土而後茂，肝之井即木之根也，而與脾土同出足大指，有土厚而木茂之義，故曰大敦。

Explanation: as the root of wood is located below [the surface], it requires the earth in order to become luxuriant; likewise, the well point of the liver is precisely the root of wood; in addition, as both [the liver-wood] and the spleen-earth [channels] emerge on the big toe, it is indicative of the meaning that the luxuriance of wood comes from the richness of earth, thus it is called Dà Dūn (Great Mound).

肝之腎病：癃，五淋，小便遺數不禁，婦人血崩不止，陰挺出，陰中痛。

Kidney diseases of the liver: dribbling block, five stranguries, frequent unrestrained enuresis, incessant flooding in women, vaginal protrusion, and pain in the genitals.

注：腎司二便，而肝實疏泄之，肝氣鬱而膀胱熱，則淋病作焉，故取此穴以散肝之鬱。《內經》云：癃，取之陰蹻及三毛上，及血絡出血，乃大敦穴也。

Explanation: while the kidneys control both urine and stool, it is in fact the liver that [allows] the free coursing and discharging of [the stool and urine]; thus, when the liver qì is depressed, there will be bladder heat; as a result, the disease of strangury will manifest, therefore, choose this point in order to disperse the depression of the liver. *The Nèijīng* states, "[To treat] dribbling block, choose the yīnqiāo [vessel] atop the three hairs, and bleed the blood network-vessels,"[378] this is [referring to] Dà Dūn (LR-1).

東垣曰：腎主閉藏，肝主疏泄，癃便取之兩經也宜矣。小便遺數，乃肝氣之脫，灸此穴以溫而收之。婦人血崩不止，皆肝氣之脫也，灸此穴以溫其下脫。陰挺出，陰中痛，皆肝氣之逆也，泄此穴以降肝之逆氣。

---

[377] For "6 respirations," *the Tóngrén* states, "10 respirations."
[378] From *Língshū* Chapter 23.

[Lǐ] Dōngyuán says, "The kidneys govern storage and the liver governs free coursing;"[379] thus, for dribbling urinary block, it is appropriate to choose these two channels. Regarding frequent enuresis, this is due to desertion of the liver qì, moxa this point in order to warm and contract it.

Regarding incessant spotting in women, in all cases, this is desertion of the liver qì, moxa this point in order to warm the sunken and deserted [qì]. For vaginal protrusion and pain in the genitals, these are both due to the counterflow of liver qì, drain this point in order to descend the counterflow qì of liver.

肝之肝病：卒疝七疝，陰頭中痛，汗出，陰上入少腹，陰偏大，腹臍中痛，悒悒不樂。

Liver diseases of the liver: sudden mounting, seven mountings,[380] pain in the glans penis, sweating, retraction of genitals towards the lower abdomen, unilateral enlargement of genitals, pain in the abdomen and umbilicus, and mental depression.

注：肝之所主者筋也，前陰爲宗筋之會，邪客肝經則筋病，故前陰諸病，先責肝之井焉。病左取右，病右取左，以肝經自橫骨之外，橫入毛際，環繞陰器，左之右，右之左，而上行也。

Explanation: that which the liver governs, it is the sinews; the front yīn [orifices][381] are the meeting place of the ancestral sinew; when evil lodges in the liver channel, there will be sinew diseases, therefore, for various diseases of the front yīn [orifices], first seek the well point of the liver.

When the disease is on the left, choose the right [point]; when the disease is on the right, choose the left [point]; this is because the liver channel [travels] horizontally to enter the pubic hair region from outside of the pubic bone,[382] it then

---

[379] We have looked through all surviving works of Lǐ Dōngyuán, as well as passages attributed to him in the *Zhēnjiǔ Jùyīng* 針灸聚英 (*Gathered Blooms of Acupuncture and Moxibustion*, 1529 CE) and the *Dàchéng*; however, we have come up short. A very similar line, "主閉藏者腎也，司疏泄者肝也。 That which governs the storage, it is the kidneys; that which governs the coursing and discharging, it is the liver;" was found in Zhū Dānxī's *Gézhì Yúlùn* 格致餘論 (*Extra Treatise Based Upon Investigation and Inquiry*, 1347 CE); however, in the original context, Zhū Dānxī is arguing for the reason why the ministerial fire occurs in the liver and kidneys. Here, based on preliminary finding, we are speculating that this quote may have been misattributed and perhaps quoted out of context by Yuè Hánzhēn.

[380] The "seven mountings" are first mentioned in the *Sùwèn*; however, it does not mention what these are. Later, *Zhūbìng Yuánhòu Lùn* 諸病源候論 (*the Origin and Indicators of Disease*, 610 CE) lists the seven mountings as: reverting mounting, concretion mounting, cold mounting, qì mounting, winding mounting, bowel mounting, and wolf mounting.

[381] I.e., the penis and vagina.

[382] Also, the name of KI-11.

encircles the yīn organs, where the left [pathway] goes right and the right [pathway] goes left; afterwards, it continues to ascend.

肝之脾病：腹脹腫，小腹痛。

Spleen diseases of the liver: distension and swelling of the abdomen, and lower abdominal pain.

注：二症皆肝氣之逆也，故取此穴，以開肝之鬱。

Explanation: both of these signs are counterflow of liver qì, thus choose this point in order to open the depression of the liver.

肝之心病：中熱喜寐，屍厥狀如死人。

Heart diseases of the liver: internal heat with tendency to sleep, and deathlike reversal that appears as a dead person.

注：邪熱中於外，而肝火應之，故屍厥如此，取此穴以泄肝之風熱。

Explanation: after evil heat strikes the exterior, liver fire further resonates with it, then deathlike reversal will occur as described, choose this point in order to drain the wind heat of the liver.

Second Point of the Liver Channel
Xíng Jiān – Moving Between (LR-2)
肝經第二穴行間

穴在足大指縫間，動脈應手，足厥陰肝經所溜爲滎火，肝實則泄之。《銅人》：灸三壯，鍼六分，留十呼。

This point is located in the space at the seam of the big toe, where the pulsating vessel resonates with the hand. The foot juéyīn liver channel gushes here, as brook and fire point. When the liver is replete, drain it. *The Tóngrén* states, "Moxa 3 cones, needle 6 fēn, and retain for 10 respirations."

注：穴名行間者，以其穴在大指、次指歧骨間，爲肝經初行之所，故曰行間。木生火，漸次而行，初至此地之義。

Explanation: regarding the point name Xíng Jiān (Moving Between), it is because the point is located Jiān (Between) the big toe and second toe, where the bones diverge. This is the place where the liver channel begins to Xíng (Move), therefore it is called Xíng Jiān (Moving Between). As wood generates fire, it carries the meaning of Xíng (Moving) in successive sequences [of the five phases] as [the channel] arrives at this location.

肝之腎病：遺溺，癃閉，莖中痛，腰痛不可俯仰，便溺難，男女小腹腫，面塵脫色，經血過多不止，崩中。

Kidney diseases of the liver: urinary incontinence, dribbling urinary block, pain in the penis, lumbar pain with inability to bend forwards and backwards, difficulty in defecating and urinating, swelling of the lower abdomen in males and females, dusty complexion with loss of colour, excessive incessant menstruation, and flooding.

注：此穴肝經所溜爲滎火。遺溺者，乃腎火之寒也，補肝火即補腎火也，故取此穴。癃閉者，乃腎火過甚也，泄肝火即泄腎火也，故取此穴。莖中痛，乃肝之氣血滯也，泄此穴以通肝之滯，而腎之滯亦消。

Explanation: this point is the place where the liver channel gushes as the brook and fire point. Urinary incontinence is due to coldness of the kidney[383] fire; supplement the liver fire, as this will supplement the kidney fire, thus choose this point. Dribbling urinary block is due to extreme or excessive kidney fire, drain the liver fire, as this will drain kidney fire, thus choose this point. Pain of the penis is stagnation of liver qì and blood, drain this point in order to free the stagnation of the liver; as a result, the stagnation of the kidneys will also be dispersed.

腰痛不可俯仰者，肝氣滯也，宜泄此穴。便溺難，氣不順也，宜泄此穴。男婦小腹腫，以經抵小腹也，宜泄其逆氣。面垢脫色，肝氣泄也，宜取此穴。崩中不止，肝氣有餘，鼓血而行也，泄肝氣之有餘，氣泄於下，則血止於上。

Lumbar pain with inability to bend forwards and backwards is liver qì stagnation, it is appropriate to drain this point. For difficulty in defecating and urinating, this is an unsmooth [flow of] qì, it is appropriate to drain this point. Regarding swelling of the lower abdomen in males and females, this is because the [liver] channel reaches the lower abdomen, it is appropriate to drain the counterflow qì.

Grimy face with loss of colour is due to leakage of the liver qì, it is appropriate to choose this point. Incessant flooding is superabundance of liver qì, which is rousing the blood to move [frenetically]; by draining the superabundance of liver qì, the qì will be drained below, and the bleeding will cease above.

肝之肝病：善怒，轉筋，小腸氣，瞑不欲視，目中淚出，太息，寒疝七疝，中風口喎，肝積肥氣，小兒急驚風。

Liver diseases of the liver: tendency to anger, cramps, small intestinal qì, dimness of vision with no desire to see, tearing of the eyes, great

---

[383] "腎 Kidney" is originally "胃 stomach" in the primary manuscript. The editors of this manuscript, Zhāng and Zhà, have amended it according to the secondary manuscript.

respiration,[384] cold mounting and seven mountings, wind stroke with deviated mouth, liver accumulation and fat qì,[385] and urgent fright wind in children.

注：善怒者，肝有火，宜泄此穴。轉筋者，寒傷筋也，宜補此穴以溫筋。小腸氣，乃肝氣逆也，宜泄之以平肝氣。瞑不欲視，目中淚出，皆肝火有餘也，宜泄此穴以降火。太息，乃肝氣鬱也，泄滎火以散肝鬱。疝病專責肝，皆肝氣中寒之所致也，補此穴以溫肝氣。口喎刺此穴，不如陽明頰車、地倉之捷也。肝積肥氣，皆肝之寒也，無寒不成積，補此穴以散肝寒。小兒急驚風，乃肝木之有餘也，急泄滎火。

Explanation: tendency to anger is the presence of fire in the liver, it is appropriate to drain this point. Cramps are because of cold damaging the sinews, it is appropriate to supplement this point in order to warm the sinews. Small intestine qì is counterflow of liver qì, it is appropriate to drain this [point] in order to balance liver qì. For dimness of vision with no desire to see and tearing of the eyes, both are superabundance of liver fire, it is appropriate to drain this point in order to descend fire. Great respiration is due to liver qì depression, drain the brook and fire point in order to disperse the liver depression.

For mounting disease, one should specifically seek the liver; it is always a result of cold striking the liver qì; thus, supplement this point in order to warm the liver qì. For deviated mouth, pierce this point; however, it is not as effective as Jiá Chē (ST-6) and Dì Cāng (ST-4) of the yángmíng [channel]. Both liver accumulation and fat qì are due to cold of the liver; in the absence of cold, accumulations cannot form; thus, supplement this point in order to disperse the liver cold. Urgent fright wind in children is due to superabundance of liver-wood, urgently drain the brook fire point.

肝之脾病：咳逆嘔血，洞泄，四肢滿，腹中脹，四肢逆冷，痎瘧。

Spleen diseases of the spleen: cough and counterflow with retching of blood, throughflux diarrhoea, fullness of the four limbs, distension of the abdomen, counterflow cold of the four limbs, and intervallic malaria.

注：咳逆嘔血，肝氣上逆也，急取此穴，以泄肝火。洞泄則肝木旺，侵脾土，宜泄此穴，以平肝。四肢滿，脾之虛也，脾之虛乃肝旺也，泄此穴以泄肝旺。腹中脹，乃肝氣有餘也，宜泄之。四肢逆冷，四肢屬脾，肝木受寒，則脾土虧而手

---

[384] "Great respiration" according to *the Practical Dictionary* is "periodic extended exhalation to relieve oppression in the chest."

[385] Fat qì is one of the five accumulations described in *Nànjīng* Difficulty 56. According to *the Practical Dictionary*, it manifests as a "glomus lump under the rib-side like an upturned cup, attributed to liver qì depression and congealing static blood."

足逆冷，急補滎火，而去肝之寒。瘧脈必弦，弦者，肝脈也。肝脈旺則脾土虧，泄此穴以平肝旺。

Explanation: cough and counterflow with retching of blood is counterflow ascent of liver qì, urgently choose this point in order to drain the liver fire. Throughflux diarrhoea is liver-wood effulgence invading spleen earth, it is appropriate to drain this point in order to balance the liver. Fullness of the four limbs is vacuity of the spleen, this vacuity of the spleen is caused by liver effulgence, drain this point in order to drain the liver effulgence.

Distension of the abdomen is due to superabundance of liver qì, it is appropriate to drain this [point]. Regarding counterflow cold of the four limbs, as the four limbs belong to the spleen, when liver-wood contracts cold, it will deplete spleen-earth; as a result, there will be counterflow cold of the hands and feet, urgently supplement the brook fire point to eliminate the cold in the liver.

The malaria pulse is always stringlike,[386] the stringlike [pulse] is the liver pulse; when the liver pulse is effulgent, spleen-earth will become depleted, drain this point in order to balance the liver effulgence.

肝之心病：肝心痛，色蒼蒼如死狀，癲疾。

Heart diseases of the liver: liver-induced heart pain, sombre deathlike complexion, and epileptic disease.

注：心痛根乎臟者有五，肝心痛則色蒼蒼，乃肝氣之上逆乎心也，泄滎火以去其有餘，又宜取肝之太衝。癲疾，心為肝氣所逆，而癲生焉，刺此穴以去母邪，而弱其子。

Explanation: there are five types of heart pain that are fundamentally caused by the zàng-viscera; for liver-induced heart pain, the complexion will be sombre, this is due to counterflow ascent of liver qì that has reached the heart, drain the brook fire point in order to eliminate the superabundance, it is also appropriate to choose Tài Chōng (LR-3) of the liver [channel].

When there is an epileptic disease, the heart is affected by the counterflow of liver qì; as a result, madness manifests, pierce this point in order to eliminate the mother's evil, so that its [influence on the] son can be weakened.

肝之肺病：消渴嗜飲，胸脇痛，短氣，嗌乾煩渴。

Lung diseases of the liver: dispersion-thirst with strong desire to drink [fluids], pain in the chest and rib-sides, shortness of breath, dry pharynx with vexation and thirst.

---

[386] Note: Also known as wiry pulse.

注：肝經有上行至肺者，肝火旺則肺熱而渴，宜泄此穴。純脇痛則責肝，胸脇痛則肝之逆上入肺而痛，宜泄此穴。肝有鬱則氣滯於肺而短，宜泄之。嗌乾煩渴，肝火逆肺也，應泄之。

Explanation: as the liver channel ascends and reaches the lung, when liver fire is effulgent, there will be thirst due to lung heat. When there is only pain in the rib-sides, blame the liver; when there is pain in [both] the chest and rib-sides, this pain is caused by counterflow ascent of the liver entering the lung, it is appropriate to drain this point. Depression of the liver will cause qì stagnation in the lung, there will be shortness [of breath], it is appropriate to drain this [point]. For dry pharynx with vexation and thirst, this is counterflow of liver fire [entering] the lung, one ought to drain this [point].

Third Point of the Liver Channel
Tài Chōng – Supreme Surge (LR-3)
肝經第三穴太衝

穴在足大指本節後二寸，或云一寸半，內間動脈應手陷中，足厥陰肝脈所注爲腧土。《銅人》：鍼三分，留十呼，灸三壯。

This point is located 2 cùn behind the base joint of the big toe; some say 1 cùn and a half; it is the depression where the pulsating vessel resonates with the hands. The foot juéyīn vessel pours here, as the stream and wood point. *The Tóngrén* states, "Needle 3 fēn, retain for 10 respirations, and moxa 3 cones."

注：《素問·水熱穴論》云：三陰之所交結於脚也，踝上各一行者，此腎脈之下行也，名曰太衝。王氏曰：腎脈與衝脈並下行，循足入盛大，故曰太衝。一云：衝脈起於氣街，衝直而通，故謂之衝。

Explanation: the "Treatise on Water and Heat Points" from *the Sùwèn* states, "The leg is the place where the three yīn [vessels] interlink; for the one pathway above the ankle on each side, this is the lower pathway of the kidney vessel, which is called Tài Chōng (Supreme Surge)." Mister Wáng says, "As the kidney vessel and the chōng vessel descend together to follow and enter the foot, they become exuberant and large, thus it is called Tài Chōng (Supreme Surge)."[387] Another [person] says,

---

[387] From Wáng Bīng's annotation of *Sùwèn* Chapter 61.

"The chōng vessel commences at Qì Jiē (ST-30),[388] it Chōng (Surges) in a straight line as it flows freely, thus it is known as the chōng [vessel]."[389]

按衝脈有三歧，一歧上脊，一歧出氣衝，循腹上行，一歧下行注於足少陰之絡。原起於腎下，出於氣街，循陰股內廉，斜入委中，伏行骭骨內廉，並少陰之經，入內踝之後，入足下。

Note by [Master Sīlián]: the chōng vessel has three branches; one branch ascends along the [interior of the] spine; another branch emerges at Qì Chōng (ST-30) to follow and ascend the abdomen; the final branch descends to pour into the network-vessels of the foot shàoyīn. From its origin, it commences from below the kidneys, it then emerges at the Qì Jiē (ST-30), follows the inner ridge on the yīn of the thigh, travels obliquely to enter Wěi Zhōng (BL-40), becomes concealed as it travels along the inside of the inner ridge of the shin bone, enters behind the inner ankle [bone] with the channel of the shàoyīn, and continues to enter the bottom of the foot.

其別者，並於少陰，滲三陰，斜入踝，伏行出屬跗屬，下循跗上，入大指之間，滲諸絡而溫足脛肌肉，故其脈常動，即此所也。

Its divergent [pathway] joins with the shàoyīn [channel] to permeate into the three yīn. It obliquely enters the ankle [bone], becomes concealed as it travels [along the ankle bone] and emerges to adjoin to the instep, descends following the surface of the instep to enter the space between the big toe [and the second toe], where it permeates into all the network-vessels in order to warm the muscles and flesh of the feet and lower leg; thus, its vessel is constantly pulsating. This is precisely referring to this place.

衝脈雖為血海，而行上行下，有氣行於其間，故曰衝。此穴在下，會於肝經，肝藏血，衝脈自腎脈下會於肝脈，至此為極盛之地，故曰太衝。

Although the chōng vessel is the sea of blood, as it travels upwards and downwards, there is qì that moves in these spaces, thus it is called Chōng (Surging). This point (LR-3) is located below and meets with the liver channel. As the liver stores the blood, when the chōng vessel descends from the kidney vessel to meet with the liver vessel, upon arriving here, it will be at its utmost exuberance, thus it is called Tài Chōng (Supreme Surging).

《素問》曰：女子二七，太衝脈盛，月事以時下，故能有子。又：診病人太衝脈有無，可以決生死。

---

388 An alternate name for ST-30, discussed in Kidney Channel.

389 In Qíjīng Bāmài Kǎo 奇經八脈考 (*An Investigation of the Eight Extraordinary Channels*, 1578 CE), this line seems to be attributed to Wáng Bīng as well; however, this line cannot be located in his annotation of the *Sùwèn*.

The Sùwèn states, "When females reach fourteen years of age, the Tài Chōng (Supreme Surging) pulse becomes exuberant; at this time, the menstruation commences, thus they are able to bear children."[390] It also states, "When diagnosing a patient, assess whether the Tài Chōng (Supreme Surging) pulse is present or absent, so that one can determine life and death."[391]

肝之腎病：腰引小腹痛，兩丸騫縮，遺溺，陰痛，小便淋，小腸疝氣痛，癀疝，小便不利，小兒卒疝，女子漏下不止，大便難，便血。

Kidney diseases of the liver: lumbar pain that radiates to the lower abdomen, retraction of both testicles, enuresis, genital pain, strangury, small intestine mounting qì with pain, slumping mounting, inhibited urination, sudden mounting in children, incessant spotting in females, difficulty in defecation, and blood in the stool.

注：肝與膂通，則膂筋之脈通於肝，而小腹又肝經所過之地，故腰引小腹痛，取肝經所注穴，以泄肝氣。兩丸騫縮，陰痛癀疝，小腸氣，小兒卒疝，皆肝氣逆也，宜泄之。

Explanation: as the liver communicates with paravertebral sinews, the vessels of the paravertebral sinews communicate with the liver as well; in addition, the lower abdomen is also the place where the liver channel traverses, thus for lumbar pain that radiates to the lower abdomen, choose the point where the liver channel pours into, so that the liver qì can be drained. For contraction of both testicles, genital pain, jaundice mounting, small intestine qì, and sudden mounting in children, these are all cases of counterflow of liver qì, it is appropriate to drain this [point].

小便淋，肝有火也，小便不利，大便難，陰痛，皆肝氣逆也，當泄焉。遺溺者，肝寒也，宜補肝之土穴以治下脫之水。便血，女子漏下不止，久則下寒而脫，當培土以澀下脫。

Strangury is presence of fire in the liver; for inhibited urination, difficulty in defecating, and genital pain, these are all counterflow of liver qì, one ought to drain [this point]. Regarding enuresis, this is liver cold, it is appropriate to supplement the earth point of the liver in order to treat the sunken and deserted water. For blood in the stools and incessant spotting in females, if they are chronic [conditions], then

---

[390] From *Sùwèn* Chapter 1.

[391] This statement cannot be found in the *Sùwèn*, rather, it seems to be a paraphrase of a quote cited by *the Tóngrén* under the entry for Tài Chōng (LR-3), which states, "凡診太衝脈可決男子病死生 when diagnosing a patient, assess the Tài Chōng pulse, so that one can determine the severity of a disease in a male." The variation of the quote that is included in this text first appeared in *the Zhēnjiǔ Jùyīng* 針灸聚英 (*Gathered Blooms of Acupuncture and Moxibustion*, 1529 CE) by Gāo Wǔ 高武.

these are desertions caused by cold in the lower [jiāo], [one] ought to bank up earth[392] in order to astringe the desertion below.

肝之肝病：跗腫內踝前痛，足寒，淫濼脛痠，腋下馬刀。

Liver diseases of the liver: swelling of the instep and pain in front of the inner ankle [bone], cold feet, pain and weakness with aching of the lower legs, and sabre lumps in the armpit.[393]

注：跗腫足內踝前痛，正本穴部分之症，泄本穴則氣散而腫痛消。足寒者，衝脈之氣滯也，泄此穴以通衝脈之滯。

Explanation: for swelling of the instep and pain in front of the inner ankle [bone], this sign is exactly in the area of this point, drain this point so that the qì will dissipate and the swelling and pain will disperse. Cold feet are due to qì stagnation of the chōng vessel, drain this point in order to free the stagnation of the chōng vessel.

淫濼脛痠，本經寒所致，補此穴以溫脛之寒。腋下馬刀，乃膽經之火，泄肝之土，以散其裏，而表火自息。

Pain and weakness with aching of the lower legs, this is a result of cold in this channel, supplement this point in order to warm the cold in the lower legs. Sabre lumps in the armpit are due to fire of the gallbladder channel, drain the earth [point] of the liver in order to dissipate the interior, so that the fire in its exterior [partner] will naturally cease.

肝之脾病：虛勞浮腫，溏泄，嘔血，嘔逆發寒。

Spleen diseases of the liver: vacuity taxation with puffy swelling, sloppy diarrhoea, retching of blood, and vomiting counterflow with chills.

注：虛勞浮腫，脾土虧矣，肝木之邪旺也，宜補此穴。溏泄，乃肝木尅土之所致也，故補肝經之土穴。

Explanation: when there is vacuity taxation with puffy swelling, spleen earth has become depleted with effulgent evil of liver wood, it is appropriate to supplement this point. Sloppy stools are a result of liver wood restraining earth, thus supplement the earth point of the liver channel.

---

[392] This is a commonly used method in herbal theory, and it is synonymous with supplementing earth.

[393] *The Practical Dictionary* defines sabre lumps "as those occurring in a configuration that looks like the shape of a sabre," these are often accompanied by 俠癭 pearl-string lumps which "occur on the neck giving the appearance of a pearl necklace."

嘔血之症，自胃而出，乃肝氣同衝脈上逆之所致也，亦宜降衝脈之上逆，而泄肝經之土穴。嘔逆發寒，皆胃氣之上逆也，泄肝土穴，以降肝氣之逆。

The sign of retching of blood originates and ejects from the stomach, it is a result of counterflow ascent of the liver qì and the chōng vessel, it is appropriate to descend the counterflow ascent of the chōng vessel; as such, drain the earth point of the liver channel. Vomiting counterflow with chills is always counterflow ascent of the stomach qì, drain the liver earth point in order to descend the counterflow liver qì.

肝之心病：心痛脈弦，心痛色蒼蒼如死狀，終日不得息。

Heart diseases of the liver: heart pain with a stringlike pulse, heart pain with sombre deathlike complexion, and inability to catch the breath all day long.

注：心痛脈弦、心痛色蒼，皆肝邪之干心也，宜泄此穴。

Explanation: for heart pain with stringlike pulse and heart pain with sombre complexion, these are both because liver evil has invaded the heart, it is appropriate to drain this point.

肝之肺病：嗌乾善渴，馬黃瘟疫，肩腫吻傷。

Lung diseases of the liver: dry pharynx with frequent thirst, [jaundice that is the] colour of a yellow horse[394] caused by scourge epidemic, swelling of the shoulder and damage to the corners of the mouth.

注：嗌乾善渴，乃肝經上行頏顙者，火逆於肺也，故宜泄肝火之子。馬黃瘟疫、肩腫吻傷，肩爲肺之府，吻乃肝經下頏環唇之所，瘟疫而至於肩腫吻傷，肝火之盛極矣，故宜泄肝火之子。

Explanation: for dry pharynx with frequent thirst, this is because the liver channel ascends to the nasopharynx [region], when there is fire counterflow in the lung, [this sign occurs], thus drain the liver by the child of fire.

Regarding [jaundice with] colour of a yellow horse caused by scourge epidemic, swelling of the shoulder, and damage to the corners of the mouth, the shoulder is the house of the lung, the corners of the mouth are indeed the place

---

[394] For this term, mǎhuáng 馬黃 (yellow-horse colour), we are not exactly sure what it means, as it is a rare term that does not show up often. We are speculating that it may refer to a severe form of jaundice disease that turns a person light orange or light brown colour that resembles a yellow horse, as this term typically appears alongside with the term jaundice; it is possible that this is describing the colour of the jaundice condition, but the term "jaundice" was dropped for reason unknown in later writings and this manuscript. Another possibility is that it refers to its homophone, mǎhuáng 馬蟥 (leech), which could have been mistakenly blamed as a transmitter of waterborne pandemic diseases (that were spread by other micro-organisms that could not be seen at the time).

where the liver channel descends the cheeks to encircle the lips; for scourge epidemic to cause swelling of the shoulder and damage to the corners of the mouth, this is an extreme exuberance of liver fire, thus it is appropriate to drain the liver by the child of fire.

Fourth Point of the Liver Channel
Zhōng Fēng – Middle Boundary[395] (LR-4)
肝經第四穴中封

一名玄泉
Alternate name: Mysterious Spring[396]

穴在足內踝前一寸筋裏宛宛中。《素》注：一寸半，仰足取陷中，伸足乃得之，足厥陰肝脈所行爲經金。《銅人》：鍼四分，留七呼，灸三壯。

This point is located in the depression between the sinews, 1 cùn in front of the inner ankle [bone]. *The Sùzhù* states, "It is 1 cùn and a half [in front of the inner ankle bone];[397] flex the foot to locate the depression, and then extend the foot to obtain [the point]." The foot juéyīn liver vessel flows here, as the river and metal point. *The Tóngrén* states, "Needle 4 fēn, retain for 7 respirations, and moxa 3 cones."

注：穴名中封者，此中字，蓋指厥陰肝而言也，以此經宜在足少陰之前，太陰之後，兩經之中，而此穴乃在兩經之前，恐人混亂不清，故指而名之曰中封。

Explanation: regarding the point name Zhōng Fēng (Middle Boundary), this character Zhōng (Middle) undoubtedly refers to the juéyīn liver [channel], because

---

[395] *Grasping the Wind* names it "Mound Center."

[396] The alternative name provided here, "Xuán Quán 玄泉 (mysterious spring)," is rendered as "Xuán Quán 懸泉 (suspended spring)" instead in all other acupuncture writings. In addition, the usage of the character "xuán 玄" here is quite peculiar, because this character was a censored character during the early Qīng dynasty, as it was part of the name of Emperor Kāngxī (1654-1722 CE), Xuányè 玄燁. In the time period, the character xuán 玄 would most often be missing its last stroke in writing in order to avoid the censorship, or converted to other characters with similar meaning, such as yuán 元 (primordial/original) and zhēn 真 (true). This leads to our speculation that this choice of character here may have been a scribal error in the manuscript or a mistaken attempt by the copyist to "restore the original character," as xuán 懸 and xuán 玄 are homophones; the copyist could have mistakenly believed this xuán 懸 to be a substitute character for the censorship.

[397] The same location of "1 cùn and a half" in front of the inner angle bone also appears in *Língshū* Chapter 2.

this channel is fittingly located[398] in front of the foot shàoyīn and behind the [foot] tàiyīn [channels]; as such, it is in the Zhōng (Middle) between the two channels. However, this point is in fact located in front of these two channels; due to the fear that people will be confused and unclear [about the placement of these channels], thus [this point] is designated by the name Zhōng Fēng (Middle Boundary).

封者，經疆也。若曰此乃足厥陰經脈之疆也，所以蠡溝絡穴之上，又名之曰中都。自中都復上一寸，而始交足太陰之後，始得其中之位而上行，足少陰在後，近足太陽，足太陰在前，近足陽明，皆相爲表裏者，肝經在兩陰經之中，膽經亦在足兩陽經之中，各用絡穴以相通焉，此中封之所以名也。

Regarding Fēng (Boundary), it is referring to the channel's boundary. Here, in this instance, it is speaking of the boundary of the foot juéyīn channel vessel. As such, above the network point, Lí Gōu (LR-5), there is another [point] named Zhōng Dū (Middle Metropolis, LR-6). At 1 farther cùn above Zhōng Dū (Middle Metropolis, LR-6), [the liver channel] intersects with and [emerges] behind the foot tàiyīn [channel]; thereupon, [the liver channel] obtains the position in the Zhōng (Middle) as it ascends. The foot shàoyīn [channel] is located behind [the liver channel] and it is nearby the foot tàiyáng [channel]; the tàiyīn [channel] is located in front [of the liver channel] and it is nearby the foot yángmíng [channel]; they all act mutually as exterior-interior [pairs]. While the liver channel is located in the Zhōng (Middle) between the two yīn channels, the gallbladder channel is also located in the Zhōng (Middle) between the two leg yáng channels; each of them utilises a network point in order to communicate with the other. This is the reasoning why it is named Zhōng Fēng (Middle Boundary).

《內經》云：使逆則宛，使和則通，搖足而得之，爲經。

The Nèijīng states, "When there is counterflow in the envoy, [the ankle] will be crooked; when the envoy is in harmony, [the ankle] can have free [movement]. [This point] can be located by moving one's foot back and forth, it is the river point."[399]

肝之腎病：五淋不得小便，足厥冷，寒疝腰中痛，筋攣陰縮入腹。

Kidney diseases of the liver: five stranguries with inability to urinate, reversal cold in the legs, cold mounting with pain in the lumbus, hypertonicity of the sinews with the testicles retracted into the abdomen.

---

[398] For "在 located," the secondary manuscript has "行 travels" instead.

[399] From *Língshū* Chapter 2. As this statement is rather ambiguous and can be interpreted in a number of different ways, we have translated it accordingly to the annotation of *the Tàisù*, "氣行曰使。宛，不伸也，塞也。 The movement of qì is namely '使 the envoy;' '宛 being crooked' means that one is not able to extend."

注：五淋不得小便，肝氣鬱也，補肝金穴，以泄肝鬱。足厥冷，肝受寒邪也，補肝金以伐肝邪。寒疝腰中痛，肝腎相通，膂筋之脈相引，補金穴以伐肝邪。筋攣陰縮入腹，乃肝腎俱受寒邪也，急補金穴。失精者，補此穴，金生水也。

Explanation: for five stranguries with the inability to urinate, it is caused by liver qì depression, supplement the liver metal point in order to drain the liver depression. Reversal cold in the legs is because the liver has contracted cold evil, supplement the liver metal [point] in order to quell the liver evil.

Regarding cold mounting with pain in the lumbus, as the liver and the kidneys communicate with each other, [the liver channel] and the vessels of the paravertebral sinews radiate towards each other, supplement the metal point in order to quell the liver evil. For hypertonicity of the sinews with the testicles retracted into the abdomen, this is because both the liver and the kidneys have contracted cold evil, urgently supplement the metal point. For seminal emission, supplement this point, because metal engenders water.

肝之肝病：痎瘧色蒼蒼振寒，小腹腫痛，繞臍痛。

Liver diseases of the liver: intervallic malaria with sombre complexion and quivering with cold, swelling and pain of the lower abdomen, and pain that encircles the umbilicus.

注：瘧症色蒼蒼，肝瘧也，小腹腫痛，繞臍痛，皆肝氣鬱也，宜補金穴。

Explanation: for malarial signs with sombre complexion, this is liver malaria; for swelling and pain of the lower abdomen and pain that encircles the umbilicus, these are both due to depression of liver qì, it is appropriate to supplement the metal point.

肝之脾病：身黃有微熱，不嗜食，身體不仁。

Spleen diseases of the liver: yellowing of the body with slight fever, no pleasure in eating, and generalised numbness.

注：以上症皆脾土虧，肝木旺也，補肝金以治肝邪，則能食而麻木愈矣。

Explanation: all of the above signs are due to spleen-earth depletion with liver-wood effulgence, supplement the liver metal [point] in order to treat the liver evil, so that one will have [pleasure] in eating and recover from the numbness.

Fifth Point of the Liver Channel
Lǐ Gōu – Woodworm Canal (LR-5)
肝經第五穴蠡溝

一名交儀

Alternate Name: Intersection Apparatus

穴在內踝上五寸，足厥陰絡別走少陽。《銅人》：鍼二分，留三呼，灸三壯。《下經》：灸七壯。穴在腨之下，踵之上，魚腹之外，蓋腨之形如魚腹，故魚腹即腨也，循其分肉，有血絡累累然，即其穴也。

This point is located 5 cùn above the inner ankle [bone]. It is the foot juéyīn network point that diverges to the foot shàoyáng [channel]. *The Tóngrén* states, "Needle 2 fēn, retain for 3 respirations, and moxa 3 cones." *The Xiàjīng* states, "Moxa 7 cones." This point is located below the calf, above the heel, outside of the fish belly;[400] undoubtedly, the shape of the calf resembles a fish belly, thus the 'fish belly' refers precisely to the calf; follow the division in the flesh, where the blood network-vessels cluster together, this is precisely this point.

注：此乃肝經之絡，而通膽經者，此經與彼經通，必有竅焉以通之，故曰溝。蠡者，蟲也，所以鑿木者，故曰蠡溝。此絡之經脛上睪，結於莖垂，其病氣逆則睪腫、卒疝。實則邪氣有餘，陰爲挺長，虛則正氣不足，而暴癢，取之本穴。

Explanation: this [point] is the network point of the liver channel; regarding its communication with the gallbladder channel, for this channel to communicate with the other channel, there must be an opening which allows such a communication, thus it is called Gōu (Canal). Lí (Woodworms), are [a type of] insects; as [this point] enables one to bore through the wood, thus it is called Lí Gōu (Woodworm Canal).

The network-vessel passes through the lower leg, ascends to the testicles, and knots at the male genitalia. For its diseases, when there is counterflow qì, there will be swelling of the testicles or sudden mounting; when it is replete, the evil qì will be superabundant, the genitals will have persistent erection; when it is vacuous, the upright qì will be insufficient, leading to fulminant itchiness; [for either case], one ought to choose this point.

肝之腎病：小腹脹滿暴痛，睪丸卒痛，實則挺長泄之，虛則暴癢補之，癃閉小便不利，臍下積氣如石，足脛寒痠屈伸難，赤白帶下，月水不調。

Kidney diseases of the liver: distention and fullness in the lower abdomen with fulminant pain, and sudden pain of the testicles; when it is replete, there

---

400 I.e., the belly of the calf muscle. It is also an alternate name for BL-57.

will be persistent erection, so drain it; when it is vacuous, there will be sudden itchiness, so supplement it; dribbling urinary block with inhibited urination, accumulated qì that resembles a stone below the umbilicus, cold aches in the feet and lower legs with difficulty in bending and stretching, red and white vaginal discharge, and irregular menstruation.

注：凡睪丸病及疝病、莖垂病，雖肝病也，而未有不由於腎氣之逆、腎氣之勞、腎氣之虛而致者，宜調肝之絡穴，相虛實而補泄之。

Explanation: for testicle diseases, mounting diseases, and diseases of the penis, although they are liver diseases, it is unprecedented that they are not caused by counterflow of kidney qì, taxation of kidney qì, or vacuity of kidney qì; it is appropriate to regulate the network point of the liver, differentiate whether it is vacuous or replete and then supplement or drain it accordingly.

小便不利，癃閉，皆肝氣之逆也，泄肝之絡，所以舒肝之逆。臍下積氣如石，以肝經上過小腹，鬱而不行，故致此症，泄此穴。足脛寒痿屈伸難，肝經中寒邪也，泄絡穴以去寒邪。赤白帶下及月水不調，而亦取此穴者，散肝火久鬱之氣，而調其氣血也。

Both inhibited urination and dribbling urinary block are due to counterflow of liver qì, drain the network point of the liver so as to course the counterflow of the liver. Regarding accumulated qì that resembles a stone below the umbilicus, the liver channel ascends to traverse the lower abdomen, when it is depressed, it will fail to move, thus it will result in this sign, drain this point.

Cold aches in the feet and lower legs with difficulty in bending and stretching are because the liver channel is struck by cold evil, drain the network point in order to eliminate the cold evil. Regarding red and white vaginal discharge as well as irregular menstruation, this point can also be chosen because it is able to regulate the qì and blood by dispersing the liver fire and chronically depressed qì.

肝之肺病：數逆，恐悸，少氣不足，悒悒不樂，咽中悶如有瘜肉，背拘急不得俯仰。

Lung diseases of the liver: frequent counterflow,[401] fearful palpitations, scantness and insufficiency of qì, mental depression, oppression in the pharynx as if there were polyps, and hypertonicity of the upper back with inability to bend forwards and backwards.

注：數逆，肝之脈上及於肺者，憂鬱於下，則氣不順於上，故取此穴，以散肝之鬱。咽中悶如有瘜肉，因肝之脈，上通頏顙，肝氣逆則有此症，宜泄絡穴，以散肝之火。

---

[401] "數逆 Frequent counterflow" is actually "數噫 frequent belching" in *the Zhēnjiǔ Dàchéng*.

Explanation: regarding frequent counterflow, as the vessel of the liver ascends to reach the lung, when the lower is afflicted by depression, qì will become unsmooth above, thus choose this point in order to disperse the depression of the liver. Regarding oppression in the pharynx as if there were polyps, it is because the vessel of the liver ascends to communicate with the nasopharynx [region]; when there is liver qì counterflow, there will be this sign, it is appropriate to drain the network point in order to disperse the fire of the liver.

背拘急不得俯仰，背者，肺之府，肝經上通於肺，肝氣上逆，而肺脈弦，遂有此症，急泄此穴，以降肝之逆。

For hypertonicity of the upper back with inability to bend forwards and backwards, the upper back is the residence of the lung; in addition, the liver channel ascends to communicate with the lung; when there is qì counterflow ascent and stringlike [quality] in the lung pulse, there will be these signs, urgently drain this point in order to descend counterflow of the liver.

Sixth Point of the Liver Channel
Zhōng Dū – Middle Metropolis[402] (LR-6)
肝經第六穴中都

一名中郄
Alternate name: Middle Cleft

穴在內踝上七寸骭骨中，與少陰相值。《銅人》：鍼三分，灸五壯。

This point is located 7 cùn above the inner ankle bone on the shin bone, where it crosses the shàoyīn [channel]. *The Tóngrén* states, "Needle 3 fēn, and moxa 5 cones."

注：穴名中都者，此穴離上一寸，遂入足太陰之後，而得其中之位，故曰中都。此中字，與前穴中封之中字相應。

Explanation: regarding the point name Zhōng Dū (Middle Metropolis), at 1 cùn above this point, [the liver channel] enters behind the foot tàiyīn [channel], hence it obtains the position in the Zhōng (Middle), thus it is called Zhōng Dū (Middle Metropolis). This character Zhōng (Middle) corresponds with the [same] Zhōng (Middle) character in the previous point of Zhōng Fēng (Middle, Boundary LR-4).

---

[402] *Grasping the Wind* names it "Central Metropolis."

肝之腎病：小腹痛不能行立，脛寒腸癖，崩中不止，產後惡露不絕。

Kidney diseases of the liver: lower abdominal pain with inability to stand or walk, cold lower legs with intestinal aggregations, incessant flooding, and persistent flow of lochia.

注：肝經十三穴，惟膝關、五里、陰廉、期門四穴不治疝病，餘九穴皆治疝病，則疝之獨責肝經，其正治也。

Explanation: among the thirteen points of the liver channel,[403] only the four points of Xī Guān (LR-7), Wǔ Lǐ (LR-10), Yīn Lián (LR-11), and Qī Mén (LR-14) do not treat mounting disease; the remaining nine points all treat mounting disease, hence for mounting, one should seek only the liver channel, as it is what [the liver channel] primarily treats.

小腹痛不能行立，肝經上行繞陰器，抵小腹，由曲骨上會任脈於關元，故取此穴，以泄肝氣於下。脛寒者，肝經中寒邪也，宜補此穴以溫之。腸癖者，肝氣滯也，取此穴以通肝之滯氣。崩中不止、惡露不絕，久則血脫於下，補此以止下脫。

Regarding lower abdominal pain with inability to stand or walk, the liver channel ascends to encircle the yīn organs, and upon reaching the lower abdomen, it ascends from the curved bone[404] to meet the rèn vessel at Guān Yuán (REN-4); thus, choose this point in order to drain the liver qì from below. Regarding cold lower legs, this is because the liver channel is struck by cold evil, supplement this point in order to warm it.

Regarding intestinal aggregations, these are liver qì stagnation, choose this point in order to free the stagnant qì of the liver. For incessant flooding and persistent flow of lochia, when these [diseases] become chronic, there will be desertion of blood below, supplement this [point] in order to stop the desertion below.

---

[403] Note: In this writing, LR-12 is not considered as a channel point of the liver channel and is discussed within the entry of LR-11.

[404] This is also the name of Qū Gǔ (REN-2).

Seventh Point of the Liver Channel
Xī Guān – Knee Pass[405] (LR-7)
肝經第七穴膝關

穴在胃經犢鼻下二寸旁陷中。《銅人》：鍼四分，灸五壯。

This point is located in the depression 2 cùn below and to the side of Dú Bí (ST-35) of the stomach channel. *The Tóngrén* states, "Needle 4 fēn, and moxa 5 cones."

注：穴名膝關者，肝經至此，上行將過膝而入股，上下骨節交折之所，有關之象焉，故曰膝關。

Explanation: regarding the point name Xī Guān (Knee Pass), upon arriving here, the ascending pathway of the liver channel is about to traverse the Xī (Knee) and enter the thigh; this is the place where the two bony joints intersect and bend; as such, it has the image of a Guān (Pass), thus it is called Xī Guān (Knee Pass).

肝之肝病：風痺膝內廉痛，引臏不可屈伸。

Liver diseases of the liver: wind impediment with pain on the inside of the knee, [pain] that radiates to the kneecap with inability to bend and stretch [the leg].

注：肝中風寒，此處皮肉薄削而先痛，至於不可屈伸，則寒中於筋，故取此穴以治寒。

Explanation: when the liver is struck by wind and cold, as the skin and flesh at this location are thin and frail, pain will manifest here first; as for inability to bend and stretch [the leg], this is because sinews have been struck by cold, thus choose this point in order to treat the cold.

肝之肺病：咽喉中痛。

Lung disease of the liver: pain in the pharynx and throat.

注：肝經上抵頏顙，氣上逆，則咽喉為之腫痛，膝關，將離膝上股之穴也，故取此穴，以泄肝氣之逆。

Explanation: as the liver channel ascends to reach the nasopharynx region, when there is counterflow qì ascent, the pharynx and throat will become swollen and painful; Xī Guān (LR-7) is the point [where the channel] is just about to leave the

---

[405] *Grasping the Wind* names it "Knee Joint."

knee and ascend the thigh, thus choose this point in order to descend the counterflow liver qì.

Eighth Point of the Liver Channel
Qū Quán – Spring at the Bend (LR-8)
肝經第八穴曲泉

穴在膝股上內側，輔骨下大筋上，小筋下陷中，屈膝橫紋頭取之，足厥陰肝木所入爲合水，肝虛則補之。《銅人》：鍼六分，留十呼，灸三壯。男子失精，膝脛冷痛，灸百壯。

This point is located on the inside of the knee and thigh, below the assisting bone, above the large sinew, in the depression below the small sinew; bend the knee to locate it at the top of the transverse crease. The foot juéyīn liver wood enters here, as the uniting and sea point. When the liver is vacuous, supplement it. *The Tóngrén* **states, "Needle 6 fēn, retain for 10 respirations, and moxa 3 cones. For seminal emission in males, cold pain in the lower legs, moxa 100 cones."**

注：穴名泉者，以肝經之合穴爲水，故有泉之名。曲者，乃以肝經初離膝而上股，正在曲折之地，故曰曲。又木曰曲直，木之水亦當名曲。肝虛則補之者，以水能生木，爲本經之母穴，補其母，所以益其子也。

Explanation: regarding the point name Quán (Spring), as it is the uniting point of the liver, which is the water point, thus it has the designation of Quán (Spring). Regarding Qū (Bend), when the liver channel begins to depart the knee and ascend the thigh, this is exactly the place that turns and Qū (Bends), thus it is called Qū (Bend). In addition, wood is said to be Qū (Bending) and straightening,[406] hence this water point of wood should also be named as Qū (Bend).

For one to supplement it when the liver is vacuous, it is because water is able to engender wood; as this is the mother point on this channel, supplement the mother in order to boost the child.

---

[406] "曲直 bending and straightening" likely refers to "洪範 Great Plan," which is ones of the earliest written records regarding the five phases found in 尚書 *the Book of History* (c. 4th to 3rd century BCE), which is the recorded oration of Jīzǐ 箕子 that supposedly took place in the 11th century BCE, "五行：一曰水，二曰火，三曰木，四曰金，五曰土。水曰潤下，火曰炎上，木曰曲直，金曰從革，土爰稼穡。The five phases: First, the water; second, the fire; third, the wood; fourth, the metal; fifth, the earth. Water means moistening and descending; fire means blazing and ascending; wood means bending and straightening; metal means conforming and reforming; earth means sowing and reaping."

肝之腎病：癩疝陰股病，陰腫，陰莖痛，女子小腹腫，陰挺出，陰癢，小便難，癃閉，房勞失精。

Kidney diseases of the liver: slumping mounting and diseases of the yīn of the thigh, genital swelling, pain of the penis, swelling of the lower abdomen in females, vaginal protrusion, pudendal itch, difficult urination, dribbling urinary block, and sexual taxation with seminal loss.

注：肝經過膝，其上行也甚速，而此穴其始也。肝之經環繞陰器，故男子癩疝、陰腫、陰莖痛，女子小腹腫、陰挺出、陰癢，皆責此穴。小便雖爲腎之所司，而肝經亦操疏泄之權，故小便難、癃閉，亦責此穴，而通肝經之滯氣。此穴爲肝之母，房勞則肝火動，失精則水不足，補此穴。

Explanation: once the liver channel traverses past the knee, it ascends [the thigh] with incredible swiftness, and this point is the beginning [of its ascent]. As the channel of the liver encircles the genitals, therefore, for slumping mounting in males, genital swelling, pain of the penis, swelling of the lower abdomen in females, vaginal protrusion, and pudendal itch, in all these cases, seek this point.

Although urine is controlled by the kidneys, the liver channel also has the power to manage the free coursing and discharge [of urine], thus for difficult urination and dribbling urinary block, also seek this point in order to free the stagnant qì in the liver channel. As this point is mother [point] of the liver, sexual taxation causes liver fire to stir, loss of essence causes insufficiency of water, supplement this point.

肝之肝病：腹脇支滿，身目眩痛，汗不出，目䀮䀮，膝關痛不可屈伸，胻腫膝脛冷痛，女子血瘕，按之如湯浸股內。

Liver diseases of the liver: propping fullness in the abdomen and rib-sides, dizzy vision with generalised body pain, absence of sweating, blurred vision, pain of the knee joint[407] with inability to bend and stretch, swelling of the lower leg with cold pain in the knee and lower leg, and female blood conglomerations, when pressed, it is as though hot water is pouring over the inner thigh to the knee.

注：腹脇支滿，肝氣上逆也，泄此穴。身目眩痛，汗不出，目䀮䀮，皆肝經之實也，宜泄此穴。膝關痛不可屈伸及胻腫膝脛冷痛，皆肝中寒邪也，宜泄此穴。血瘕，肝氣滯而血鬱也，宜泄此穴。

Explanation: propping fullness of the abdomen and rib-sides is due to counterflow ascent of liver qì, drain this point. For dizzy vision with generalised

---

[407] This is also the name of Xī Guān (LR-7).

body pain, absence of sweating, and blurred vision, all these are repletion of the liver channel, it is appropriate to drain this point.

For pain of the knee joint with inability to bend and stretch, as well as swelling of the shin with cold pain in the knee and lower leg, all these are because the liver is struck by cold evil, it is appropriate to drain this point. For blood conglomerations, this is blood depression caused by the liver qì stagnation, it is appropriate to drain this point.

肝之脾病：泄利，四肢不舉，少氣，泄水，下利膿血，身體極痛。

Spleen diseases of the liver: diarrhoea, inability to lift the limbs, scantness of qì,[408] watery diarrhoea, diarrhoea with pus and blood, and extreme pain in the body.

注：泄利，四肢不舉，少氣，脾土虧，肝木忌旺，急泄肝母穴。泄水、下利膿血至於身體極痛，血虧極矣，急補此穴，以生肝血。

Explanation: for diarrhoea, inability to lift the four limbs, and scantness of qì, these are due to depletion of spleen-earth; as such, it is unfavourable for liver-wood to be effulgent, urgently drain the liver mother point. For watery diarrhoea and diarrhoea with pus and blood that has caused extreme pain of the body, the blood has become severely depleted, urgently supplement this point in order to engender liver blood.

肝之心病：發狂。

Heart disease of the liver: mania.

注：狂而新發，先取曲泉，左右動脈及盛者見血，有頃已，不已，以法取之，灸骶骨二十壯。肝盛上逆，而有是症，肝爲心之母，而此穴又爲肝之母，急宜泄之。

Explanation: for a new onset of mania, initially choose Qū Quán (LR-8); when its vessel is pulsating in exuberance, let the blood; in a short moment, [the mania] will cease. If it does not cease, choose this point according to the [previous] method, and in addition, moxa 20 cones on the sacrum.[409] When the liver is exuberant with counterflow ascent, there will be this sign; as the liver is the mother of the heart, and as this point is also the mother [point] of the liver, it is appropriate to urgently drain this [point].

---

[408] "Scantness of qì" can also be translated as "scantness of breath," as this is categorised under the spleen, we chose the former in this instance.

[409] Note: Yuè Hánzhēn also lists Dǐ Gǔ 骶骨 (Sacrum) as an alternate name for DU-1.

肝之肺病：衄血，喘呼，小腹痛引咽喉。

Lung diseases of the liver: nosebleeds, panting, and lower abdominal pain that radiates to the throat.

注：衄血雖爲陽明經及肺經熱症，而肝之上逆亦助之，宜泄。喘呼雖爲肺症，肝氣不逆則上喘不甚，宜泄。下而小腹，上而咽喉，皆肝經所至之地，小腹痛引咽喉，肝氣上逆也，宜泄。

Explanation: although nosebleeds is a heat sign of the yángmíng channel and lung channel, yet, it is also assisted by the counterflow ascent of liver, it is appropriate to drain. Although panting is a lung sign, in the absence of liver qì counterflow, the panting will not be severe, it is appropriate to drain. As the liver channel reaches both the lower abdomen below and the throat above, lower abdomen pain that radiates to the throat is due to the counterflow ascent of liver qì, thus it is appropriate to drain.

Nineth Point of the Liver Channel
Yīn Bāo – Enveloped Yīn[410] (LR-9)
肝經第九穴陰包

穴在膝上四寸，內廉兩筋間，蹺足取之，內側必有槽中。《銅人》：鍼六分，灸三壯。《下經》：鍼七分。

This point is located 4 cùn above the knee, in the space between the two sinews on the inside ridge, which is located by curling the leg, where there must be a groove on the inner [thigh]. *The Tóngrén* states, "Needle 6 fēn, and moxa 3 cones." *The Xiàjīng* states, "Needle 7 fēn."

注：穴名陰包者，蓋肝經過膝，而行乎兩陰之中，爲太陰、少陰所包，故曰陰包。又以穴在股之槽中，亦象包形。

Explanation: regarding the point name Yīn Bāo (Enveloped Yīn), undoubtedly, as the liver channel traverses the knee, it travels in the middle between the two Yīn (Yīn) channels, where it is Bāo (Enveloped) by the tàiyīn and shàoyīn [channels], thus it is called Yīn Bāo (Enveloped Yīn). In addition, as this point is located in the groove on the thigh, it has the image of being Bāo (Enveloped) in its physical form.

---

[410] *Grasping the Wind* names it "Yīn Womb."

肝之腎病：腰尻引小腹痛，小便難，遺溺不禁，月水不調。

Kidney diseases of the liver: pain that radiates from the lumbus and sacrum to the lower abdomen, difficult urination, unrestrained enuresis, and irregular menstruation.

注：腰尻小腹，皆肝經之地，肝氣逆乃相引而痛，宜泄。小便難，乃肝氣滯也，宜泄。遺溺不禁，乃肝寒也，宜補。肝主血，月水不調，過期則泄此穴，不及期則補此穴。

Explanation: the lumbus, sacrum, and lower abdomen, these are the places of the liver channel; when there is liver qì counterflow, there will be pain that radiates between [these areas], it is appropriate to drain. Difficult urination is due to liver qì stagnation, it is appropriate to drain. Unrestrained enuresis is due to liver cold, it is appropriate to supplement. As the liver governs blood, when there is irregular menstruation, if it is delayed, drain this point; if it is early, supplement this point.

Tenth Point of the Liver Channel
Wǔ Lǐ – Five Lǐ (LR-10)
肝經第十穴五里

穴在氣衝下三寸，陰股中，動脈應手。《銅人》：鍼六分，灸五壯。

This point is located 3 cùn below Qì Chōng (ST-30), on the yīn of the thigh, where the pulsating vessel resonates with the hand. *The Tóngrén* states, "Needle 6 fēn, and moxa 5 cones."

注：穴名五里者，言其遠也，肝經自大敦起，過足指、足跗、足踝、足腑、足膝、足股至此，乃有動脈應手，將入腹，故曰五里。

Explanation: regarding the point name Wǔ Lǐ (Five Lǐ), that is speaking of its vast distance. The liver channel commences from Dà Dūn (LR-1), it traverses the big toe, the instep, the ankle [bone], the calf, the knee, and finally the thigh to arrive at this [point]; it is also where the pulsating vessel resonates with the hand and where [the liver channel] is about to enter the abdomen, thus it is called Wǔ Lǐ (Five Lǐ).

肝之腎病：腸滿，熱閉不得溺。

Kidney diseases of the liver: intestinal fullness, and heat block with inability to urinate.

注：上症，肝經之逆也，急泄其將入腹之穴。

Explanation: the above signs are due to counterflow of the liver channel, urgently drain the point that is about to enter the abdomen.

肝之肝病：風勞嗜臥。

Liver disease of the liver: wind taxation with somnolence.

注：肝血不足，則筋無血以養之，則不能久坐立也，宜補此穴，以生肝血。

Explanation: when the liver blood is insufficient, it will lack the blood to nourish the sinews, thus there will be inability to sit or stand for long periods, it is appropriate to supplement this point in order to engender the liver blood.

Eleventh Point of the Liver Channel
Yīn Lián – Yīn Corner (LR-11)
肝經第十一穴陰廉

穴在羊矢下，去氣衝下二寸動脈中。《銅人》：鍼八分，留七呼，灸三壯。

This point is located below the goat faeces,[411] on the pulsating vessel, 2 cùn below Qì Chōng (ST-30). *The Tóngrén* states, "Needle 8 fēn, retain for 7 respirations, and moxa 3 cones."

注：肝經將入腹矣，廉者，言其隅也，銳也，離股而入腹，有廉之象焉，肝經爲陰，故曰陰廉。

Explanation: as the liver channel is about to enter the abdomen, for Lián (Corner), it is referring to the pointed edge of a border; as [the liver channel] departs the thigh to enter the abdomen, there is the image of a Lián (Corner); in addition, as the liver channel is Yīn (Yīn), thus it is called Yīn Lián (Yīn Corner).

《内經》云：厥陰毛中急脈各一。言肝經有急脈在陰毛中，上引小腹，下引陰丸，寒則爲痛，其脈甚急，故曰急脈，乃睾丸之系也。可灸而不可刺，然灸書無此穴，當在睾丸直衝之上，即歸來等穴之所，然偏墜吊痛者，果有急脈引痛。

---

[411] I.e., anterior superior iliac crest. It is also designed as an extra point Yáng Shǐ (UEX-LE-1). *Grasping the Wind* translates this term as "goat arrow" and lists it as an alternate name for LR-12; in addition, it notes that its name "is derived from the hard arrow-shaped sinew located just below this [LR-12]." However, Yuè Hánzhēn seems to have a different interpretation and renders this term as "goat faeces," see the first extra point listed in the Extra Points Associated with the Rèn Channel.

The Nèijīng states, "The juéyīn has an urgent pulse[412] on each [side] in the pubic hair."[413] This is speaking of the urgent pulse of the liver channel that is located within the pubic hair [region]; it extends to the lower abdomen above, and extends to the testicles below; when there is cold, there will be pain, and the pulse will become extremely tense,[414] thus it is called the urgent pulse. It is the connector to the testicles.

While moxibustion can be performed [on the urgent pulse], it cannot be pierced; yet, many moxibustion texts do not contain this point; it should be located directly above the testicles, precisely where points such as Guī Lái (ST-29) are located; hence, for those with hemilateral sagging or suspended pain of the testicle, there will be pain that radiates towards the urgent pulse.

肝之腎病：婦人絕產，若未經生產者，灸三壯，即有子。

Kidney diseases of the liver: for infertility in women, if they have never become pregnant, moxa 3 cones, they will have child promptly.

注：肝主血，婦人受胎，以血爲主，從未生產，非肝氣之滯，即肝氣之寒，灸此穴以暖其血，而通其滯。

Explanation: the liver governs blood, when women become pregnant, it is the blood that governs [the pregnancy]; for those who have never become pregnant, if it were not caused by the stagnation of liver qì, then it would have been caused by the coldness of liver qì, moxa this point in order to warm the blood, so that the stagnation can be freed.

---

[412] I.e., Jí Mài 急脈 (Urgent Pulse, LR-12).

[413] From *Sùwèn* Chapter 59.

[414] Jí 急 can be translated as "urgent" or "tense" based on the context. In prior incidences, it was translated as "urgent," as "Urgent Pulse" is an established translation for the point name; but for here, "tense" fits the context better, as a tense pulse quality tends to manifest in the presence of a cold invasion.

Twelfth Point of the Liver Channel
Zhāng Mén – Timber Gate[415] (LR-13)[416]
肝經第十二穴章門

一名長平
Alternate name: Long Level

一名脇髎
Alternate name: Lateral Costal Bone-Hole

穴在大橫外，直季脇肋端，當臍上二寸，兩旁六寸，側臥屈上足，伸下足，舉臂取之。又云：肘尖盡處是穴。脾之募，足少陰、厥陰之會。《銅人》：鍼六分，灸百壯。《明堂》：灸七壯，止五百壯。《素》注：鍼八分，留十呼，灸三壯。《千金》：賁豚積聚，堅滿脹痛，吐逆不下食，腰脊冷痛，小便白濁，灸脾募百壯，三報之。又治狂走癲癇，灸三十壯。又溺血，灸百壯。

This point is located outside of Dà Héng (SP-15), directly at the edge of the floating rib, at precisely 2 cùn above the umbilicus, and 6 cùn on each side [of the midline]; lie on one's side, bend the top leg while extending the bottom leg, and raise the arm to locate it. Another states, where the tip of the elbow [rests], that is the point. It is the collecting point of the spleen. It is the meeting of the foot shàoyīn and juéyīn [channels]. *The Tóngrén* states, "Needle 6 fēn, and moxa 100 cones." *The Míngtáng* states, "Moxa 7 cones, and up to 500 cones."

The Sùzhù states, "Needle 8 fēn,[417] retain for 10 respirations,[418] and moxa 3 cones."[419] *The Qiānjīn* states, "For running piglet with accumulations and gatherings, hardened fullness with distension and pain, vomiting counterflow with inability to ingest food, cold pain in the lumbar spine, and turbid white urine, moxa 100 cones on the spleen collecting point for 3 sessions. In addition, to treat manic walking with epilepsy, moxa 30 cones. Moreover, [to treat] bloody urine, moxa 100 cones."

---

[415] *Grasping the Wind* names it "Camphorwood Fate."

[416] LR-12 is absent as an individual entry in this text; however, it is discussed above in the explanation of the name of LR-11. We have kept the modern numbering standards here as to avoid confusion, but it must be noted that the last two points were the 12th point (LR-13) and 13th point (LR-14) in Yuè Hánzhēn's arrangement.

[417] For "8 fēn," *the Sùzhù* actually states "6 fēn."

[418] For the "10 respiration," it is "6 respiration" in *the Sùzhù* and the secondary manuscript instead.

[419] For the "3 cones," it is actually "5 cones" in *the Sùzhù* instead.

注：《難經》：臟會章門。疏云：臟病治此。臟者，心肝脾肺腎也。按肝之行於臍下者八寸，即交出足太陰脾經之後，則與脾會矣。

Explanation: *the Nánjīng* [states], "Zàng-viscera meet at Zhāng Mén (Timber Gate)." *The [Nánjīng] Shū* states, "For zàng-viscera diseases, treat this [point]." Regarding the "zàng-viscera," they are the heart, liver, spleen, lung, and kidneys.

Note by [Master Sīlián]: at 8 cùn below the umbilicus,[420] the [left and right] pathways of the liver intersect and emerge behind the foot tàiyīn spleen channel, hence it meets with the spleen.

此穴又為脾之募，上行而入胸也，上注肺，則與肺會矣。下行在小腹者，中極、關元，皆任經、足少陰腎經所會之處，注於肺則及於心矣，故此穴為肝經入腹之要穴，而曰臟會章門也。

Furthermore, as this point is the collecting point of the spleen, its pathway ascends to enter the chest; since it ascends to pour into the lung, hence it meets with the lung. The pathway descends to the lower abdomen, to Zhōng Jí (REN-3) and Guān Yuán (REN-4), both of which are locations where the rèn channel and the foot shàoyīn kidney channel meet. Moreover, as [its ascending pathway] pours into the lung, it will also reach the heart; therefore, this point is a pivotal point where the liver channel enters the abdomen; as such, it is said that the zàng-viscera meet at Zhāng Mén (Timber Gate).

章者何？草曰本，木曰章，肝陰木，膽陽木也，脅肋正肝膽所治之部分，故曰章門。肝經在腹，止有二穴，皆以門稱。以木性曲直，而有啟閉之義，故曰門。

What is meant by Zhāng (Timber)? Plants are said to have roots, wood is said to offer Zhāng (Great Timber);[421] while the liver is yīn wood, the gallbladder is yáng wood; the rib-sides are exactly the area where the liver and gallbladder govern, thus it is called Zhāng Mén (Timber Gate). The liver channel only has two

---

[420] Note: this "8 cùn below the umbilicus" brings to the level of Qì Chōng (ST-30); however, according to the pathway description, the liver channel does not intersect with that point, and does not provide any point or landmark at that level. So, we are offering three possibilities here: The first is simply a location along the liver channel that is 8 cùn below the umbilicus, possibly around the genitals. Second, it could be a scribal error. Third, it could be LR-12, which is located above LR-11 (which is 2 cùn below ST-30) yet with an undefined location in this writing.

[421] This is an uncommon definition for zhāng 章 in early usages, before the publication of *Shuōwén Jiězì* 説文解字 (*Explaining Graphs and Analysing Characters*, c. 2nd century CE), which was the first comprehensive dictionary that came to define Chinese characters. A textual example could be found in 史記貨殖列傳 the *Records of the Grand Historian*: "Chronicles of the Trades and Merchants" (91 BCE), "山居千章之材 in the mountains, there lies the resource of thousands of great timbers."

points on the abdomen, both of which are denoted as Mén (Gate). As it is said that the nature of wood is bending and straightening,[422] it has the meaning of opening blockages, thus it is called Mén (Gate).

大橫乃脾經穴，在腹哀下三寸五分，去腹中行各寸半，此穴在大橫之外，臍上二寸，正任經下脘之穴，與此穴平直，正在季脇肋端，側臥取其端，非如此取不可也。

Dà Héng (SP-15) is a spleen channel point, it is located 3 cùn 5 fēn below Fù Āi (SP-16) on the abdomen, 1 cùn and a half on each side of the abdominal midline. This point is located outside of Dà Héng (SP-15), 2 cùn above the umbilicus, exactly in a horizontal line with the point Xià Wǎn (REN-10) of the rèn channel; it is exactly at the edge of the floating rib; lie on the side to find the edge, without following this [method], one will be unable to locate it.

肝之腎病：腰痛不得轉側，腰脊冷痛，溺多白濁，賁豚積聚，脊強，四肢懈惰，疝病。

Kidney diseases of the liver: lumbar pain with inability to turn to the sides, cold pain in the lumbar spine, urine that is often white and turbid, running piglet with accumulations and gatherings, stiffness of the spine, slackness and laxness of the four limbs, and mounting disease.

注：腰者，腎之府也，肝氣逆於腰，則痛不得轉側，宜泄此穴。腰脊冷痛，乃肝經受寒所致，宜泄以去寒邪。溺多白濁，乃下焦有濕熱所致，宜泄以去濕熱。

Explanation: the lumbus is the residence of the kidneys, when there is counterflow liver qì in the lumbus, there will be pain with inability to turn to the sides, it is appropriate to drain this point. Cold pain in the lumbar spine is because the liver channel has contracted cold, it is appropriate to drain this point in order to eliminate the cold evil. Urine that is often white and turbid is a result of damp-heat in the lower jiāo, it is appropriate to drain in order to eliminate the damp-heat.

賁豚積聚，雖宜責腎，亦肝經之氣滯所致，宜泄以舒肝氣。肝附着於脊，受寒邪則脊強，而四肢之筋不能榮，則懈惰，宜泄。

For running piglet with accumulations and gatherings, although it is appropriate to blame the kidneys, it can also be a result of qì stagnation in the liver channel, it is appropriate to drain in order to course the liver qì. As the liver attaches

---

[422] For "the nature of wood is bending and straightening," see footnote 406.

itself to the spine,[423] when it contracts cold evil, there will be stiffness of the spine as well as the inability to flourish the sinews of the four limbs, hence there will be slackness and laxness, it is appropriate to drain.

疝病乃寒在下焦，東垣曰：氣在於腸胃者，取之太陰、陽明，不下，取三里、章門、中脘。又疝病自臍下上至於心，脹滿嘔吐，煩悶，不進飲食，此寒在下焦，灸章門、氣海有驗。

Mounting disease is due to cold in the lower jiāo; [Lǐ] Dōngyuán says, "For qì located in the intestines and stomach, choose the tàiyīn and yángmíng [channels], do not precipitate, choose Sān Lǐ (ST-36), Zhāng Mén (LR-13), and Zhōng Wǎn (REN-12)."[424] In addition, for mounting disease that ascends to affect the heart from below the umbilicus, [it will cause] distension and fullness, vexation and oppression, and stoppage of food and drink, this is cold in the lower jiāo, it is effective to moxa Zhāng Mén (LR-13) and Qì Hǎi (REN-14).

肝之肝病：脇痛不得臥，善恐少氣，厥逆，肩臂不舉。

Liver diseases of the liver: rib-side pain with inability to lie down, susceptibility to fear with scantness of qì, reverse flow, and inability to raise the shoulder and arm.

注：脇痛不得眠臥，肝氣逆也，宜泄。善恐少氣，肝氣怯也，宜補。厥逆、肩臂不舉，肝經受寒邪也，宜灸。

Explanation: rib-side pain with inability to lie down is liver qì counterflow, it is appropriate to drain. Susceptibility to fear with scantness of qì is liver qì timidity, it is appropriate to supplement. For reverse flow and inability to raise the shoulder and arm, this is because the liver channel has contracted cold evil, it is appropriate to moxa.

肝之脾病：腸鳴食不化，煩熱口乾，不嗜食，吐逆飲食都出，傷飽身黃。

Spleen diseases of the liver: rumbling intestines with indigestion, heart vexation with dry mouth, no pleasure in eating, vomiting with counterflow

---

[423] This statement does not appear to be located in the canons, it appears to first be discussed in *Shísìjīng Fāhuī* 十四經發揮 (*Elucidation of the Fourteen Channels*, 1341 CE) by 滑壽 Huá Shòu, which states, "肝之為臟……其臟在右脅右腎之前，並胃貫脊之第九椎 For the liver zàng-viscus, the location of the this zàng-viscus is in front of the right kidney on the right rib-side, where it stands side by side with the stomach and further links with the 9th vertebra of the spine."

[424] From the chapter titled, "胃氣下溜五臟氣皆亂其為病互相出見論 Cross-Referencing the Disease of the Stomach Qì Flowing Downward with the Complete Chaos of the Qì of the Five Zàng-Viscera," in *the Píwèi Lùn* 脾胃論 (*the Treatise on the Spleen and Stomach*, 1249 CE) by Lǐ Dōngyuán.

ejection of all food and drink, and generalised yellowing caused by satiation damage.[425]

注：肝氣受寒，入逆於腸，則腸鳴而食不化，宜泄，更宜灸。煩熱口乾、不嗜食，乃肝氣滯而火動，肝木旺而尅脾土也，宜泄。吐逆飲食都出，肝尅脾土所致也，宜泄。傷飽身黃，脾弱而木旺矣，宜泄。

Explanation: when liver qì contracts cold, it enters to cause counterflow in the intestines; as a result, there will be rumbling intestines with indigestion of food, it is appropriate to drain, it is even more appropriate to moxa. For heart vexation with dry mouth and no pleasure in eating, these are due to liver qì stagnation leading to fire stirring; when liver-wood is effulgent, it will restrain spleen-earth, it is appropriate to drain.

Regarding vomiting with counterflow and ejection of all food and drink, this is a result of liver restraining spleen earth, it is appropriate to drain. For generalised yellowing caused by satiation damage, the spleen has become weak while the liver is effulgent, it is appropriate to drain.

肝之肺病：胸脇支滿，喘息心痛而嘔。

Lung diseases of the liver: propping fullness in the chest and rib-sides, and panting with retching due to heart pain.

注：胸者，肺之室也。胸滿者，肝邪中於肺也，宜泄。喘息心痛而嘔，肝邪上干於肺也，宜泄。

Explanation: regarding the chest, it is the chamber of the lung; fullness in the chest is because liver evil has struck the lung, it is appropriate to drain. For panting with retching due to heart pain, this is because liver evil has ascended to interfere with the lung, it is appropriate to drain.

Thirteenth Point of the Liver Channel
Qī Mén – Arranged Gate[426] (LR-14)
肝經第十三穴期門

穴在直乳上二肋端，不容旁一寸五分。又曰乳旁一寸半，直下又一寸半，肝之募，足厥陰、太陰、陰維之會。《銅人》：鍼四分，灸五壯。

---

[425] For "傷飽身黃 generalised yellowing caused by with satiation damage," the *Zhēnjiǔ Dàchéng* has "傷飽身黃瘦 generalised yellowing and slimness caused by satiation damage" instead.

[426] *Grasping the Wind* names it "Cycle Gate."

This point is located in the second intercostal space directly [below] the breast, 1 cùn 5 fēn to the side of Bù Róng (ST-19). Another says, it is 1 cùn and a half to the side of the breast, and 1 cùn and a half directly below. It is the collecting point of the liver. It is the meeting of the foot juéyīn, tàiyīn [channels], and yīnwéi [vessel]. *The Tóngrén* states, "Needle 4 fēn, and moxa 5 cones."

注：穴名期門者，與太陰脾經、陰維相會，陰維自足少陰築賓穴發脈，循股內廉上行入腹，既會足太陰、厥陰、少陰、陽明於府舍，而又會太陰、厥陰於此，若有所期約而然也，故曰期門。

Explanation: for this the point to be named Qī Mén (Arranged Gate), this is because it meets with the tàiyīn spleen channel and yīnwéi [vessel]; the yīnwéi vessel emerges from Zhù Bīn (KI-9) of the foot shàoyīn [channel], it follows the inside ridge of the thigh and ascends to enter the abdomen, thereupon arriving at Fǔ Shè (SP-13), where it meets the foot tàiyīn, juéyīn, shàoyīn, and yángmíng [channels]; it further meets with the tàiyīn and juéyīn [channels] at this place (LR-14), as though it has done so by having Qī (Arranged) engagements [with all these channels], thus it is called Qī Mén (Arranged Gate).

肝之腎病：賁豚上下，目青而嘔。

Kidney diseases of the liver: running piglet that moves up and down, and clear-eye [blindness] with retching.

注：賁豚上下，本腎積也，目青而嘔，則肝邪助之矣，宜泄之以散肝邪。

Explanation: running piglet that moves up and down is fundamentally the kidney accumulation;[427] when there is clear-eye [blindness] with retching [in addition to the running piglet], liver evil is involved in this [condition], it is appropriate to drain it in order to disperse the liver evil.

肝之肝病：脇下積氣，傷寒過經不解，熱入血室。

Liver diseases of the liver: qì accumulations under the rib-side, cold damage that has failed to resolve after channel passage, and heat entering the blood chamber.

注：脇下積氣，宜責肝之募。傷寒過經不解，男子則由陽明而入，婦人血水適來，邪盛及產後餘疾，則患熱入血室，宜刺期門。

Explanation: for qì accumulations under the rib-side, it is appropriate to seek the collecting point of the liver. Regarding cold damage that has failed to resolve after channel passage, in men, it originates in yángmíng and proceeds deeper; in women, when the menstruation happens to arrive, when the evil is

---

[427] Note: running piglet is the kidney accumulation described in *Nànjīng* Difficulty 56.

exuberant, or when they suffer from various postpartum illnesses, they will further suffer from "heat entering the blood chamber, it is appropriate to pierce Qī Mén (LR-14)."[428]

肝之脾病：霍亂泄利，腹堅硬不得臥，嘔吐酸，食飲不下，食後吐水。

Spleen diseases of the liver: sudden turmoil with diarrhoea, abdominal hardness with inability to lie down, retching and vomiting of sour [fluids], inability to get food and drink down, and vomiting of water after eating.

注：霍亂泄利，乃肝氣之逆也，宜泄。酸者，木之味也。嘔酸者，肝寒也，宜灸以溫之。

Explanation: sudden turmoil with diarrhoea is due to counterflow of the liver qì, it is appropriate to drain. Sour is the flavour of wood; vomiting of sour [fluids] is due to liver cold, it is appropriate to moxa in order to warm it.

肝之肺病：胸脇支滿，男婦血結，胸滿，面赤火燥，口乾消渴，胸中痛，太陽、少陽並病，胸中煩熱。

Lung diseases of the liver: propping fullness in the chest and rib-sides, blood bind in men and women, chest fullness, fiery and dry red face, dry mouth with dispersion-thirst, pain in the chest, tàiyáng and shàoyáng combined disease, and heat vexation in the chest.

注：胸脇支滿，乃肝氣自脇而上逆於胸也，急泄肝募以舒之。男婦血結等症，皆肝氣載血上逆也，急泄肝募。太陽與少陽並病，頭項強痛或眩，如血結心下硬痞者，當刺肺腧、肝腧，慎不可發汗，發汗則譫語，五六日不止，當刺期門。胸中煩熱，乃肝火上逆於肺也，宜刺肝募，以降肝火。

Explanation: propping fullness in the chest and rib-sides is due to the counterflow ascent of liver qì from the rib-sides into the chest, urgently drain the liver collecting point in order to soothe it. For signs of blood bind in men and women, in all cases, this is the blood carried by the counterflow ascent of liver qì, urgently drain the liver collecting point.

"For tàiyáng and shàoyáng combined disease, there will be headache and stiff painful nape or possibly dizziness, as if there is bound blood with a hard glomus below the heart, one ought to pierce Fèi Shù (BL-13) and Gān Shù (BL-18); one should be cautious as to not cause sweating; if one causes sweating, there will be delirious speech; if it does not cease after five or six days, one ought to pierce Qī Mén (LR-14)."[429] Heat vexation in the chest is due to counterflow ascent of liver fire

---

[428] *Shānghán Lùn* Lines 143 & 216, as well as *Jīnguì Yàolüè* Chapter 22.
[429] *Shānghán Lùn* Line 142.

into the lung, it is appropriate to pierce the collecting point of the liver in order to descend the liver fire.

肝之心病：傷寒心切痛。

Heart disease of the liver: cold damage with sharp pain in the heart.

注：上症乃肝邪上干於心也，急泄肝慕，以散肝邪。

Explanation: the above sign is because liver evil has ascended to interfere with the heart, urgently drain the liver collecting point in order to disperse the liver evil.

Extra Points Associated with the Foot Juéyīn Liver Channel
足厥陰肝經奇穴

Yīn Yáng Point (UEX-LE 34)
Yīn Yáng Xué – 陰陽穴

在足大拇指下，橫紋頭，白肉際。主治婦人漏下赤白，注泄，灸隨年壯，三報之。

This point is located underneath the big toe, at the top of the transverse crease at the border of the white flesh. It governs the treatment of red and white spotting in women as well as outpour diarrhoea; moxa according to one's age for 3 sessions.

Midpoint of the Transverse Crease Underneath the Big Toe (UEX-LE 33)
Zú Dà Zhǐ Xià Héng Wén Zhōng – 足大指下橫紋中

治癩疝，卵腫如瓜，入腹欲死，即腫邊，灸隨年壯，神效。又治卒中惡，悶熱毒欲死，隨年壯。

To treat downfall mounting, swollen testicles that resemble a melon and ascend into the abdomen with desire to die; only one side is swollen; moxa according to one's age, it is miraculously effective. In addition, to treat sudden malignity strike, oppression due to heat toxin with desire to die, [moxa] according to one's age.

Within the Gathering of Three Hairs (UEX-LE 29)
Sān Máo Jù Zhōng – 三毛聚中

治癩疝，灸七壯。鼻衄時癢，灸十壯，劇者灸百壯。又治陰腫，治魘不醒者，灸三七壯。

To treat downfall mounting, moxa 7 cones. [To treat] nosebleeds with periodic itchiness, moxa 10 cones; for severe cases, moxa 100 cones. In addition, to treat genital swelling and nightmares with confusion, moxa 21 cones.

Foot Tàiyīn Point (UEX-LE 11)
Zú Tài Yīn Xué – 足太陰穴

在內踝後白肉際，骨陷宛宛中。婦人逆產足先出，刺入三分，足入乃出鍼。

This point is located at the border of the white flesh behind the inner ankle [bone], in the bony depression. For a breech birth where the baby presents feet first, pierce to a depth of 3 fēn; [once] the feet retract, remove the needle.

Four Points of Nutritive Pool (UEX-LE 21)
Yíng Chí Sì Xué – 營池四穴

穴在內踝前後兩邊池上脈，一名陰陽穴。治婦人下血，漏下赤白，灸三十壯。

These points are located on the vessels in the pools[430] in front and behind the inner ankle [bone]. An alternate name is Yīn Yáng Xué.[431] To treat precipitation of blood in women,[432] red and white spotting, moxa 30 cones.

Leaky Yīn (UEX-LE 24)
Lòu Yīn Xué – 漏陰穴

在內踝下五分，微動脈上。治漏下赤白，四肢痠軟，灸三十壯。

---

[430] I.e., the depressions on the inner ankle, which are close to the location of LR-4 and KI-3, which add up to four points on both sides.

[431] I.e., "Yīn Yáng Point;" however, this is not the same as the previously mentioned point UEX-LE 34.

[432] I.e., bloody stool.

This point is located 5 fēn below the inner ankle [bone], on the faint pulsating vessel. To treat red and white spotting, fatigue and lack of strength in the four limbs, moxa 30 cones.

内踝下稍斜向前有穴。《外臺》云：向前一指。治反胃吐食，灸三壯。

There is another point located below the inner ankle [bone] and slightly obliquely towards the front. *The Wàitái* states, "It is one finger-width in front [of the angle bone]." To treat stomach reflux vomiting, moxa 3 cones.

内踝尖上一穴，灸七壯，或鍼出血。治下牙痛，内廉轉筋，脚氣寒熱。

On the tip of the inner ankle bone, there is another point, moxa 7 cones, or needle to let blood. It treats pain in the lower teeth, cramping of the inside ridge [of the leg], and leg qì[433] with chills and fevers.

Life Support (UEX-LE 12)
Chéng Mìng Xué – 承命穴

在内踝後上行三寸動脈中。治狂邪驚癇，灸三十壯。

This point is located behind the inner ankle [bone], on the pulsating vessel 3 cùn above. To treat mania evil with fright epilepsy, moxa 30 cones.

Long Grain (UEX-CA 37)
Cháng Gǔ – 長谷

穴在挾臍兩旁相去五分，一名循際。《千金》：主治下利，不嗜食，食不消化，灸五十壯，三報之。

This point clasps the two sides of the umbilicus at 5 fēn[434] each side; an alternate name is Xún Jì.[435] *The Qiānjīn* states, "To govern the treatment of diarrhoea, no pleasure in eating, and indigestion of food, moxa 50 cones for 3 sessions."

---

[433] According to *the Practical Dictionary*, leg qì is "a disease characterized by numbness, pain, limpness, and in some cases any of a variety of possible signs such as hypertonicity, swelling, redness, or wilting of or heat in the calf, and in advanced stages by abstraction of spirit-mind, heart palpitations, panting, oppression in the chest, nausea and vomiting, and deranged speech".

[434] For "5 fēn," *the Qiānjīn* actually states "5 cùn."

[435] According to *the Practical Dictionary* it is translated as "Cycle Border," which is listed as an alternate name for ST-25.

Head of the Rib (UEX-CA 4)

Lè Tóu Xué – 肋頭穴

《千金翼》：治瘕癖，患左灸左，患右灸右，第一肋頭近第二肋下，即是灸處，第二肋頭近第三肋下，向肉翅前，亦是灸處，初日灸三壯，次日五壯，後七壯，周而復始，至十日止，惟忌大蒜。

The Qiānjīn Yì states, "To treat conglomerations and aggregations, if one suffers it on the left, treat the left side; if one suffers it on the right treat the right;[436] at the bottom of the head of the first rib near the second rib,[437] that is precisely the location to moxa; at the bottom of the head of the second rib near the third rib[438] and towards the fleshy wing,[439] that is also a location to moxa. On the first day, moxa 3 cones; the next day, [moxa] 5 cones; the day after, [moxa] 7 cones; after completing this cycle, repeat it again and again until the tenth day. The only contraindication is to avoid garlic.

Rib Fissure (UEX-CA 5)

Lè Xià – 肋罅

《千金翼》云：治飛屍諸注，以繩量病人兩乳間，中屈之，乃從乳頭向外量，使當肋罅，於繩頭盡處是穴，灸隨年壯。又云：灸三壯或七壯，男左女右。

The Qiānjīn Yì states, "It treats flying corpse with various infixations. Use a string to measure [the distance] between the patient's nipples. Fold the string by half, then apply that distance outwards from the nipple, so that it should be precisely at the rib fissure; where the string ends, that is the point, moxa according to one's age. It also states, "Moxa 3 cones or 7 cones, on the left for males and on the right for females."

又云：凡中屍者，飛屍、遁屍、風注也，其狀皆腹脹痛，急不得息，氣上衝心胸、兩脇，或踝湧起，或牽引腰脊，灸乳後三寸，男左女右，二七壯，如不止，多其壯數愈。

It further states, "For all those struck by corpse [diseases], such as flying corpse, concealed corpse, and wind infixation, these all manifest with

---

[436] Note: In the primary manuscript, the treatment is conducted on both sides; in the secondary manuscript, the treatment is conducted on the opposite side instead. The editors of this manuscript, Zhāng and Zhà, have amended it according to the Qiānjīn Yì, which treats the condition on the same side.

[437] I.e., the medial corner of the first intercostal space.

[438] I.e., the medial corner of the second intercostal space.

[439] I.e., pectoralis major.

distending pain in the abdomen, urgent breathing with inability to catch one's breaths, qì surging upwards into the heart and both rib-sides, or rushing upwards from the ankle, or pulling[440] pain that radiates towards the lumbar spine; moxa 3 cùn to the side of the breast, on the left for males and on the right for females, 14 cones; if it does not cease, continue to increase the number of moxa cones until recovery."

---

[440] For "牽 pulling," *the Qiānjīn Yì* actually states "攣 hypertonicity."

Overview of the Extraordinary Channels

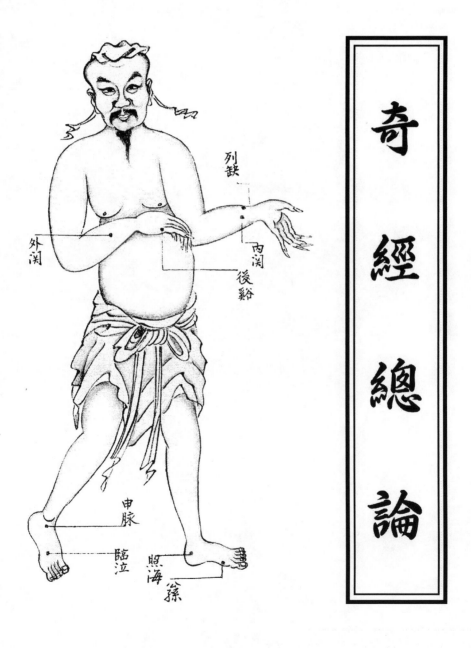

Overview of the Extraordinary Channels

奇經總論

思蓮子曰：十二經之外，又有奇經八脈，不在十二經，一陰一陽表裏配合，接諸灌輸之中，而無不周貫約束維接於十二經之脈，而又各有陰陽，各有約結，雖非十二經之屬絡臟腑，而十二經離之不能。

Master Sīlián says, besides the twelve channels, there are also the eight vessels of extraordinary channels; they are not located within the twelve channels, nor is there the arrangement where each yīn [vessel] pairs up with one yáng [vessel] as the interior and exterior.

After receiving [the overflow of qì] from all [of the twelve channels], [the eight extraordinary vessels] irrigate and transport to the within;[441] as such, without exception, all of them encompass and interlink the twelve channels together, by keeping them within bounds and linking them together. Furthermore, they can also be either yīn or yáng, [so that] they can restrain one another; although they do not network to the zàng-viscera and fǔ-bowels like the twelve channels, yet, the twelve channels are unable to be detached [from them].

其各奇經，穿交於十二正經之穴，其所治病，則當並其所穿結之經之症而治。醫不明此，鍼灸醫藥，茫無下手處矣。欲疏各經之起止，經過各正經之詳，而先總議各奇經起止之略。八奇之名，督、任、衝、帶、陽維、陰維、陽蹻、陰蹻也。

Regarding each of the extraordinary channels, they pass through and intersect with points of the twelve principal channels; for what diseases they treat, they should treat the same signs of the channel where they pass through and knot.

When a physician is ignorant of this, whether by acupuncture, moxibustion, or medicinals, that person has absolutely no [idea] where to commence [the treatment]. Therefore, I wish to discuss in detail on the beginnings and endings of each of the channels, as well as where they pass through each of the

---

441 Note: For this sentence, based on whether the character, shū 輸, is interpreted as a verb (transport) or as a noun (acupuncture points), the meaning can be drastically different. The current translation takes the interpretation of the character as a verb, but an alternative is equally valid, "After receiving from all [twelve channels], they irrigate into the acupuncture points."

primary channels; as such, let me first briefly discuss the beginning and ending of each of the extraordinary channels.

The names of the eight extraordinary [vessels] are the dū, rèn, chōng, dài, yángwéi, yīnwéi, yángqiāo, and yīnqiāo.

督脈起於會陰，循背而上行於身之後，爲陽脈之總督，故曰陽脈之海。

The dū vessel commences at Huì Yīn (REN-1) and follows the back to ascend on the rear of the body. It is the Dū (Governor) General[442] of the yáng vessels, thus, it is called the sea of the yáng vessels.[443]

任脈起於會陰，循腹而行於身之前，爲陰脈之承任，故曰陰脈之海。

The rèn vessel commences at Huì Yīn (REN-1), it follows the abdomen and travels on the front of the body. It is the Rèn (Controlling) Councillor[444] of the yīn vessels, thus, it is called the sea of yīn vessels.

衝脈亦起於會陰，挾臍而上行，直衝於上，爲諸脈之衝要，故曰十二經之海。督主身後之陽，任、衝主身前之陰，以南北言也。

The chōng vessel also commences at Huì Yīn (REN-1), ascends as it clasps the umbilicus, Chōng (Surging) vertically towards the above. It serves as the strategic Chōng (Hub) among all the vessels, thus, it is called the sea of the twelve channels.

While the dū [vessel] governs the yáng on the rear of the body, the rèn and chōng [vessels] govern the yīn on the front of the body;[445] as such, they represent the north-south [orientation of the human body].[446]

---

[442] Note: "總督 Governor-General" is an imperial official title, the holder of which is delegated to oversee provincial jurisdictions and manage regional military affairs.

[443] This, and the following passages are all from *the Qíjīng Bāmài Kǎo* 奇經八脈考 (*An Investigation of the Eight Extraordinary Channels*, 1578 CE).

[444] Note: unlike that of the dū vessel in the previous footnote, "承任 Controlling Councillor," is not a historical official title. While "chéng 承 (councillor)" is a general term for aides, assistants, or ministers in the imperial court, "rèn 任" does not represent any official title. Based on the parallelism, we have created a fictional title here as "Controlling Councillor" for the rèn vessel, so that it can serve as a contrast with "Governor-General" of the dū vessel. Otherwise, one may simply read this line literally as, "It is what the yīn vessels chéng (employ) and rèn (control)." Nevertheless, it does read to be ill-fitting for the context.

[445] For this line, "任衝主身前之陰 the rèn and chōng govern the yīn on the front of the body," the secondary manuscript has "任脈主身前之陰 the rèn vessel governs the yīn on the front of the body" instead.

[446] *Sùwèn* Chapter 6 states, "聖人南面而立 facing the south, the sage stands erect." Thus, in the context of this passage, the rèn and chōng are orientated in the south, whereas the dū vessel is oriented in the north.

帶脈則橫圍於腰，狀如束帶，所以總約諸脈者也，凡奇經之脈，上下往來於身前後者，無不約而聯束之。

The dài vessel horizontally encircles the waist; as its shape resembles a Dài (Sash), that is why it manages and restrains all the vessels. For all [other] vessels of the extraordinary channels, when they come and go from the above and below, in the front and the rear of the body, without exception, they are all restrained and conjoined together by it.

陽維起於諸陽之會，由外踝而上行於衛分，所以主一身之表。陰維起於諸陰之交，由內踝而上行於營分，主一身之裏。陽維、陰維，以乾堃言也。

The yángwéi [vessel] commences at the meeting of all yáng [channels]; from the outer ankle [bone], it ascends in the wèi-defence aspect, that is why it governs the exterior of the whole body.

The yīnwéi [vessel] commences at the intersection of all yīn [channels]; from the inner ankle [bone], it ascends in the yíng-nutritive aspect, [that is why] it governs the interior of the whole body.

The yángwéi and yīnwéi [vessels] represent the qián and kūn [of the human body].[447]

陽蹻起於跟中，循外踝而上行身之左右，而主一身左右之陽。陰蹻起於跟中，循內踝而上行於身之左右，而主一身之陰，所以使一身機關之蹻捷，以東西也。帶脈而橫束之，以六合言也。

The yángqiāo [vessel] commences from within the heel, follows the outer ankle [bone], and ascends on the left and right sides of the body; thus, it governs the yáng on the entire left and right sides of the body.

The yīnqiāo [vessel] commences from within the heel, follows the inner ankle [bone], and ascends on the left and right sides of the body; thus, it governs the yīn [aspect] of the entire body. That is why [the qiāo vessels] enable all the joints of the body to be vigorous and agile; they represent the east-west [orientation of the human body].[448]

The dài vessel horizontally encircles them; as such, it represents [the pivotal axis of] the six directions [in the human body].[449]

---

[447] Qián 乾 and kūn 堃/坤 are trigrams that represent pure yáng (☰) and pure yīn (☷), respectively

[448] As the front and rear are oriented as south and north, the left and right sides are oriented as east and west.

[449] The six directions refer to the four cardinal directions of north, south, east and west with the addition of up and down. In this context, as rèn, chōng, dū, yángwéi, and yīnwéi serve the four cardinal directions, the dài vessel serves as the pivotal axis (up and down) that binds and interlinks all of them into an integral system.

The Rèn Channel & Points

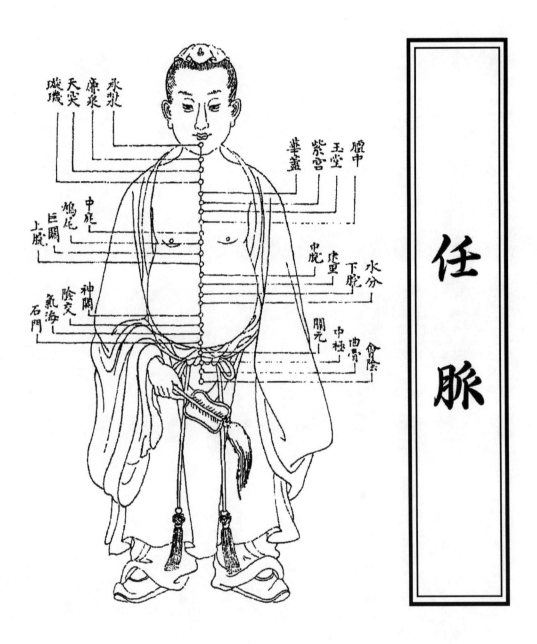

任脈

The Rèn Channel & Points
任經

Overview of the Rèn Channel
任經總論

思蓮子曰：此脈爲陰脈之海，以人之脈絡，周流於諸陰之分者，譬猶水也，而任脈則爲之總會，故名曰陰脈之海焉。

Master Sīlián says, this vessel is the sea of the yīn vessels because when the vessels and network-vessels of a human being flow and circulate in the various yīn aspects, they resemble rivers; and the rèn vessel is where all of them converge together; therefore, it is called the sea of the yīn vessels.

其始行也，同督、衝二脈，出自小腹之內，至兩陰中間，穴名會陰之處分，遂分三歧，督上行脊裏，衝上行本經之兩旁，本經遂中上行，而外循本經橫骨上毛際陷中曲骨穴，上毛際至本經之臍下四寸，膀胱幕之中極穴，

For its pathway from the origin, it is the same as two other vessels, the dū and chōng, it emerges from within the lower abdomen and arrives between the yīn [orifices], at the area of this point named Huì Yīn (REN-1); thereupon, it divides into three paths: while the dū [vessel] ascends on the interior of the spine and the chōng [vessel] ascends on two sides of this channel, this channel ascends in the middle. It then moves outwards to Qū Gǔ (REN-2) of this channel, which is in the depression at the pubic hair region, above the transverse bone.

It ascends the pubic hair region to arrive at Zhōng Jí (REN-3) of this channel, the collecting point of the bladder, at 4 cùn below the umbilicus.

至此處則同足厥陰肝經、足太陰脾經、足少陰腎經並行於腹之裏，至本經臍下三寸關元穴，而與足三陰經俱會於此穴。

Arriving at this place, it travels together with the foot juéyīn liver channel, foot tàiyīn spleen channel, and foot shàoyīn kidney channel on the interior of the abdomen, and it arrives at Guān Yuán (REN-4) of this channel, at 3 cùn below

the umbilicus, where [the rèn vessel] meets with all three foot yīn channels at this point.

又上歷本經臍下二寸，三焦募之石門穴，又上行臍下一寸半，男子生氣之海，名氣海穴。

It continues to ascend to pass through Shí Mén (REN-5) of this channel, the collecting point of the sānjiāo, at 2 cùn below the umbilicus. It continues to ascend to Qì Hǎi (REN-6), the sea of engendering qì in males, at 1 and a half cùn below the umbilicus.

又上行會足少陰、衝脈於臍下一寸，當膀胱上際，亦爲三焦募之陰交穴，又上循臍中本經之神闕穴，

It continues to ascend to Yīn Jiāo (REN-7), which is at 1 cùn below the umbilicus, where it meets with the foot shàoyīn and chōng vessels, directly on the upper border of the bladder; [this point] is also the collecting point of the sānjiāo. It continues to ascend to pass through Shén Què (REN-8) of this channel at the centre of the umbilicus.

遂過臍而上行臍上一寸，小腸下口，本經之水分穴，又上行會足太陰於本經之臍上二寸之下脘穴，

Thereupon, it traverses the umbilicus and ascends to Shuǐ Fēn (REN-9) of this channel, which is at 1 cùn above the umbilicus, by the lower mouth of the small intestine. It continues to ascend to Xià Wǎn (REN-10) of this channel, at 2 cùn above the umbilicus, where it meets with the foot tàiyīn [vessel].

又歷本經臍上三寸之建里穴，遂會手太陽小腸經、手少陽三焦經、足陽明胃經於臍上四寸，胃之募，本經之中脘穴，

It continues to follow this channel to Jiàn Lǐ (REN-11), at 3 cùn above the umbilicus. Thereupon, it ascends to Zhōng Wǎn (REN-12) of this channel, the collecting point of the stomach, at 4 cùn above the umbilicus, where it meets with the hand tàiyáng small intestine channel, hand shàoyáng sānjiāo channel, and foot yángmíng stomach channel.

又上過臍上五寸，本經之上脘穴，又上行本經鳩尾穴下一寸，本經心之募巨闕穴，遂過心前，蔽骨下五分之鳩尾穴，遂入胸，過本經膻中下一寸六分陷中，本經之中庭穴，

It continues to traverse to Shàng Wǎn (REN-13) of this channel, at 5 cùn above the umbilicus. It continues to ascend to Jù Què (REN-14) of this channel, the collecting point of the heart, at 1 cùn below Jiū Wěi (REN-15) of this channel. Thereupon, it traverses to Jiū Wěi (REN-15), which is in front of the heart, 5 fēn below the sheltered bone.[450] **Thereupon, it enters the chest and traverses to Zhōng Tíng (REN-16) of this channel, in the depression 1 cùn 6 fēn below Dàn Zhōng (REN-17) of this channel.**

又上過本經橫直兩乳之膻中穴，自此而上一寸六分，爲本經之玉堂穴，再一寸六分本經之紫宮穴，

It continues to traverse this channel to Dàn Zhōng (REN-17), which is on the horizontal line [between] the two nipples. From here, it ascends 1 cùn 6 fēn to Yù Táng (REN-18) of this channel. A further 1 cùn 6 fēn [above] is Zǐ Gōng (REN-19) of this channel.

再上一寸六分，爲本經之華蓋穴，其上再一寸六分，爲本經之璇璣穴，再一寸六分，爲本經之天突穴，遂離胸而上喉嚨，會陰維於結喉下四寸宛宛中之天突穴，

A further 1 cùn 6 fēn above is Huá Gài (REN-20) of this channel. A further 1 cùn 6 fēn above is Xuán Jī (REN-21) of this channel. A further 1 cùn 6 fēn [above] is Tiān Tū (REN-22) of this channel. Thereupon, it departs the chest and ascends the throat, where it meets with the yīnwéi [vessel] at Tiān Tū (REN-22) in the depression 4 cùn below the laryngeal prominence.[451]

又過結喉，而上舌中央之廉泉穴，遂上頤，與手陽明大腸、足陽明胃並督脈，會於唇下之承漿穴，

It traverses the laryngeal prominence and ascends to Lián Quán (REN-23), which is in the midline [below] the tongue. Thereupon, it ascends the chin to Chéng Jiāng (REN-24) below the lip, where it meets with the hand yángmíng large intestine, foot yángmíng stomach, and dū vessel.

遂環唇上至下齒齦交，復出分行，循面系兩目之下，中央七分，直瞳子陷中，至足陽明胃經兩承泣而終。

Thereupon, it encircles the [lower] lip and ascends to arrive at Yín Jiāo (DU-28) at the bottom teeth. There, a branching pathway re-emerges and follows the face to connect with and terminate at Chéng Qì (ST-1) of the foot yángmíng stomach channel, which is below each of the two eyes, in the depression 7 fēn directly below the pupil.

其別絡曰尾翳，即前本經之膏之原鳩尾穴，下散於腹。實則腹皮痛，虛則搔癢。

Its diverging network-vessel is Wěi Yì (REN-15), which is precisely the aforementioned Jiū Wěi (REN-15) of this channel and the source point of the

---

[450] The xiphoid process.

[451] Note: this last line seems to be misplaced. This could be either a scribal error in the manuscript or it could be yet another case of inline annotation that is absorbed into the main text.

gāo;[452] it descends to dissipate in the abdomen; when it is replete, the abdominal skin will be painful; when it is vacuous, there will be itchiness.[453]

任脈之爲病也，男子內結七疝，女子帶下瘕聚。女子二七而天癸至，太衝脈盛，月事以時下，七七任脈虛，太衝脈衰，天癸竭，地道不通，故形壞而無子。

When the rèn vessel is diseased, in males, there will be internal binding and seven mountings;[454] in females, there will be vaginal discharge, conglomerations and gatherings.[455]

"When females are fourteen years of age, the heavenly water arrives, the great chōng vessel is exuberant, and menstruation[456] begins[457]... at forty-nine years of age, the rèn vessel is vacuous, the great chōng vessel is debilitated, the heavenly water is exhausted, the earthly pathway no longer flows, thus as the form declines, they are no longer able to bear child."[458]

又上氣有音者，治其缺盆中，謂天突穴也，乃陰維、任脈之會。刺一寸，灸三壯。然一寸則太深矣，五分可也。

Also, "When there is audible qì ascent, treat what is in between Quē Pén (ST-12),"[459] this is speaking of Tiān Tū (REN-22), because it is the meeting of the yīnwéi and rèn vessels; "pierce it 1 cùn, and moxa 3 cones."[460] Yet, as [piercing] 1 cùn is too deep, 5 fēn is acceptable.

若其脈之見於寸口，如緊細實長至關者，任脈也，此脈若見，則苦小腹繞臍，下引橫骨中切痛，取本經關元穴治之。

When its pulse appears at the cùnkǒu, if the incoming [pulse] at the guān [position] is tight, fine, replete, and long, this is the rèn vessel [pulse]; if this pulse appears, one will suffer from stabbing pain in the lower abdomen that encircles the umbilicus and radiates downwards to the transverse bone; choose Guān Yuán (REN-4) of this channel to treat it.[461]

---

[452] See *Língshū* Chapter 1.

[453] Paraphrased from *Língshū* Chapter 10.

[454] For "seven mountings," see footnote 380.

[455] From *Sùwèn* Chapter 60; in addition, *Nànjīng* Difficulty 28 also has similar phrases.

[456] Lit. monthly matters/affairs.

[457] *Sùwèn* Chapter 1 finishes this clause with "故有子 thus, they are able to bear a child."

[458] This passage is from *Sùwèn* Chapter 1.

[459] This is paraphrased from *Sùwèn* Chapter 60, which states "其上氣有音者，治其喉，中央在缺盆中者 When there is audible qì ascent, treat the larynx, it is located in the centre between Quē Pén (ST-12).

[460] From *the Qíjīng Bāmài Kǎo* 奇經八脈考 (*An Investigation of the Eight Extraordinary Channels*, 1578 CE).

[461] From *the Màijīng* Vol. 2, Chapter 4.

又如見寸口邊橫丸丸者，亦任脈也，此脈如見則苦腹中有氣，如指上搶心，不得俯仰拘急。

Also, if one observes [a pulse] that resembles rolling pellets at the border of the cùnkǒu [pulse], this is also the rèn vessel [pulse]; when this pulse appears, one will suffer from qì within the abdomen that is shaped like a finger, which surges upwards to prod the heart, with an inability to bend forwards and backwards due to the hypertonicity.[462]

任之病，脈兩見於寸口者，一爲緊細直，實長至關，一爲寸口橫丸丸，蓋此兩脈爲任之病脈。

For diseases of the rèn [vessel], there are two types of pulse that appear at the cùnkǒu; one [pulse] is tight and fine across [all the positions], replete and long at the guān [position]; another one resembles rolling pellets to the side of the cùnkǒu; undoubtedly, both of these two pulses represent diseased pulses of the rèn [vessel].

任爲十二經之海，此經之脈見，則十二經不復朝於寸口，而單見此脈，則知任經之爲病也。

As the rèn [vessel] is the sea of the twelve channels, when the pulse of this [rèn] channel appears, the twelve channels will no longer assemble at the cùnkǒu [positions], and only this pulse will be observed; as such, one knows the rèn channel has become diseased.

其取穴之法也，臍之上下，皆以臍計。自會陰、曲骨穴而上，臍下四寸爲中極，臍下三寸爲關元，臍下二寸爲石門，臍下一寸五分爲氣海，臍下一寸爲陰交，臍之中爲神闕，

As for the method of locating the points above and below the umbilicus, they are all determined by the umbilicus. [The rèn channel] ascends from Huì Yīn (REN-1) and Qū Gǔ (REN-2) to Zhōng Jí (REN-3) at 4 cùn below the umbilicus, to Guān Yuán (REN-4) at 3 cùn below the umbilicus, to Shí Mén (REN-5) at 3 cùn below the umbilicus, to Qì Hǎi (REN-6) at 1 cùn 5 fēn below the umbilicus, to Yīn Jiāo (REN-7) at 1 cùn below the umbilicus, and to Shén Què (REN-8) at the centre of the umbilicus.

臍上一寸爲水分，臍上二寸爲下脘，臍上三寸爲建里，臍上四寸爲中脘，臍上五寸爲上脘，臍上五寸六分爲巨闕，鳩尾則蔽骨下五分焉。

Shuǐ Fēn (REN-9) is 1 cùn above the umbilicus, Xià Wǎn (REN-10) is 2 cùn above the umbilicus, Jiàn Lǐ (REN-11) is 3 cùn above the umbilicus, Zhōng Wǎn (REN-12) is 4 cùn above the umbilicus, Shàng Wǎn (REN-13) is 5 cùn above the

---

[462] A paraphrase from the Màijīng Vol. 2, Chapter 4.

umbilicus, Jù Què (REN-14) is 5 cùn 6 fēn above the umbilicus, and Jiū Wěi (REN-15) is 5 fēn below the sheltered bone.

胸中之穴，則以膻中計，以膻中與兩乳橫直也，膻中下一寸六分爲中庭，膻中之上一寸六分爲玉堂，膻中上三寸二分爲紫宮，膻中上四寸八分爲華蓋，膻中上六寸四分爲璇璣，璇璣上一寸爲天突，而胸之穴終矣。

As for the points on the chest, they are determined by Dàn Zhōng (REN-17); Dàn Zhōng (REN-17) is located on a horizontal line between the two nipples, Zhōng Tíng (REN-16) is 1 cùn 6 fēn below Dàn Zhōng (REN-17), Yù Táng (REN-18) is 1 cùn 6 fēn above Dàn Zhōng (REN-17), Zǐ Gōng (REN-19) is 3 cùn 2 fēn above Dàn Zhōng (REN-17), Huá Gài (REN-20) is 4 cùn 8 fēn above Dàn Zhōng (REN-17), Xuán Jī (REN-21) is 6 cùn 4 fēn above Dàn Zhōng (REN-17), and Tiān Tū (REN-22) is 1 cùn above Xuán Jī (REN-21); as such, chest points [of the rèn channel] terminate here.

天突在結喉下四寸，廉泉則在頤之下尖骨之中，承漿則在頤之前，唇棱之下宛宛中，此任脈取穴法也，由下而上，以本經自下而上，爲腹之中行故也。

Tiān Tū (REN-22) is located 4 cùn below the laryngeal prominence, Lián Quán (REN-23) is located within the sharp bone below the chin, and Chéng Jiāng (REN-24) is located in front of the chin, in the depression below the edge of the [lower] lip.

This is the method to locate the points of the rèn vessel, from the below to the above, just as this channel ascends from below on the midline of the abdomen.

凡二十四穴，臍下除會陰共五穴，臍上除神闕共六穴，胸上除鳩尾共七穴，項上二穴，唇下一穴。

For the twenty-four points, there are a total of 5 points below the umbilicus excluding Huì Yīn (REN-1), a total of 6 points above the umbilicus excluding Shén Què (REN-8), a total of 7 points on the chest excluding Jiū Wěi (REN-15), 2 points on the neck, and 1 point below the [lower] lip.

First Point of the Rèn Channel
Huì Yīn – Meeting of the Yīn (REN-1)
任經第一穴會陰

一名屏翳
Alternate name: Shrouded Screen[463]

---

[463] *Grasping the Wind* names it "Screen."

穴在兩陰間，任、督、衝三脈所起，督由會陰而行背，衝由會陰而行上下，在腹在股之足少陰經，任則由會陰而上行腹之中行。《銅人》：灸三壯。指微：禁鍼。非卒死溺死者不可鍼。

This point is located between the two yīn [orifices], where the three vessels of the rèn, dū, and chōng commence; from Huì Yīn (REN-1), the dū [vessel] travels to the back; from Huì Yīn (REN-1), the chōng [vessel] travels along the foot shàoyīn channel to the abdomen above and to the thigh below; from Huì Yīn (REN-1), the rèn [vessel] ascends on the midline of the abdomen. *The Tóngrén* states, "Moxa 3 cones." *The Zhǐwēi* states, "Needling is contraindicated, except for those who resemble a state of near death, or after nearly being drowned, when it can be needled."

注：穴名會陰者，以其處在二陰之間，又爲衝、任、督相會之所，故曰會陰。禁鍼者，以此處乃大小便所行之處，恐鍼傷孔道也。

Explanation: regarding the point name Huì Yīn (Meeting of the Yīn), [this point] is situated in between the two yīn [orifices]; in addition, it also is where the chōng, rèn, and dū [vessels] meet with one another; therefore, it is called Huì Yīn (Meeting of the Yīn). Regarding the contraindication of needling, it is because this location is where the urine and stool pass through, it is for the fear that needling could damage these narrow passages.

任之腎病：陰汗，陰頭痛，女子陰中諸症，前後相引痛，不得大小便，男子陰端寒衝心，竅中熱，皮痛，穀道搔癢，久痔相通，女子經水不通，陰門腫痛，卒死者，鍼一寸補之。溺死者，令人倒拖出水，鍼此穴溺屎出則活，餘不可鍼。

Kidney diseases of the rèn: genital sweating,[464] pain in the head of the penis, various genital signs in females, pain that radiates between the front and rear,[465] inability to urinate or defecate, cold that surges to the heart from the tip of the penis, heat in the orifice,[466] pain in the skin, itchiness of the anus,[467] chronic haemorrhoids that connect [the internal and external haemorrhoids] together, amenorrhoea in females, and swelling and pain of the yīn door.[468] For a state that resembles death, needle 1 cùn and supplement it. For near drowning, drag the person out of water upside down,[469] if the person discharges urine and stool after this point is needled, that person will live; for all other signs, [this point] cannot be needled.

---

[464] Lit. yīn sweating.

[465] I.e., genitals and anus.

[466] I.e., the genitals.

[467] Lit. grain path.

[468] I.e., the vulva.

[469] I.e., drag the person out of water by their feet, with the person facing downwards, likely causing the person to eject some water naturally while dragging.

注：此穴所治，皆前後二陰之症，以穴在二便之間也。卒死者補之，補其氣使上通也。溺死者補之，亦使其氣通，大小便出則水行矣，而其要猶在倒拖出水。

Explanation: the entirety of what this point treats are signs of both yīn [orifices] in the front and rear, because this point is located between [where the] urine and stool [pass through]. For a state that resembles death, supplement it, because by supplementing the qì, it will allow [the qì] to flow freely in the above. For a near drowning, supplement it, because this will also allow the qì to flow freely; if the urine and stool are discharged, this means the water is now flowing [properly]; yet, the key is still to drag the person out of water upside down.

Second Point of the Rèn Channel
Qū Gǔ – Curved Bone (REN-2)
任經第二穴曲骨

穴在橫骨上，中極下一寸，毛際陷中，動脈應手，乃足厥陰肝經環陰器，與任脈相會之所。《銅人》：灸七壯至七七壯，鍼二寸。《素》注：鍼六分，留七呼。又云：鍼一寸。《千金》云：水腫脹，灸百壯。

This point is located on the transverse bone, 1 cùn below Zhōng Jí (REN-3), in the depression within the pubic hair region, where the hand resonates with the pulsating vessel. After encircling the genitals, the foot juéyīn liver channel meets with the rèn vessel here. *The Tóngrén* states, "Moxa 7 to 49 cones, and needle 2 cùn." *The Sùzhù* states, "Needle 6 fēn, and retain for 6 respirations." Another source states, "Needle 1 cùn." *The Qiānjīn* states "Moxa 100 cones for water swelling and distension."

注：中行自鳩尾，豎懸於上，此穴橫置骨於上中行之中，餘無骨焉。曰曲者，其形彎曲非直也。

Explanation: as the midline is suspended vertically from Jiū Wěi (REN-15)[470] above, a Gǔ (Bone) is horizontally placed at this point, in the middle of the ascending pathway on the midline, no Gǔ (Bone) is found in any other [locations]. As for the meaning of Qū (Curved), this is because its shape is curved and not straight.

任之腎病：五臟虛弱，失精，虛乏冷極，小腹脹滿，小便淋瀝不通，癀疝小腹痛，婦人赤白帶下。

Kidney diseases of the rèn: weakness and vacuity of the five zàng-viscera, seminal loss, vacuity and exhaustion with extreme cold, distension and

---

[470] Lit. "Turtle-Dove's Tail," it is the xiphoid process.

fullness in the lower abdomen, strangury with inhibited and blocked urination, slumping mounting and pain of the lower abdomen, red and white vaginal discharge in women.

注：虛冷者補之灸之，餘症俱宜泄之，所治諸症，皆其部分。小腹脹滿，氣滯也，宜泄其氣。小便不通，亦宜泄以通其氣。癀疝乃肝病也，此穴正肝經相會之地，故取此穴。

Explanation: for vacuity cold, supplement it and moxa it; for all the other signs, drain this [point]. The various signs [this point] treats are all located in the area [of this point]. Distension and fullness of the lower abdomen is qì stagnation, it is appropriate to drain the qì. For urinary blockage, it is also appropriate to drain it in order to free the qì. For slumping mounting, it is a liver disease, as this point is exactly the place where the liver channel meets with [the rèn vessel], thus choose this point.

Third Point of the Rèn Channel
Zhōng Jí – Middle Pole (REN-3)
任經第三穴中極

一名玉泉
Alternate name: Jade Spring

一名氣原
Alternate name: Qì Source

穴在關元下一寸，臍下四寸，膀胱之募，足三陰、任脈之會。《銅人》：鍼八分，留十呼，得氣即泄，灸百壯至三百壯。《明堂》：灸不及鍼，日三七壯。《下經》：灸五壯。

This point is located 1 cùn below Guān Yuán (REN-4), 4 cùn below the umbilicus. It is the collecting point of the bladder. It is the meeting of the three foot yīn [channels] and rèn vessel. *The Tóngrén* states, "Needle 8 fēn, retain for 10 respirations, obtain qì then promptly drain, and moxa 100 to 300 cones." *The Míngtáng* states, "Moxa is inferior to needling, and moxa 21 cones daily." *The Xiàjīng* states, "Moxa 5 cones."

注：此穴一名玉泉，一名氣原，一名中極。名玉泉者，以爲膀胱募也；玉泉者，爲水而言也。名氣原者，爲生氣之原也。

Explanation: this point is named Yù Quán (Jade Spring), Qì Yuán (Qì Source), and Zhōng Jí (Middle Pole). Regarding the name Yù Quán (Jade Spring), this is because it is the collecting point of the bladder; Yù Quán (Jade Spring) is simply referring to water. Regarding the name Qì Yuán (Qì Source), this is because it is the Yuán (Source) of where Qì (Qì) is engendered.

名中極者，中指任脈在腹之中也。極者，自承漿而下，此爲極處也。又自下而上，曲骨猶在骨，此則初入腹之第一穴也，故曰中極。合三名而參之，而此穴命名之義始全。

Regarding the name Zhōng Jí (Middle Pole), the Zhōng (Middle) is referring to the rèn vessel that is located on the Zhōng (Middle) of the abdomen. Regarding Jí (Pole), from Chéng Jiāng (REN-24), [the rèn vessel] descends to this [point], which is the location of a Jí (Pole). Moreover, as it ascends from below, Qū Gǔ (REN-2) is still located on the bone; thus, this is the first point (REN-3) that has entered onto the abdomen, therefore, it is called Zhōng Jí (Middle Pole). It is only by juxtaposing these three names together, that a full [understanding] of the intention behind this point's naming can be acquired.

任之任病：冷氣積聚，時上衝心，腹中熱，臍下結塊，奔豚搶心，陰汗水腫，陽氣虛憊，小便頻數，失精絕子，婦人疝瘕，產後惡露不下，胎衣不下，月事不調，血結成塊，子門腫痛不端，小腹苦寒，陰癢而熱，陰痛，恍惚屍厥，饑不能食，臨經行房，羸瘦寒熱，轉脬不得溺，婦人斷緒，四度鍼即有子。

Rèn diseases of the rèn: accumulation and gathering of cold qì that periodically surges into the heart, heat in the abdomen, bound lumps below the umbilicus, running piglet that rushes into the heart, genital sweating with water swelling, yáng qì vacuity and fatigue, frequent urination, seminal loss with childlessness, mounting-conglomeration in women, retention of lochia, postpartum retention of the placenta, irregular menstruation, bound blood and formation of clots, incessant swelling and pain of the infant's gate,[471] discomfort and cold in the abdomen, genital itchiness with heat, genital pain, abstraction and deathlike reversal, hunger yet with inability to eat, marked weakness and emaciation with chills and fever induced by having sexual intercourse on the brink of menstruation, and shifted bladder with inability to urinate; for breaking lineage in women,[472] after four sessions of needling, they will become fertile.

注：其所治男子婦人病，皆其本經所行臍下部分應有之症。寒者灸之補之，結者鍼之泄之，皆正治也。惟恍惚屍厥、饑不能食之症，乃下元虛極而有是症，除鍼之補之，續灸三百壯外，還宜用藥補之可也。婦人斷緒者，無子也，鍼四度即有子，調其下焦不足之氣也。

Explanation: for all diseases of men and women this [point] treats, they are all signs that correspond to the area below the umbilicus, where this channel

---

[471] I.e., the opening of the uterus.
[472] I.e., infertility.

travels. For cold, moxa it to supplement it; for bindings, needle it to drain it, both of these are straight treatments.

Only for the signs of abstraction and deathlike reversal, as well as hunger yet with an inability to eat, such signs occur when there is the utmost vacuity of the lower source; besides needling it to supplement it, one should continue with 300 cones of moxa, in addition, it is appropriate for one to further utilize herbs to supplement [the person]. Regarding [the sign of] breaking lineage in females, this is childlessness; after four sessions of needling, they will become fertile, because [this point] regulates the insufficient qì of the lower jiāo.

Fourth Point of the Rèn Channel
Guān Yuán – Origin Pass (REN-4)
任經第四穴關元

一名次門
Alternate name: Second Gate

一名下紀
Alternate name: Lower Regulator

又名三結交
Alternate name: Triple Intersection[473]

穴在臍下三寸，小腸之募，足三陰並足陽明胃與任脈之會。《素》注：鍼一寸二分，留七呼，灸七壯。又云：鍼二寸。《銅人》：鍼八分，留三呼，泄五吸，灸百壯，止三百壯。《明堂》：孕婦禁鍼。若鍼而落胎，胎多不出，鍼外足太陽經崑崙穴立出。

This point is located 3 cùn below the umbilicus. It is the collecting point of the small intestine. It is the meeting of the three foot yīn [vessels] together with the foot yángmíng stomach [channel] and rèn vessel.

The Sùzhù states, "Needle 1 cùn 2 fēn, retain for 7 respirations, and moxa 7 cones." Another source states, "Needle 2 cùn." *The Tóngrén states,* "Needle 8 fēn, retain for 3 respirations, drain for 5 inhalations, and moxa 100 to 300 cones." *The Míngtáng states,* "Needling is contraindicated for pregnant women. If foetus drop[474] occurs after [this point] is needled, usually, the placenta will be retained; in that case, needle Kūn Lún (BL-60) of the tàiyáng channel on the outer foot and [the placenta] will be discharged immediately.

---

[473] Note: this name can be literally translated as "Knot and Intersection of the Three."
[474] I.e., abortion and loss of foetus.

注：足三陰上行入腹者，必會於此處，有關之象焉，以任脈在中，而三陰共會之，有元之義焉，故曰關元。又曰下紀，乃綱紀諸脈於臍之下者也。又名三結交，三結交者，陽明胃、太陰脾也，言三經俱會於此，故謂三結交。所治病身有所傷，血出多及中風寒。若有所墮墜，四肢懈惰不收，名曰體倦之病也。

Explanation: for the three foot yīn [vessels] that ascend to enter the abdomen, they have to meet at this place; hence, there is an image of a Guān (Pass). Since the rèn vessel is in the middle, and all the three yīn meet with it, thus, it has the meaning of [acting as a] Yuán (Origin); therefore, it is called Guān Yuán (Origin Pass). It is also called Xià Jì (Lower Regulator) because it administrates all vessels below the umbilicus.

Regarding its name Sān Jié Jiāo (Triple Intersection), the Sān Jié Jiāo (Triple Intersection) refers to the three channels, the yángmíng stomach, tàiyīn spleen, and [rèn channel], all of which meet at this point; that is why it is called Sān Jié Jiāo (Triple Intersection). The diseases treated by [this point] are bodily injuries, profuse bleeding, and strike by wind and cold. If there is any laziness and sagging, sluggishness and slackening of the four limbs with inability to contract them, this is named the disease of fatigued body.

任之任病：積冷虛乏，臍下絞痛，流入陰中，發作無時，冷氣結塊痛，寒氣入腹痛，失精白濁，溺血七疝，轉脬閉塞，小便不通，黃赤勞熱，石淋五淋，泄利，奔豚搶心，臍下結血，狀如覆杯，婦人帶下，月經不通，絕嗣不生，胞門閉塞，胎漏下血，產後惡露不止。

Rèn diseases of the rèn: accumulated cold with vacuity and exhaustion, sporadic episodes of gripping pain below the umbilicus that flows into the genitals, cold qì with painful bound lumps, cold qì that enters the abdomen and causes pain, seminal loss and white turbidity,[475] bloody urine and seven mountings, shifted bladder with blockage [of urine], urinary blockage, yellowing and reddening with taxation heat [effusion], stone strangury and five stranguries, diarrhoea, running piglet that rushes into the heart, bound blood below the umbilicus that is shaped like an upturned cup, vaginal discharge in women, absence of menses, infertility, blocked uterine gate, foetal bleeding, and persistent flow of lochia after childbirth.

注：任之所主者血也，血病責此穴者，以此穴爲足三陰所聚，皆主血者，故男子婦人血病皆責也，按其寒熱而補泄之。

Explanation: what the rèn governs is the blood, for blood diseases, seek this point. As this point is where the three foot yīn [channels] congregate, all [three] of

---

[475] According to *the Practical Dictionary*, this is either "murky urine that is white in colour" or "discharge of murky white substance from the urethra, associated with inhibited urination with clear urine."

which govern blood, thus for blood diseases in males and females, always seek [this point], supplement or drain it in accordance with whether it is a hot or cold [disease].

又：主風虛頭眩。

Also: it governs wind vacuity with dizzy head.[476]

注：此症亦責此穴者，風行於上，而泄之在下故也。

Explanation: for these signs, also seek this point, because when wind travels above, one should drain it from below.

Fifth Point of the Rèn Channel
Shí Mén – Stone Gate (REN-5)
任經第五穴石門

一名命門
Alternate name: Mìng Mén (Life Gate)

一名精露
Alternate name: Essence Reveal[477]

一名丹田
Alternate name: Dān Tián (Cinnabar Field)

一名利機
Alternate name: Crux Disinhibitor

穴在臍下二寸，三焦募也。《銅人》：灸二七壯，止一百壯。《甲乙》：鍼八分，留三呼，得氣即泄。《千金》：鍼五分。《下經》：灸七壯。《素》註：鍼六分，留七呼。婦人禁灸，犯之絕子。

This point is located 2 cùn below the umbilicus. It is the collecting point of the sānjiāo. *The Tóngrén* states, "Moxa 14 to 100 cones." *The Jiǎyǐ* states, "Needle 8 fēn, retain for 3 respirations, and obtain qì then promptly drain." *The Qiānjīn* states, "Needle 5 fēn." *The Xiàjīng* states, "Moxa 7 cones." *The Sùzhù* states, "Needle 6 fēn, and retain for 7 respirations. Moxa is contraindicated for women; if one infringes upon [the contraindication], [the woman] will become infertile."

---

[476] For "dizzy head," both the secondary manuscript and the *Dàchéng* have "headache" instead.
[477] *Grasping the Wind* names it "Essential Dew."

注：此穴一名利機，一名精露，一名丹田，一名命門，乃三焦之募。此穴部分，在臍下僅二寸，故以丹田名之，乃人身最要之地，故又以命門名之。

Explanation: this point is named Lì Jī (Crux Disinhibitor), Jīng Lù (Essence Reveal), Dān Tián (Cinnabar Field), Mìng Mén (Life Gate), and it is the collecting point of the sānjiāo. As the location of this point is only 2 cùn below the umbilicus, that is why it is named Dān Tián (Cinnabar Field). Furthermore, as it surely is the place of utmost importance within the human body, that is why it is named Mìng Mén (Life Gate).

其曰利機、曰精露者，皆言其下爲總筋，乃一身機關發動之本，而精之下出者，於此已爲露。此穴之貴要如此，故命曰石門，着其禁也，甚言此穴之不可輕鍼也。至婦人犯之絕子，的有至驗，不可忽也。

For the names Lì Jī (Crux Disinhibitor) and Jīng Lù (Essence Reveal), both are referring to the assembled sinew[478] below this [point], which surely is the foundation to initiate movement in the joints of the entire body. As for that which discharges the Jīng (Essence) in the below,[479] it has already been Lù (Revealed) here. Such is the value and importance of this point, thus, it is named Shí Mén (Stone Gate). Moreover, [this name] is also touching upon its contraindications; specifically, it is indicating that this point should not be needled recklessly. As for the statement, "after infringing [the contraindication of moxa], the woman will become infertile," this has indeed been proven and verified, one must not ignore it.

任之任病：傷寒，小便不利，泄利不禁，小腹絞痛，陰囊入腹，奔豚搶心，腹皮堅硬，卒疝繞臍，氣淋血淋，小便黃，小腹皮敦敦然氣滿，婦人因產後惡露不止，結成塊，崩中漏下。

Rèn diseases of the rèn: cold damage, inhibited urination, unrestrained diarrhoea, gripping pain in the lower abdomen, retraction of the yīn sac[480] into the abdomen, running piglet that rushes into the heart, hardening and firming of the abdomen skin, sudden mounting that encircles the umbilicus, qì strangury and blood strangury, yellow urine, swelling and distension of the skin of the lower abdomen with qì fullness, persistent flow of lochia after childbirth, binding and formation of lumps, flooding and spotting.

注：小便、陰囊、小腹絞痛，奔豚繞臍，卒疝，皆本經所應部分之病，故責之。氣淋、血淋、小便黃亦宜責之者，亦本經本穴所過之部分也。

Explanation: for the urine, yīn sac, gripping pain in the lower abdomen, running piglet that encircles the umbilicus, and sudden mounting, all of these are

---

[478] Note: this could refer to its homophone, 宗筋 (ancestral sinew), the gathering point of the three yīn and three yáng channel sinews at the pubic region.

[479] I.e., the penis.

[480] I.e., the scrotum.

diseases that correspond to the areas of this channel, thus seek this [point]. For qì strangury, blood strangury, and yellow urine, it is appropriate to seek this [point], as these are also places where points of this channel traverse.

水腫水氣行皮膚，嘔吐血，不食穀，穀不化。

Water swelling with water qì moving through the skin, retching and vomiting of blood, no desire to eat grain, and indigestion of grain.

注：水氣行皮膚，而責此穴者，泄之在下，使水歸膀胱也。嘔吐血，胃病也，有火而後有此病，宜責此穴以降上焦之火。食穀者胃也，化穀者脾也，下焦之火不上，而寒爲之不化，宜補此穴以溫之，使胃暖而食化。

Explanation: when water qì is moving through the skin, seek this point as to drain it from below, so that water will return to the bladder. Retching and vomiting of blood is a stomach disease; when this disease occurs after the presence of fire, it is appropriate to seek this point in order to descend the fire of the upper jiāo.

The stomach is that which consumes grain, the spleen is what transforms grain; when the fire of the lower jiāo fails to ascend, there will be cold, which halts the transformation, it is appropriate to supplement this point in order to warm it; once the stomach is warm, food will be transformed.

Sixth Point of the Rèn Channel
Qì Hǎi – Sea of Qì (REN-6)
任經第六穴氣海

一名脖胦
Alternate name: The Navel

一名下肓
Alternate name: Lower Huāng

穴在臍下一寸半宛宛中，男子生氣之海。《銅人》：鍼八分，得氣即泄，泄後宜補之，灸百壯。《明堂》：灸七壯。

This point is located in the depression 1 cùn and a half below the umbilicus, it is the sea of engendering qì in males. _The Tóngrén_ states, "Needle 8 fēn, obtain qì then promptly drain; after draining, it is appropriate to supplement it, and moxa 100 cones." _The Míngtáng_ states, "Moxa 7 cones."

注：此穴雖爲男子生氣之海，抑婦人之氣別有所生乎？當爲人身生氣之海，人身之氣生於此穴，而會於腹中，概男女而通言之也。

Explanation: although this point is the Hǎi (Sea) of engendering Qì (Qì) in males, is the Qì (Qì) of women engendered in a different place? It should be the Hǎi (Sea) of engendering Qì (Qì) in the human body. After the Qì (Qì) of the human body is engendered at this point, it meets in the middle of the abdomen; surely, this is a general statement for both men and women.

任之任病：一切氣疾久不瘥，肌體羸瘦，四肢力弱，冷病面赤，臟虛氣憊，真氣不足，傷寒飲水過多，腹腫脹，氣喘心下痛，奔豚七疝，小腸膀胱腎餘，癥瘕結塊狀如覆杯，腹暴脹按之不下，臍下冷氣痛，中惡脫陽欲死，陰症卵縮，四肢厥冷，大便不通，小便赤，卒心痛，婦人臨經行房，羸瘦，崩中，赤白帶下，月事不調，產後惡露不止，繞臍疞痛，閃著腰痛，小兒遺溺。

Rèn diseases of the rèn: all chronic and recalcitrant qì diseases, marked emaciation of the muscles and body, weakened strength of the four limbs, cold diseases[481] with red face, vacuity of the zàng-viscera with exhaustion of qì, insufficiency of true qì, cold damage with drinking excessive amounts of water, swelling and distension of the abdomen, panting with pain below the heart, running piglet and seven mountings [due to] superabundance in the small intestine, bladder, and kidney, concretions and conglomerations with bound lumps that are shaped like an upturned cup, sudden abdominal distension that does not yield upon pressing, cold qì and pain below the umbilicus, malignity strike with yáng desertion with desire to die, yīn [organ] signs with retracted testicles, reversal cold of the four limbs, constipation, red urine, sudden heart pain, women's marked emaciation and weakness induced by having sexual intercourse on the brink of menstruation, flooding, red and white vaginal discharge, irregular menstruation, persistent flow of the lochia after childbirth, tense pain that encircles the umbilicus, lumbar pain from wrenching, and enuresis in children.

注：下利、昏仆目上視，便注汗泄脈大，此陽暴脫，當灸此穴。按任之為脈，所主者血也，而血中不能無氣，此穴為氣海，其所主者，又為一身之氣，病如日久，氣疾不瘥者責之。臟虛氣憊者，亦責之。傷寒飲水過多，水漬於下，不入膀胱者，亦責之。

Explanation: when there is diarrhoea, clouding collapse with upward gazing eyes, faecal incontinence, sweating and a large pulse, this is sudden desertion of the yáng, one ought to moxa this point. From my observation, the vessel of the rèn is what governs the blood; yet, qì cannot be absent within blood. As this point is Qì Hǎi (REN-6), what it governs is also the qì of the whole body; if when a disease is prolonged, or when a qì disease fails to recover, seek this [point].

---

481 "Cold diseases" is originally "冷氣 cold qì" in the primary manuscript. The editors of this manuscript, Zhāng and Zhà, have amended it in accordance with the secondary manuscript and the Dàchéng.

For vacuity of the zàng-viscera with exhaustion of the qì, also seek this [point]. For cold damage with drinking excessive amounts of water, this water does not enter the bladder and instead saturates the lower, also seek this [point].

奔豚搶心，氣也；腹暴脹，氣也；七疝，亦氣也。結塊雖為血，氣滯而後血凝焉。陽暴脫亦氣也，卵縮亦氣也。大便不通，氣滯也；小便赤，氣熱也，卒心痛，亦氣也。無不責此穴者，總以此穴所主者氣症耳。

Running piglet surging into the heart is a qì [sign]; sudden abdominal distension is a qì [sign]; the seven mountings are also qì [signs]. Although bound lumps are blood [signs], blood only becomes congealed after the qì stagnates. Sudden yáng desertion is also a qì [sign]; retraction of the testicles is also a qì [sign]. Constipation is due to qì stagnation; red urine is due to qì heat, sudden heart pain is also a qì [sign]. Without exception, this point is always sought, because qì signs are governed by this point.

Seventh Point of the Rèn Channel
Yīn Jiāo – Yīn Intersection (REN-7)
任經第七穴陰交

一名少關
Alternate name: Scarce Pass

一名橫户
Alternate name: Horizontal Door

穴在臍下一寸，當膀胱上際，三焦之募，任脈、足少陰腎脈、衝脈之會。《銅人》：鍼八分，得氣即泄，泄後宜補，灸百壯。《明堂》：灸不及鍼，日三七壯，止百壯。《神農》：治臍下冷痛，可灸二十一壯。

This point is 1 cùn below the umbilicus, it is directly on the upper border of the bladder. It is the collecting point of the sānjiāo.[482] It is the meeting of the rèn vessel, foot shàoyīn kidney vessel, and chōng vessel. *The Tóngrén* states, "Needle 8 fēn, obtain qì then promptly drain; after draining it is appropriate to

---

[482] Note: This statement appeared first in *the Zhēnjiǔ Jùyīng* 針灸聚英 (*Gathered Blooms of Acupuncture and Moxibustion*, 1529 CE) by Gāo Wǔ 高武, and was later compiled into *the Zhēnjiǔ Dàchéng* in 1601 CE and *the Lèijīng Túyì* 類經圖翼 (*the Illustrated Wings of the Classified Canon*, 1624 CE), both of which Yuè Hánzhēn drew heavily from. Gāo Wǔ did not provide any reasoning as to why he also listed REN-7 as the collecting point of the sānjiāo, in addition to REN-5 listed as the collecting point of the sānjiāo in *the Tóngrén*. We speculate that this may in fact be an error by Gāo Wǔ, as REN-5 has always been listed as the sole collecting point of the sānjiāo ever since *the Jiǎyǐ Jīng* in 259 CE.

supplement, and moxa 100 cones." *The Míngtáng* states, "Moxa is inferior to needling, and moxa 21 to 100 cones daily." *The Shénnóng* states, "One can moxa 21 cones to treat cold pain below the umbilicus."

注：穴名陰交者，以足少陰同衝脈自下而上，共會於此處，故曰陰交。臍上下任經之穴，有兩三焦募也，石門既爲三焦募於下，而此穴又爲三焦募於上。三焦爲上下中主氣之經，而其募則結於任主血之經，而氣血相關紐者如是。

Explanation: regarding the point name Yīn Jiāo (Yīn Intersection), the foot shàoyīn and the chōng vessels ascend together from below to meet at this place, thus it is called Yīn Jiāo (Yīn Intersection). Among points of the rèn channel above and below the umbilicus, there are two sānjiāo collecting points: Shí Mén (REN-5) is the collecting point of the sānjiāo below, and this point is the collecting point of the sānjiāo above. As the sānjiāo is the channel that governs the qì in the upper, lower, and middle, its collecting points are bound to the rèn [vessel], which is the channel that governs the blood; as such, [these two collecting points] are hubs that are pertinent to both the qì and blood.

任之任病：奔豚上腹，氣痛如刀攪，腹脹堅痛，下引陰中，不得小便，兩丸騫疝痛，陰汗濕癢，腰膝拘攣，臍下熱，婦人血崩，月事不絕，帶下，產後惡露不止，繞臍冷痛，絕子陰㿉，小兒顋陷，鬼擊鼻出血。

Rèn diseases of the rèn: running piglet that ascends into the abdomen, qì pain that resembles twisting the knife [in the wound], bloating, hardness, and pain in the abdomen that radiates downwards to the genitals, inability to urinate, retraction of the testicles with mounting and pain, genital sweating with damp itchiness, hypertonicity of the lumbus and knees, heat below the umbilicus, flooding in women, incessant menstruation, vaginal discharge, persistent flow of lochia after childbirth, cold pain that encircles the umbilicus, infertility with genital impediment,[483] depressed fontanel in infants, and attack by ghosts with nosebleeds.

注：所治奔豚小腹痛，皆本經過臍下之正病，內屬膀胱，其治小便不利，乃行氣也。臍下熱，當泄之。腰膝拘攣，氣之滯也，亦當泄之。

Explanation: for its treatment of running piglet with pain in the lower abdomen, this is a principal disease of this channel as it traverses [the area] below the umbilicus. As [this point] internally adjoins to the bladder, it treats inhibited urination by simply moving the qì. For heat below the umbilicus, one ought to drain it. Hypertonicity of the lumbus and knees is due to the stagnation of qì, one should also drain it.

---

[483] For "陰㿉 genital impediment," it is "陰癢 pudendal itchiness" in *the Zhēnjiǔ Dàchéng*.

陰汗、陰痺、兩丸騫疝，乃任經之正通前陰而下之橫骨穴，正肝經環陰之處，固宜灸以通其滯而散其寒。所治婦人月事諸病，按其寒熱而補泄之，多以灸爲宜。

For genital sweating, genital impediment, and retraction of the testicles with mounting [and pain], it is precisely because the rèn channel communicates with Héng Gǔ (KI-11) located below the anterior yīn [orifice]; in addition, it is also located exactly at the place where the liver channel encircles the [anterior] yīn [orifice]; thus, it is appropriate to moxa this point in order to unblock the stagnation and disperse the cold. As for its treatment of various menstrual diseases in women, supplement or drain it in accordance with whether it is a hot or cold [condition]; but in general, it is appropriate to moxa to warm it.

小兒顖陷，宜灸以昇其下陷之氣。鬼擊鼻出血，則無理以解之，其以穴名陰交，乃陰氣之所聚，爲招鬼之所歟，鬼擊何以知。止鼻出血，而取此穴，想有驗者，必非無稽之談也。

For depressed fontanel in infants, it is appropriate to moxa in order to raise the qì that has fallen downwards. There is no logical explanation as to [why it treats] attacks by ghosts with nosebleeds; as the name of this point is Yīn Jiāo (REN-7), this is where the yīn qì gathers, could it possibly be [a place] that summons ghosts? But then, how could one recognize an attack by ghost? Regarding choosing this point to stop nosebleeds, I suppose that it must have been reproduced and certainly not an unfounded statement.

Eighth Point of the Rèn Channel
Shén Què – Spirit Gate Towers[484] (REN-8)
任經第八穴神闕

一名氣舍
Alternate name: Qì Abode

穴在當臍中。《素》注：禁鍼。鍼之使人惡瘡發潰後，屎出者死。《銅人》：灸百壯。《千金》：納鹽臍中，灸三壯，治淋瀝。又云：凡霍亂，納鹽臍中，灸二七壯，並治脹滿。

This point is located exactly at the centre of the umbilicus. *The Sùzhù* states, "Needling is contraindicated. Needling will cause malign sores; when [the

---

484 *Grasping the Wind* names it "Spirit Gate."

sore] erupts, those who discharge stool[485] will die." *The Tóngrén* states, "Moxa 100 cones." The Qiānjīn states, "To treat dripping sweat, place salt at the centre of the umbilicus and moxa 3 cones." It also states, "Whenever there is sudden turmoil, place salt at the centre of the umbilicus and moxa 14 cones; it also treats distension and fullness."

注：此穴一名氣舍，乃腹之中上下氣所舍之地。名神闕者，以任脈上直乎心，心之所藏者神，此穴有隙焉，如王者宮門之有闕，故曰神闕，決不可鍼者也。

Explanation: this point is also named Qì Shè (Qì Abode), as it is the location where the Qì (Qì) of the upper, middle, and lower abdomen Shè (Abides). Regarding the name Shén Què (Spirit Gate Towers), the rèn vessel ascends vertically into the heart, and the heart is where the Shén (Spirit) is stored; in addition, there is a cleft at this point, which resembles the Què (Gate Towers) by the gate of the emperor's imperial palace, thus it is called Shén Què (Spirit Gate Towers). On no account can it be needled.

任之任病：腹中虛冷，臟腑泄利不止。

Rèn diseases of the rèn: vacuity cold in the abdomen, incessant diarrhoea of the zàng-viscera and fǔ-bowels.

注：此症乃腹寒也，宜灸溫之。

Explanation: these signs are due to cold in the abdomen, it is appropriate to moxa to warm it.

又，水腫鼓脹，腸鳴狀如流水聲。

Also, water swelling with drum distension, and rumbling intestines that sounds like flowing water.

注：此症乃脾虛不能運水抵膀胱，而止在腸中作聲，亦宜灸以溫之。

Explanation: these signs are all due to spleen vacuity and its failure to transport water to the bladder; as a result, [water] lodges inside the intestines and creates sounds; it is also appropriate to moxa it in order to warm it.

又，中風不省人事，風癇角弓反張。

Also, wind strike with loss of consciousness, and wind epilepsy with arched-back rigidity.

---

[485] "Those who discharge stool" is originally "those who discharge urine" in the primary manuscript. The editors of this manuscript, Zhāng and Zhà, have amended it in accordance with *the Sùzhù* and *the Dàchéng*.

注：兩症皆氣爲痰滯，上下閉塞，前後氣血反亂，宜灸百壯，以溫其氣，而助其正。

Explanation: both these signs are qì stagnation caused by phlegm, which [creates] a blockage between the above and below; as a result, the qì and blood in the front and rear are in chaos; it is appropriate to moxa 100 cones in order to warm the qì and assist the upright [qì].

Nineth Point of the Rèn Channel
Shuǐ Fēn – Water Divide (REN-9)
任經第九穴水分

一名分水
Alternate name: Divided Waters

一名中守
Alternate name: Central Guard

穴在下脘下一寸，臍上一寸，正當小腸下口。《素》注：鍼一寸。《銅人》：鍼八分，留三呼，泄五吸，水病禁鍼，鍼之水盡則死。《明堂》：水病灸七七壯，止四百壯，鍼三分，留三呼。《資生》云：不鍼爲是。

This point is located 1 cùn below Xià Wǎn (REN-10), 1 cùn above the umbilicus, exactly on the lower opening of the small intestine. *The Sùzhù* states, "Needle 1 cùn." *The Tóngrén* states, "Needle 8 fēn, retain for 3 respirations, and drain for 5 inhalations. It is contraindicated to needle in the presence of water diseases; upon needling, the person will die as water becomes exhausted." *The Míngtáng* states, "For water diseases, moxa 49 to 400 cones, needle 3 fēn, and retain for 3 respirations." *The Zīshēng* states, "Do not needle it, that is the proper way."

注：此穴當小腸下口，小腸爲受盛之官，至是而始泌別清濁，水液入膀胱，滓渣入大腸，故曰水分。

Explanation: this point is located exactly at the lower opening of the small intestine; the small intestine is the official of receiving and holding, upon arriving here, it begins to separate the clear and turbid; hence, the Shuǐ (Water) and fluid enter the bladder, the dregs and waste enter the large intestine, therefore it is called Shuǐ Fēn (Water Divide).

任之任病：水病腹堅腫如鼓，腸胃虛脹，繞臍痛衝心，腰脊急強，腸鳴狀如雷聲，上衝心，鬼擊鼻出血，小兒顖陷。

Rèn diseases of the rèn: water disease with abdomen that is swollen and hardened like a drum, vacuity distension of the intestines and stomach, pain that encircles the umbilicus and surges into the heart, tension and stiffness of the lumbar spine, rumbling intestines that sound like thunder and surge into the heart, attack by ghosts with nosebleeds, and depressed fontanel in infants.

注：水不能入膀胱，故腹爲之堅，宜灸以通其氣，令其仍入膀胱，由小便而出，此潔淨府之正治也。如鍼之自外出，則水終不入胱膀，而水猶然汛溢於周身則危矣，所以禁鍼。

Explanation: as water fails to enter the bladder, the abdomen will become hardened, thus it is appropriate to moxa this point in order to unblock the qì and allow [the water] to enter the bladder, so that it will be discharged as urine; this is the straight treatment to cleanse the fǔ-bowel.[486] If it is needled, while the water will discharge to the outside, it will never enter the bladder; as such, the water will still flood and spill out into the entire body, which can lead to peril. This is the reason why needling [this point] is contraindicated.

審之腸胃虛脹而非水，及腸鳴如雷上衝心，的確是氣，乃鍼此以泄腸胃之滯氣。

Upon examining, if it is vacuity distension of the intestines and stomach and not due to water, or if there are rumbling intestines that sound like thunder and surge upwards into the heart, both of these are indeed qì [signs]; as such, needle it in order to drain the stagnant qì of the intestines and stomach.

鬼擊鼻出血，臍下取陰交，臍上取水分之義，終不可解。鼻出血而取陽明經，此穴在胃之下，取之以降逆上之氣，此可理解者，但鬼擊則無着耳。小兒顖陷，灸之使氣上行。

For attack by ghosts with nosebleeds, I have never understood the reason why one chooses Yīn Jiāo (REN-7) below the umbilicus and Shuǐ Fēn (REN-9) above the umbilicus. For nosebleeds, [one should] choose the yángmíng channel; as this point is located below the stomach, I can understand the reason that by choosing [this point], it can descend the counterflow ascent of qì; however, I am a completely at loss about [why it treats] attack by ghosts. For depressed fontanel in infants, moxa it to cause the qì to ascend.

---

486 For "潔淨府 cleanse the fǔ-bowel," according to the annotation of *Sùwèn* Chapter 14 from the *Sùzhù*, "謂寫膀胱水去也 this refers to draining the urinary bladder and thereby removing the water."

Tenth Point of the Rèn Channel
Xià Wǎn – Lower Duct[487] (REN-10)
任經第十穴下脘

穴在建里下一寸，臍上二寸，當胃下口，小腸上口，水穀於是入焉，足太陰、任脈之會。《銅人》：鍼八分，留三呼，泄五吸，灸二七壯，止二百壯。

This point is located 1 cùn below Jiàn Lǐ (REN-11), 2 cùn above the umbilicus, exactly at the lower opening of the stomach and upper opening of the small intestine, where the water and grain enter [the small intestine]. It is the meeting of the foot tàiyīn [channel] and rèn vessel. *The Tóngrén* states, "Needle 8 fēn, retain for 3 respirations, drain for 5 inhalations, and moxa 14 to 200 cones."[488]

注：胃有三脘，此穴正當其內下脘，紆曲於腸之下，上小而中大，下脘仍微小於中，下口則愈小，以交於小腸，水穀至此，已為脾之真火磨化已融，方下入小腸，而分清獨，故曰下脘。

Explanation: The stomach has three Wǎn (Ducts), this point is exactly at the place where the Xià Wǎn (Lower Duct) is internally, which winds underneath the [large] intestine. [Of the three Wǎn (Ducts)], the upper [duct] is small, the middle [duct] is large, and the Xià Wǎn (Lower Duct) is slightly smaller than the middle [duct] and with an even smaller lower opening, where it intersects with the small intestine. When the water and grain arrive here, they are already dissolved after being grinded and transformed by the true fire of the spleen; it is only in such a state that they descend to enter the small intestine, where they are further divided into the clear and turbid; therefore, [this point] is called Xià Wǎn (Lower Duct).

任之任病：臍下厥氣動堅硬，痞塊連臍上厥氣動，日漸羸瘦，胃脹羸瘦腹痛，六腑之氣寒，穀不轉化，不嗜食，脈厥動，翻胃。

Rèn diseases of the rèn: stirring of reverse qì below the umbilicus with [abdominal] hardening and firming, glomus lumps that connects to the top of the umbilicus with stirring of reverse qì, progressively marked emaciation with each passing day, distension of the stomach with marked emaciation and abdominal pain, cold qì in the six fǔ-bowels, indigestion, no pleasure in eating, reversal and stirring of the vessels, and stomach reflux.

注：脘中氣滯，遂有臍上動氣、臍下動氣之症，胃脹亦氣也，皆宜泄之，以舒其氣。六腑之氣寒，穀不轉化，宜灸以溫之。翻胃乃氣上逆也，宜泄其氣。

---

[487] *Grasping the Wind* names it "Lower Venter."
[488] For "14 cones," *the Tóngrén* actually states "49 cones."

Explanation: when there is qì stagnation within the [stomach] duct, there will be signs of stirring of qì above the umbilicus and stirring of qì below the umbilicus; in addition, stomach distension is also due to qì [stagnation]; for all [three signs], it is appropriate to drain [this point] in order to soothe the qì. When there is cold qì in the six fǔ-viscera, grains will fail to transform, it is appropriate to moxa in order to warm it. Stomach reflux is due to counterflow qì ascent, it is appropriate to drain the qì.

Eleventh Point of the Rèn Channel
Jiàn Lǐ – Fortifying the Interior[489] (REN-11)
任經第十一穴建里

穴在中脘下一寸，臍上三寸。《銅人》：鍼五分，留十呼，灸五壯。《明堂》：鍼一寸二分。《千金》：主腸鳴霍亂腹脹，可刺八分，泄五吸，疾出鍼，日灸二七壯至百壯。

This point is located 1 cùn below Zhōng Wǎn (REN-12), 3 cùn above the umbilicus. *The Tóngrén* states, "Needle 5 fēn, retain for 10 respirations, and moxa 5 cones." *The Míngtáng* states, "Needle 1 cùn and 2 fēn." *The Qiānjīn* states, "To govern [the treatment of] intestinal rumbling, sudden turmoil, and abdominal distension, one can pierce 8 fēn, drain for 5 inhalations, swiftly remove the needle, or moxa 14 to 100 cones daily."

注：里者，土也；建者，厚之之意。以內所當者，正在胃中脘之下，恐其弱也，故命曰建里。

Explanation: Lǐ (Interior) is the earth; Jiàn (Fortifying) is the concept of consolidating [the earth]. This is because what is on the interior [of this point] is exactly below the middle duct of the stomach; owing to the fear of its weakness, thus it is named Jiàn Lǐ (Fortifying the Interior).

任之任病：腹脹身腫，心痛上氣，腸中冷，嘔逆不嗜食。

Rèn diseases of the rèn: abdominal distension with generalised swelling, heart pain with qì ascent, cold in the intestines, and vomiting counterflow with no pleasure in eating.

注：以上病，皆氣滯症也，宜泄以通其氣。

Explanation: all of the above diseases are signs of qì stagnation, it is appropriate to drain [this point] in order to unblock the qì.

---

[489] *Grasping the Wind* names it "Interior Strengthening."

Twelfth Point of the Rèn Channel
Zhōng Wǎn – Middle Duct[490] (REN-12)
任經第十二穴中脘

一名太倉
Alternate name: Supreme Granary

一名胃脘
Alternate name: Stomach Duct

一名上紀
Alternate name: Upper Regulator

穴在上脘下一寸，臍上四寸，居心蔽骨與臍之中，手太陽小腸、手少陽三焦、足
陽明胃經與任脈之會。《銅人》：鍼八分，留七呼，泄五吸，疾出鍼，灸二七
壯，止二百壯。《明堂》：灸二七壯，止四百壯。《素》注：鍼一寸二分，灸七
壯。

**This point is located 1 cùn below Shàng Wǎn (REN-13), 4 cùn above the
umbilicus; it is situated between the sheltered bone [below] the heart and the
umbilicus. It is the meeting of hand tàiyáng small intestine, hand shàoyáng
sānjiāo, foot yángmíng stomach channels, and rèn vessel. *The Tóngrén* states,
"Needle 8 fēn, retain for 7 respirations, drain for 5 inhalations, swiftly take the
needle out, and moxa 14 to 200 cones."[491] *The Míngtáng* states, "Moxa 14 to
400 cones." *The Sùzhù* states, "Needle 1 cùn 2 fēn, and moxa 7 cones."**

注：上紀者，中脘也，胃之募也。《難經》云：腑會中脘。腑病治此穴。
蓋六腑以胃爲本，而胃又以中脘爲要，故曰上紀，乃綱紀諸脈於臍之上者也。

Explanation: Shàng Jì (Upper Regulator) refers to the Zhōng Wǎn (Middle
Duct), which is the collecting point of the stomach. *The Nànjīng* states, "The fǔ-
bowels meet at Zhōng Wǎn (Middle Duct)."[492] [*The Nànjīng Shū* states], "For fǔ-
bowels diseases, treat this point." Undoubtedly, the stomach is the foundation of the
six fǔ-bowels, and likewise, the Zhōng Wǎn (Middle Duct) is the crux of the stomach,
thus it is called Shàng Jì (Upper Regulator) because it administrates all vessels above
the umbilicus.[493]

東垣曰：氣在於腸胃者，取之足太陰、陽明不下，取胃之三里、肝之章
門、任之中脘。又曰：胃虛而致太陰無所稟者，於足陽明募穴中引導之。據此則知

---

[490] *Grasping the Wind* names it "Central Stomach Duct."

[491] For "100 cones," *the Tóngrén* actually states "200 cones."

[492] From *Nànjīng* Difficulty 45.

[493] Note: this point should be read in conjunction with REN-4, which is also called 下紀
Lower Regulator, as the point that administrates all vessels below the umbilicus.

此穴所主皆胃病也。穴正在任之中行，而實爲在內胃之中腕，乃胃氣所結之地，故曰胃募。

[Lǐ] Dōngyuán says, "Regarding the qì located in the intestines and stomach, if it fails to descend after choosing the foot tàiyīn and yángmíng [channels], one should choose Sān Lǐ (ST-36) of the stomach [channel], Zhāng Mén (LR-13) of the liver, and Zhōng Wǎn (Middle Duct) of the rèn [channel]."[494]

He also says, "When the tàiyīn is no longer endowed due to the stomach vacuity, guide and abduct by the collecting point of the foot yángmíng."[495]

According to [these statements], one knows that all [diseases] this point governs are stomach diseases. This point is located exactly on the midline on the rèn [vessel], and in fact, the Zhōng Wǎn (Middle Duct) of the stomach is located on the interior [to this point], which is the place where the stomach qì binds; that is the reason why it is called the stomach collecting point.

任之胃病：五膈，喘息不止，腹暴脹。

Stomach diseases of the rèn: five occlusions [of qì],[496] incessant panting, and sudden abdominal distension.

注：此症乃胃氣滯而不下，故取此穴，以降胃氣。

Explanation: these signs are due to stagnant stomach qì that is unable to descend, thus choose this point in order to descend the stomach qì.

中惡脾痛，飲食不進，翻胃。

Malignity stroke with pain of the spleen, inability to ingest food and drink, and stomach reflux.

注：此症乃胃有寒邪，宜灸以溫之。

Explanation: these signs are due to presence of cold evil in the stomach, it is appropriate to moxa in order to warm it.

---

[494] From the chapter titled, "胃氣下溜五臟氣皆亂其爲病互相出見論 Cross-Referencing the Disease of the Stomach Qì Flowing Downward with the Complete Chaos of the Qì of the Five Zàng-Viscera," of *the Píwèi Lùn 脾胃論 (the Treatise on the Spleen and Stomach*, 1249 CE) by Lǐ Dōngyuán.

[495] Also from the aforementioned chapter from the previous footnote.

[496] *The Zhūbìng Yuánhòu Lùn 諸病源候論 (the Origin and Indicators of Disease*, 610 CE) states, "五膈氣者，謂憂膈、恚膈、氣膈、寒膈、熱膈也 the five occlusions of qì are occlusion due to worry, occlusion due to rage, occlusion due to qì, occlusion due to heat, and occlusion due to cold."

赤白痢，寒澼。

Red and white dysentery, and cold afflux.[497]

注：此症，胃有積滯，宜灸以溫之。

Explanation: these signs are due to the presence of accumulation and stagnation in the stomach, it is appropriate to moxa it in order to warm it.

氣心痛，伏梁，心下如覆杯，心下膨脹，面色痿黃。

Qì pain in the heart, deep-lying beam, [water-rheum] below the heart that is shaped like an upturned cup,[498] bloating and distension below the heart, wilted and yellow facial complexion.

注：胃中氣滯也，而後有積，積久而後面色黃，宜鍼以散之，灸以溫之。

Explanation: when there is qì stagnation in the stomach, accumulations will form afterwards; when the accumulations remain for an extended period of time, there will be a wilted and yellow facial complexion afterwards; thus, it is appropriate to needle in order to dissipate it, and moxa in order to warm it.

天行傷寒，熱不已。

Cold damage due to seasonal current with incessant fevers.

注：此症乃邪在陽明經也，宜鍼以泄其邪熱。

Explanation: these signs are due to evil in the yángmíng channel, it is appropriate to needle in order to disperse the evil heat.

溫瘧，先腹痛先泄。

Warm malaria with either abdominal pain or diarrhoea at the onset.

注：此症乃胃有熱，宜泄以去熱。

Explanation: these signs are due to the presence of heat in the stomach, it is appropriate to drain in order to eliminate the heat.

霍亂，泄出不知，飲食不化。

Sudden turmoil, unconscious discharge of diarrhoea, and indigestion.

---

[497] According to *the Practical Dictionary*, afflux is synonymous with dysentery.
[498] Refer to *Jīnguì Yàolüè* Lines 14.31 and 14.32.

注：此氣亂於胃所致，宜泄此穴，以正其亂氣。

Explanation: these are caused by the chaos of qì in the stomach, it is appropriate to drain this point in order to rectify the qì in chaos.

心痛身寒，不可俯仰，氣發噎。

Heart pain with generalised chills with inability to bend forwards and backwards, and hiccoughs.

注：二症皆胃有寒氣所致，宜灸以溫之。

Explanation: both of these signs are a result of the presence of cold qì in the stomach, it is appropriate to moxa in order to warm it.

Thirteenth Point of the Rèn Channel
Shàng Wǎn – Upper Duct[499] (REN-13)
任經第十三穴上脘

穴在巨闕下一寸半，臍上五寸，上脘、中脘屬胃絡脾，足陽明胃、手太陽、任脈之會。《銅人》：鍼八分，先補後泄，風癎熱病，先泄後補，立愈。日灸二七壯至百壯，未愈倍之。《明下》：灸三壯。

This point is located 1 cùn and a half below Jù Quē (REN-14), 5 cùn above the umbilicus. Both Shàng Wǎn (REN-13) and Zhōng Wǎn (REN-12) adjoin to the stomach and network to the spleen. It is the meeting of the foot yángmíng stomach, hand tàiyáng, and rèn vessel. *The Tóngrén* states, "Needle 8 fēn, initially supplement then subsequently drain. For wind epilepsy and febrile disease, initially drain then subsequently supplement, and there will be immediate recovery. Moxa 14 to 200 cones daily; if they have not yet recovered, double the number [of cones]." *The Míngxià* states, "Moxa 3 cones."

注：此穴在內爲飲食初入於胃之所，故曰上脘。

Explanation: this point is located at the place where the food and drink first enter the stomach on the interior, thus it is called Shàng Wǎn (Upper Duct).

任之任病：腹中雷鳴相逐，食不化，腹疼刺痛。

Rèn diseases of the rèn: thunderous rumbling in the abdomen that comes and goes, indigestion, tension and stabbing pain in the abdomen.

---

[499] *Grasping the Wind* names it "Upper Venter."

注：前症乃胃之氣不和，宜鍼泄其氣，而後灸以溫之。

Explanation: the above signs are due to disharmony of the stomach qì, it is appropriate to needle to drain the qì, and moxa it afterwards in order to warm it.

霍亂吐利腹痛。

Sudden turmoil, vomiting with diarrhoea, and abdominal pain.

注：上症且吐且利，而腹爲之痛，胃中之氣亂也，亦宜鍼以泄而灸以溫之。

Explanation: the above signs are abdominal pain with simultaneous vomiting and diarrhoea, this is due to the chaos of qì within the stomach, it is appropriate to needle in order to drain it, and moxa afterwards in order to warm it.

身熱汗不出。

Generalised heat [effusion] with absence of sweating.

注：上症乃身以前熱，陽明經之邪也，宜泄其邪而汗自出。

Explanation: the above sign is heat in the anterior body, which is caused by evil in the yángmíng channel, it is appropriate to drain the evil; as such, sweating will naturally occur.

翻胃嘔吐，食不下。

Stomach reflux and inability to ingest food.

注：前症乃胃之氣上逆也，宜泄以散其上逆之氣。

Explanation: the above sign is due to counterflow qì ascent of the stomach, it is appropriate to drain [this point] in order to dissipate the counterflow ascent of qì.

腹脹氣滿。

Abdominal distension with qì fullness.

注：上症乃胃氣逆也，宜泄此穴，以散其上逆之氣。

Explanation: the above sign is due to counterflow of the stomach qì, it is appropriate to drain this point in order to dissipate the counterflow ascent of qì.

心忪驚悸，時嘔血痰，多涎沫。

Heart agitation with fright palpitations, periodic vomiting of blood and phlegm, and [vomiting] of copious drool and foam.

注：胃有疾則心爲驚悸，嘔血痰者，胃中有鬱血也，宜泄此穴以散之。

Explanation: when the stomach has a disease, there will be fright palpitations in the heart; vomiting of blood and phlegm is due to depressed blood within the stomach, it is appropriate to drain this point in order to dissipate it.

奔豚伏梁，卒心痛。

Running piglet with deep-lying beam, and sudden heart pain

注：奔豚者，氣積也；伏梁者，心積也。素無心痛而暴痛者，謂之卒心痛，非冷即熱，或痰或氣所致，皆宜泄此穴。

Explanation: running piglet is due to accumulation of qì; deep-lying beam is an accumulation [disease] of the heart.[500] For someone who does not normally have heart pain, but suddenly, there is now heart pain, this is what is called sudden heart pain; if it is not caused by cold, then it would be caused by heat; sometimes, it can also be caused by phlegm or qì; for all cases, it is appropriate to drain this point.

風癎熱病，五毒症不能食。

Wind epilepsy with febrile disease, and five toxic infixations[501] with inability to eat.

注：痰積胃中而上膈，遂爲癎，宜泄此穴以降之。五毒症，皆胃有痰也，並宜泄之。

Explanation: when phlegm accumulates within the stomach, it will ascend the diaphragm; consequently, there will be epilepsy, it is appropriate to drain this point in order to descend it. All five toxic infixations are caused by phlegm within the stomach, it is also appropriate to drain this [point].

馬黃黃疸。

Jaundice that is the colour of a yellow horse.

注：胃有濕熱而黃生焉，泄此穴以去其濕熱之氣。

Explanation: when there is a presence of damp heat in the stomach, it will cause yellowing, drain this point in order to eliminate the qì of damp heat.

---

[500] This refers to *Nànjīng* Difficulty 56 which discusses the accumulation diseases of the five zàng-viscera.

[501] For "五毒症 five toxic infixations" here, the manuscript has "五毒痔 five toxic haemorrhoids" instead. The editors of this manuscript, Zhāng and Zhà, have amended it in accordance with *the Dàchéng*. Sidenote: the "five toxins" typically refer to the five poisonous creatures (scorpion, viper, centipede, house lizard, and toad).

積聚堅大如盤。

Accumulations and gatherings that are hardened and enlarged like a dish.

注：此乃胃有積也，宜泄此穴，以破其積。

Explanation: this is due to accumulations within the stomach, it is appropriate to drain this point in order to break up the accumulations.

虛勞吐血。

Vacuity taxation with vomiting of blood.

注：此症乃鬱血積胃也，宜鍼以散之。

Explanation: this sign is due to the accumulation of depressed blood in the stomach, it is appropriate to needle in order to dissipate it.

Fourteenth Point of the Rèn Channel
Jù Quē – Great Gate Towers[502] (REN-14)
任經第十四穴巨闕

穴在鳩尾下一寸，臍上六寸五分，心之募。《銅人》：鍼六分，留七呼，得氣即泄，灸七壯，止七七壯。《神農》：治心腹積氣，可灸十四壯。又治小兒諸癇病，如口噤吐沫，可灸三壯，艾炷如小麥。

This point is located 1 cùn below Jiū Wěi (REN-15), 6 cùn 5 fēn above the umbilicus. It is the collecting point of the heart. *The Tóngrén* states, "Needle 6 fēn, retain for 7 respirations, obtain qì then promptly drain, and moxa 7 to 49 cones." *The Shénnóng* states, "To treat accumulated qì in heart and abdomen, one can moxa 14 cones. In addition, to treat various types of epilepsy in children with [signs] such as dry retching and vomiting of foam, one can moxa 3 cones; the cones should be the size of a wheat grain."

---

[502] *Grasping the Wind* names it "Great Tower Gate." Note: regarding the character, quē 闕, found in REN-8 and REN-14, we have translated it as "gate towers" because historically speaking, quē 闕 are the towers that stand on the two sides of a gate. It can be a pair of small ceremonial pillars that stand on the two sides of the gate to a temple, a pair of stone columns that stand at the entrance of a mausoleum, a pair of small watch towers erected above the city wall, or massive protruded towered fortifications like the Meridian Gate of the Forbidden City in Beijing. These towers typically come in pairs; thus, we have translated the character, quē 闕, in the plural case instead of the singular case.

注：穴名巨闕者，心爲一身之主，在乎上之內，此穴在胸之下，兩脇在其旁，有闕象焉，故曰巨闕。巨者，大也，尊稱也。心募者，心之氣結於此也。

Explanation: for the point name Jù Quē (Great Gate Towers), the heart is the governor of the whole body and it is located on the interior above; this point is located below the chest, with the ribs on its two sides, which resemble the image of Quē (Gate Towers), thus it is called Jù Quē (Great Gate Towers). Jù (Great) is large, it is a respectful form of address. Regarding the heart collecting point, this is because the qì of the heart binds at this place.

任之心病：數種心痛冷痛，蚘蟲痛，蠱毒貓鬼，胸中痰飲，先心痛先吐，驚悸傷寒，煩心喜嘔，發狂，五臟氣相干，卒心痛，屍厥，妊娠子上衝心。

Heart diseases of the rèn: numerous kinds of heart pain and cold pain, pain due to roundworms, gǔ toxin with [attack by] ghosts of cats, phlegm-rheum in the chest with either heart pain or vomiting at its onset, fright palpitations with cold damage, vexation of the heart with frequent retching, mania, mutual invasion among qì of the five zàng-viscera, sudden heart pain, deathlike reversal, and [sensation of] foetus that surges up into the heart during pregnancy.

注：前症皆氣之干於心者，故取此穴。冷痛宜灸以溫之。蚘蟲痛宜鍼以止之。蠱毒宜鍼。貓鬼，心氣之虛，爲邪所干也，宜灸之。

Explanation: all above signs are invasions of the qì into the heart, thus choose this point. For cold pain, it is appropriate to moxa it in order to warm it. For pain due to roundworms, it is appropriate to needle to stop [the pain]. For gǔ toxin, it is appropriate to needle. [Attack by] ghosts of cats is an invasion by evil due to vacuity of the heart qì, it is appropriate to moxa it.

胸中痰飲、先心痛先吐者，乃痰逆於上也，宜鍼以泄之，灸以溫之。驚悸亦心氣之虛也，宜灸以補之。

Phlegm-rheum in the heart with heart pain or vomiting on its onset, this is due to counterflow phlegm in the above, it is appropriate to needle to drain it, and moxa in order to warm it. Fright palpitations is also due to vacuity of the heart qì, it is appropriate to moxa it in order to supplement it.

傷寒，邪入於肺而心爲煩，宜泄此穴。五臟氣相干，卒心痛，亦宜泄此穴。屍厥，心氣不達於肢體也，宜鍼此穴以通之。

[For this type of] cold damage, the evil has entered the lung to cause vexation in the heart, it is appropriate to drain this point. For mutual invasion among qì of the five zàng-viscera and sudden heart pain, it is also appropriate to drain this point. Regarding deathlike reversal, it is the failure of heart qì to reach the limbs, it is appropriate to needle this point in order to unblock it.

任之肺病：胸滿短氣，背痛胸痛，痞寒，咳嗽煩熱，膈中不利。

Lung diseases of the rèn: fullness in the chest and shortness of breath, upper back pain and chest pain, cold glomus, cough with heat vexation, and inhibition within the chest.

注：此皆胃之氣上逆，而干於肺也，宜泄此穴，以降其逆上之氣。

Explanation: all of these are counterflow ascent of the stomach qì, which invades the lung, it is appropriate to drain this point in order to descend the counterflow ascent qì.

任之胃病：霍亂不識人，腹脹暴痛，恍惚不止，吐逆不食，少氣腹痛，黃疸急疸，急疫，上氣咳逆。

Stomach diseases of the rèn: sudden turmoil with inability to recognise people, abdominal distension with sudden pain, continuous abstraction, vomiting counterflow with no desire to eat, scantness of breath with abdominal pain, jaundice and acute jaundice,[503] **acute epidemic disease, qì ascent with cough and counterflow.**

注：前症皆胃氣之亂也，宜泄此穴，以散其亂氣。黃疸急疸，濕熱鬱於胃也，亦宜泄此穴，以散濕熱。急疫亦邪氣干胃也，亦宜泄此穴。上氣咳逆，乃胃氣鬱也，宜泄此穴以開之。

Explanation: all the above signs are caused by the chaos of stomach qì, it is appropriate to drain this point in order to disperse the chaotic qì. Jaundice and acute jaundice are caused by depression of damp-heat in the stomach, it is appropriate to drain this point in order to dissipate the damp-heat.

Acute epidemic disease is also due to evil qì invasion of the stomach, it is also appropriate to drain this point. Qì ascent with cough and counterflow is also caused by the depression of the stomach qì, it is appropriate to drain this point in order to open [the depression].

任之肝病：狐疝，小腹脹，噫。

Liver diseases of the rèn: fox-like mounting,[504] **distension of the lower abdomen, and belching.**

---

503 For "黃疸急疸 jaundice and acute jaundice," it is originally "黃疸急黃 jaundice with acute yellowing" in the primary manuscript. The editors of this manuscript, Zhāng and Zhà, amended it according to the secondary manuscript, *the Dàchéng*, and the subsequent explanation section.

504 According to *Practical Dictionary*, fox-like mounting is a disease "characterized by protrusion of the small intestine into the scrotum. The intestine retracts periodically of

注：肝氣鬱於下而爲疝，然疝乃本經之正症也，任經鬱而爲疝。小腹之脹噫，皆本經之氣不順也，飽食氣滿而有聲爲噫，鬱在上者，泄其上以散之。

Explanation: when the liver qì is depressed in the lower, it will cause mounting; surely, mounting is a principal sign of this channel, as when the rèn channel is depressed, it will cause mounting. Regarding distension of the lower abdomen and belching, they are both due to adverse flow of qì in this channel. When there is qì fullness with audible belching after eating, this is depression located above,[505] disperse the above to dissipate it.

Fifteenth Point of the Rèn Channel
Jiū Wěi – Turtledove Tail (REN-15)
任經第十五穴鳩尾

一名尾翳
Alternate name: Tail Screen

一名𩩲骬[506]
Alternate name: Breastbone

穴在兩歧骨下一寸，臍上七寸五分，脈之別。《銅人》：禁灸，灸之令人少心力。又云：大妙手方鍼，不然，鍼取氣多令人夭。鍼三分，留三呼，泄五吸，肥人倍之。《明堂》：灸三壯。《素》注：不可灸刺。

This point is 1 cùn below where the bones diverge, 7 cùn 5 fēn above the umbilicus. It is where the [rèn] vessel diverges. *The Tóngrén* states, "Moxa is contraindicated; if one performs moxibustion on it, it will cause a reduction of strength in the person's heart." It also states, "Only a skilled practitioner can needle it; otherwise, if [the patient] inhales deeply after being needled, it will cause premature death of that person. Needle 3 fēn, retain for 3 respirations, drain for 5 inhalations, and double [the depth] for obese people." *The Míngtáng* states, "Moxa 3 cones." *The Sùzhù* states, "One cannot moxa or needle it."

注：穴名鳩尾者，以其骨之下垂如鳩尾也。灸多少心力，鍼取氣多令人夭，《素》禁鍼灸，確宜遵之。《靈樞》云：膏之原，出於鳩尾。

---

its own accord, and can be drawn back in by the patient himself in lying posture. It is usually attributed to cold qì congealing in the juéyīn channel."

505 For "上 above" here, the secondary manuscript has "下 below."

506 Note: the Chinese font set that we have used throughout this text does not contain these two rare characters; hence, we have been forced to use a different font.

Explanation: this point is named Jiū Wěi (Turtledove Tail) because the bone that hangs down here resembles a Jiū Wěi (Turtledove Tail). If excessive moxa is performed on it, it will cause a reduction of strength in the heart; if [the patient] inhales deeply after being needled, it will cause premature death of that person. As needling and moxa are contraindicated in *the Sù[zhù]*, it is truly appropriate for one to abide by it.

The Língshū states, "The source point of the gāo[507] emerges at Jiū Wěi (Turtledove Tail)."

任之肺病：息賁，噫喘喉鳴，胸滿咳嘔，喉痹咽腫，水漿不下。

Lung diseases of the rèn: rushing respiration, belching and panting with rales in the throat, fullness in the chest with coughing and retching, throat impediment with swollen pharynx, and inability to get water or fluids down.

任之心病：癲癇，不擇語言，心中氣悶，不喜聞人語，咳唾血，心驚悸，精神耗散。

Heart diseases of the rèn: epilepsy, unfiltered speech, qì oppression in the heart, dislike of hearing people talk, coughing with spitting of blood, fright palpitations in the heart, wasting and dissipation of the essence and spirit.

任之肝病：熱病偏頭痛，引目外眥痛。

Liver disease of the rèn: febrile disease with hemilateral headache with pain that radiates to the outer canthus.

任之腎病：少年房勞，短氣少氣。

Kidney diseases of the rèn: bedroom taxation in young people, shortness of breath and scantness of breath.[508]

注：以上諸症，雖爲本穴所司，然灸多則令人心力少，鍼取氣多則令人夭，雖曰非大妙手不可鍼，然總不如以他穴代之可也。

Explanation: regarding the various signs above, although they are commanded by this point, yet if one performs moxibustion excessively, it will cause a reduction of strength in the person's heart; if [the patient] inhales deeply after being needled, it will cause premature death of that person. Even though it is said that "only a skilled practitioner can needle it," yet, it is still much better to use other points as a substitute for it.

---

[507] See BL-43 in Vol.1 for explanation of both gāo and huāng.
[508] This could also be read as "shortness of qì and scantness of qì."

Sixteenth Point of the Rèn Channel
Zhōng Tíng – Centre Courtyard[509] (REN-16)
任經氣十六穴中庭

穴在膻中下一寸六分。《銅人》：灸五壯，鍼三分。《明堂》：灸三壯。

This point is located 1 cùn 6 fēn below Dàn Zhōng (REN-17). *The Tóngrén* states, "Moxa 5 cones, and needle 3 fēn." *The Míngtáng* states, "Moxa 3 cones."

注：中庭者，爲心之庭也，心在內，而此穴爲外見之庭，自此穴而上至天突穴，凡七穴皆以一寸六分取之。

Explanation: Zhōng Tíng (Centre Courtyard) is the Tíng (Courtyard) of the heart; as the heart is located on the interior, this point is the Tíng (Courtyard) [of the heart] that is visible on the exterior. From this point to Tiān Tū (REN-22) above, all of these 7 points are located [with a distance of] 1 cùn 6 fēn [apart].

任之肺病：脅胸支滿，噎塞，食飲不下，嘔吐食出，小兒吐奶。

Lung diseases of the rèn: propping fullness in the chest and rib-side, dysphagia, inability to get food and drink down, vomiting of food, and vomiting of breast milk in children.

注：此在胸上，所治者乃胸氣塞逆之症，宜泄此穴，散而降之。

Explanation: this point is located on the chest, so what it treats are signs of blockage and counterflow of qì in the chest, it is appropriate to drain this point in order to dissipate [the blockage] and descend [the counterflow].

Seventeenth Point of the Rèn Channel
Dàn Zhōng - Chest Centre (REN-17)
任經第十七穴膻中

一名元兒
Alternate name: Original Child

一名上氣海
Alternate name: Upper Sea of Qì

---

[509] *Grasping the Wind* names it "Centre Palace."

穴在玉堂下一寸六分，橫量兩乳間陷中，仰而取之，足太陰脾、少陰腎、手太陽小腸、少陽三焦與任脈共會之所，灸五壯。《明堂》：灸七壯，止二七壯，禁鍼。此氣之會也，凡上氣不下，及氣噎、氣膈、氣痛之類，均宜灸之。

This point is located 1 cùn 6 fēn below Yù Táng (REN-18), in the depression on the horizontal line between the nipples; lie supine to locate it. This is the place where the foot tàiyīn spleen, shàoyīn kidney, hand tàiyáng small intestine, shàoyáng sānjiāo, and rèn vessel meet together. Moxa 5 cones. *The Míngtáng* **states, "Moxa 7 to 14 cones, and needling is contraindicated." This [point] is the meeting of qì; in general, for any type of [sign] such as qì ascent that does not descend, as well as qì dysphagia, qì occlusion, and qì pain, it is always appropriate to moxa it.**

注：此穴內直心包絡，故心之包絡，一名膻中，爲臣使之官，喜樂出焉。《難經》云：氣會膻中，蓋指脾、腎、小腸、三焦俱會於此所也，氣病治此穴，禁鍼者，與心近也。

Explanation: this point connects directly inwards with the pericardial network. Another name for the pericardiac network of the heart is "Dàn Zhōng (Chest Centre), which holds the office of minister and envoy, joy and happiness emanate from it."[510] *The Nànjīng* states, "The qì meets at Dàn Zhōng (Chest Centre);"[511] undoubtedly, this is referring to the meeting of the spleen, kidney, small intestine and sānjiāo [channels] at this place; as such, [*The Nànjīng Shū* states], "For qì diseases, treat this point." Needling is contraindicated because it is nearby the heart.

任之肺病：上氣氣短，咳逆噫氣，膈氣喉鳴，喘嗽不下氣，胸中如塞，心胸痛，風痛咳嗽，肺癰唾膿，嘔吐涎沫，婦人乳汁少。

Lung diseases of the rèn: qì ascent with shortness of breath, cough and counterflow with belching, qì occlusion with rales in the throat, panting and cough with inability to inhale as though there is a blockage in the chest, pain of the heart and chest, wind pain with cough, pulmonary welling-abscess with spitting of pus, vomiting and retching of drool and foam, and scant breast milk.

注：以上皆肺分之病，肺主一身之氣，氣病亦貴此穴，惟用灸爲宜。

Explanation: all of the above are diseases in the lung aspect; as the lung governs the qì of the whole body, when there is a qì disease, seek this point; however, it is appropriate to only utilise moxibustion.

---

[510] From *Sùwèn* Chapter 8.
[511] From *Nànjīng* Difficulty 45.

Eighteenth Point of the Rèn Channel
Yù Táng – Jade Hall (REN-18)
任經第十八穴玉堂

一名玉英

Alternate name: Jade's Beauty

穴在紫宮下一寸六分陷中。《銅人》：灸五壯，鍼三分。

This point is located in the depression 1 cùn 6 fēn below Zǐ Gōng (REN-19). *The Tóngrén* states, "Moxa 5 cones, and needle 3 fēn."

注：玉堂者，心之堂也，心在內，而此其堂也。

Explanation: regarding Yù Táng (Jade Hall), [it is referring to] the Táng (Hall) of the heart; while the heart is located on the interior, this is its Táng (Hall) [on the exterior].

任之肺病：胸腋疼痛心煩，咳逆上氣，胸滿不得息，喘急嘔吐寒痰。

Lung diseases of the rèn: pain in the chest and armpit with vexation in the heart, cough with qì counterflow ascent, chest fullness with inability to catch one's breath, and rapid panting with retching and vomiting of cold phlegm.

注：此穴與肺近，故所治皆肺有逆氣之症。

Explanation: as this point is nearby the lung, thus what it treats are all signs of counterflow qì of the lung.

Nineteenth Point of the Rèn Channel
Zǐ Gōng – Purple Palace (REN-19)
任經第十九穴紫宮

穴在華蓋下一寸六分，仰而取之。《銅人》：灸五壯，鍼三分。《明堂》：灸七壯。

This point is 1 cùn 6 fēn below Huá Gài (REN-20), lie supine to locate it. *The Tóngrén* states, "Moxa 5 cones, and needle 3 fēn." *The Míngtáng* states, "Moxa 7 cones."

注：紫宮者，紫微之宮也，心正在內，此穴爲宮。

Explanation: regarding Zǐ Gōng (Purple Palace), it is the Gōng (Palace) of the Zǐwéi;[512] as the heart is located directly on the interior [to this point], this point is the Gōng (Palace) [of the heart].

任之肺病：胸脇支滿，胸膺骨痛，飲食不下，嘔逆上氣，煩心咳逆，吐血，唾如白膠。

Lung diseases of the rèn: propping fullness in the chest and rib-sides, pain of the anterior chest bones, inability to get food and drink down, vomiting with qì counterflow ascent, vexation of the heart with cough and counterflow, vomiting of blood, and spittle that resembles white glue.

注：前症皆肺病也，任之經至此，而肺有鬱所生諸疾，皆取此穴治之。

Explanation: all the above signs are diseases of the lung; as the rèn channel arrives at this place, when various diseases manifest as a result of depression in the lung, one should always choose this point in order to treat them.

Twentieth Point of the Rèn Channel
Huá Gài – Florid Canopy (REN-20)
任經第二十穴華蓋

穴在璇璣下一寸六分，仰而取之。《銅人》：鍼三分，灸五壯。《明堂》：灸三壯。

This point is located 1 cùn 6 fēn below Xuán Jī (REN-21), lie supine to locate it. *The Tóngrén* states, "Needle 3 fēn, and moxa 5 cones." *The Míngtáng* states, "Moxa 3 cones."

注：此穴則在心之上，故爲華蓋，如蓋之覆乎人頂也。

Explanation: as this point is located above the heart, thus it is the Huá Gài (Florid Canopy), which resembles a Gài (Canopy) that covers the top of a person.

任之肺病：喘急上氣，咳逆咳嗽，喉痹咽腫，水漿不下，胸脇支滿痛。

Lung diseases of the rèn: rapid panting with qì ascent, coughing and counterflow, throat impediment with swollen pharynx, inability to get water or fluids down, and propping fullness with pain in the chest and rib-sides.

---

512 I.e., the north star (α Ursae Minoris), or the "帝星 star of the emperor." As the Zǐwéi sits on the north pole with all celestial bodies revolving around it, it exemplifies the role of an emperor in celestial movements. It is also a term often used to refer to the emperor.

注：以上皆肺病，此穴在心上，正抵肺，故肺病皆取之。

Explanation: all the above are lung diseases; as this point is located above the heart and exactly on the lung, thus for all lung disease, choose this [point].

Twenty-First Point of the Rèn Channel
Xuán Jī – Jade Swivel (REN-21)
任經第二十一穴璇璣

穴在天突下一寸六分陷中，仰頭取之。《銅人》：鍼三分，灸五壯。

This point is in the depression 1 cùn 6 fēn below Tiān Tū (REN-22), raise the head to locate it. *The Tóngrén states, "Needle 3 fēn, and moxa 5 cones."*

注：璇璣者，乃紫微垣之星，在華蓋之上，此穴亦在華蓋之上，故名。

Explanation: regarding Xuán Jī (Jade Swivel), it is the [group of four] stars within the Zǐwéi enclosure[513] located above [the constellation] Huá Gài;[514] likewise, this point is located above [the point] Huá Gài (REN-20), that is why it is named as such.

任之肺病：胸脇支滿痛，咳逆上氣，喉鳴喘不能言，喉痺咽癰，水漿不下。

Lung diseases of the rèn: propping fullness in the chest and rib-sides, cough and counterflow with qì ascent, rales in the throat with panting and inability to speak, throat impediment or pharynx paralysis, and inability to get water or fluids down.

注：此穴當肺系之上，肺有氣鬱之症，取之以泄其有餘之氣。

Explanation: as this point is directly above the lung connector, when there are signs of qì depression in the lung, choose this [point] in order to drain the superabundance of qì.

任之胃病：胃中有積。

Stomach disease of the rèn: accumulations in the stomach.

---

[513] The Zǐwéi enclosure is a collection of thirty-nine stars around the north pole, all of which can be observed throughout the year in the northern hemisphere. Xuán Jī (Jade Swivel) is the collective name of the four stars that constitute the "bowl" of the big dipper (α Ursae Majoris, β Ursae Majoris, γ Ursae Majoris, and δ Ursae Majoris).

[514] Note: this constellation Huá Gài carries the same name as Huá Gài (Florid Canopy, REN-20). It is roughly equivalent to the Cassiopeia constellation in western astrology.

注：胃中有積亦取之，胃之脘當在肺系之後，取之則覺遠矣。

Explanation: when there are accumulations in the stomach, one can also choose this point; as the stomach duct is directly behind the lung connector, by choosing this [point], [the patient] will notice its remote [effect].[515]

Twenty-Second Point of the Rèn Channel
Tiān Tū – Celestial Chimney (REN-22)
任經第二十二穴天突

一名天瞿
Alternate name: Celestial Polearm[516]

一名玉戶
Alternate name: Jade Door

穴在頸結喉下四寸宛宛中，陰維、任脈之會。《銅人》：鍼五分，留三呼，得氣即泄，灸亦得，不及鍼。若下鍼當直下，不得前。低手即泄五臟之氣，傷人短壽。《明堂》：灸五壯，鍼一分。《素》注：鍼一寸，留七呼，灸五壯。《神農》：治咳嗽，灸五壯。

This point is located on the neck, in the depression 4 cùn below the laryngeal prominence. It is the meeting of the yīnwéi and rèn vessels. *The Tóngrén* **states, "Needle 5 fēn, retain for 3 respirations, and obtain qì then promptly drain; one can also use moxa, [yet it is] inferior to needling. If it is needled, it ought to be needled vertically downwards,[517] not inwards.[518] Once [this point is utilized by] an unskilled practitioner, it will promptly drain the qì of the five zàng-viscera; it will injure the person and shorten their life."**

The Míngtáng **states, "Moxa 5 cones, and needle 1 fēn."** *The Sùzhù* **states, "Needle 1 cùn, retain for 7 respirations, and moxa 5 cones."** *The Shénnóng* **states, "To treat cough, moxa 5 cones."**[519]

---

515 I.e., the effect will take place at the stomach duct (oesophagus), which is located behind both the needling site and the lung connector (trachea).

516 *Grasping the Wind* names it "Celestial Alarm." Note: Qú 瞿 is a rare type of ancient polearm held by court attendants as a ceremonial weapon during the Zhou dynasty. It resembles a dagger-axe in appearance, but with a straightened and symmetrical blade, a curved striking edge, and a thicker and larger body than that of a typical dagger-axe.

517 I.e., needling downwards towards the feet.

518 For "不得前 not inwards," *the Tóngrén* actually states, "橫下不得 one may not insert horizontally."

519 For "moxa 5 cones," it is "moxa 7 cones" in the secondary manuscript.

注：突猶曲突徙薪之突，乃實而有隙通氣之稱。天者，言其高處也，任脈入胸穴者在於骨，至此穴乃爲空隙之處，而所在又甚高，故名天突。

Explanation: Regarding Tū (Chimney), it refers to the Tū (Chimney) from [the idiom] "making the Tū (Chimney) vent crooked and moving the firewood,"[520] which is namely a solid [object] with a gap so that it is able to vent air. Regarding Tiān (Celestial), it is referring to the elevated position [of this point]. After the rèn vessel enters the chest, the points are on bone; upon arriving here, it is a place with a hollow gap, and it is situated at a highly elevated place, thus it is named Tiān Tū (Celestial Chimney).

許氏曰：此穴一鍼四效，凡下鍼後良久，先脾磨食，覺鍼動爲一效。次鍼破病根，腸中作聲爲二效。次覺流入膀胱爲三效。然後覺氣流入腰後腎堂間爲第四效，總言氣滯而散之狀。

Mister Xǔ[521] says, "With one needle at this point, one can bring about four effects. In general, after needling [and retaining] it for a long time, the spleen will begin to grind the food, and [the patient] will notice a movement at the needle; this is the first effect. Next, as the needle breaks up the root of the disease, the intestines will create a sound; this is the second effect. Next, [the patient] will notice something flowing into the bladder; this is the third effect. Lastly, [the patient] will notice qì flowing into the waist on the rear, between the halls of kidneys; this is the fourth effect." In summary, [its effect] will appear as though the stagnant qì is dissipated.

任之肺病：上氣咳逆，氣暴喘，咽腫咽冷，聲破喉中生瘡，喉猜猜喀膿血，瘖不能言，身寒熱頸腫，哮喘，喉中噛噛如水鷄聲，胸中氣梗梗，挾舌下青脈，瘿瘤。

---

520 "曲突徙薪 making the chimney vent crooked and moving the firewood" comes from 漢書霍光金日磾傳 the Book of Hàn, "Biographies of Huò Guāng and Jīn Mìdī" (82 CE), "客有過主人者，見其灶直突，傍有積薪，客謂主人，更爲曲突，遠徙其薪，不者且有火患，主人嘿然不應。俄而家果失火。 A guest passed by the [residence] of the host. He saw the hearth had a horizontal chimney vent, [which opened] next to a pile of firewood. The guest told the host that he should modify the chimney vent to a crooked one and move the firewood far away [from the vent]; otherwise, there would be a fire. The host stayed silent without making any response. Later, there was indeed a fire." It means taking preventive measures against future disasters.

521 We do not know who this person may be, as the following quote seems to first appear in the Zhēnjiǔ Jùyīng 針灸聚英 (Gathered Blooms of Acupuncture and Moxibustion, 1529 CE) by Gāo Wǔ 高武, where it is simply attributed to "許氏 Mister Xǔ." Nevertheless, as Gāo Wǔ cited a number of quotes from Xǔ Xī 許希, a famous acupuncturist who lived in early Sòng dynasty with the nickname "許神針 Xǔ the Miracle Needle," it is possible that he was citing from Xǔ's lost work, Shényìng Zhēnjiǔ Yàojué 神應針灸要訣 (Essential Acupuncture Rhymes of Miraculous Responses, c. 11th century CE).

Lung diseases of the rèn: qì ascent with counterflow and cough, fulminant qì panting, swollen and cold pharynx, cracked voice due to manifestation of sores in the larynx, cāi cāi [noises] in the throat[522] with spitting pus and blood, loss of voice, generalised chills and fevers and swelling of the neck, wheezing and panting, wheezing noises in the throat [that resemble] the sound of a frog, qì hindrance in the chest, blue-green veins under the tongue, goitre and tumour.

注：前症皆肺有餘之症，泄此穴以散肺氣。

Explanation: all the above signs are signs of superabundance in the lung, drain this point in order to dissipate the lung qì.

任之心病：心與背相控而痛。

Heart disease of the rèn: pain and [tension] that resemble the drawing of a bow between the heart and upper back.

注：背者，心肺之室也，相控而痛，乃氣滯於內也，泄此穴以散其滯氣。

Explanation: the upper back is the chamber of the heart and lung; when there is pain and [tension] that resemble the drawing of a bow, this is due to qì stagnation in the interior, drain this point in order to dissipate the stagnated qì.

任之胃病：面皮熱，五噎，黃疸，醋心多唾，嘔吐。

Stomach diseases of the rèn: heat in the facial skin, the five dysphagias,[523] jaundice, heartburn with copious spittle, retching and vomiting.

注：胃中熱則面皮熱，宜泄此穴以散胃中之熱。噎者，氣爲痰滯也，泄此穴以通氣。黃疸，胃有濕熱也，泄此穴以去胃中濕熱之氣。醋心多唾、嘔吐，皆胃有痰也，泄此穴，氣散而痰下。

Explanation: with heat in the stomach, there will be heat in the facial skin, it is appropriate to drain this point in order to dissipate the heat in the stomach. A dysphagia occurs when qì is stagnated by phlegm, drain this point to unblock the qì. Jaundice is due to the presence of damp-heat in the stomach, drain this point in order to eliminate the damp-heat qì of the stomach. For heartburn with copious spittle, and retching and vomiting, they are all caused by phlegm within the stomach, drain this point; once the qì dissipates, the phlegm will descend.

---

[522] Though we are not completely certain, we believe this "cāi cāi" noise is most likely a sound generated by frequent dry cough.

[523] The five dysphagias are first mentioned in *Zhūbìng Yuánhòu Lùn* 諸病源候論 (*the Origin and Indicators of Disease*, 610 CE), which are namely the dysphagia due to qì, dysphagia due to worry, dysphagia due to food, dysphagia due to taxation, and dysphagia due to thought.

Twenty-Third Point of the Rèn Channel
Lián Quán – Ridge Spring (REN-23)
任經第二十三穴廉泉

一名本池
Alternate name: Root Pool

一名舌本
Alternate name: Tongue Root

穴在頸下結喉上中央，仰面取之，陰維、任脈之會。《素》注：低鍼取之，鍼一寸，留七呼。《銅人》：灸三壯，鍼三分，得氣即泄。《明堂》：鍼二分。

This point is located in the centre of the neck, above the laryngeal prominence, face upward to locate it. It is the meeting of the yīnwéi and rèn vessels. *The Sùzhù* states, "Lower the needle [to pierce it],[524] needle 1 cùn, and retain for 7 respirations."[525] *The Tóngrén* states, "Moxa 3 cones, and needle 3 fēn, obtain qì then promptly drain." *The Míngtáng* states, "Needle 2 fēn."

注：穴名廉泉者，乃舌下生津液之本也，舌下津液，由此而生，乃任脈自下行者，入交於舌之下，而生津液，有泉之象焉。

Explanation: this point is named Lián Quán (Ridge Spring) because it is the source of the fluid engenderment below the tongue; as such, the fluids below the tongue are engendered from this place. For the rèn vessel that travels here from the below, it enters to intersect below the tongue; as a result, the fluids are engendered; thus, it has the image of a Quán (Spring).

所得不多，非在外之水，乃一身經脈所成。修養者，吞咽之水，即此泉之水也，故曰廉泉。又《內經》云：足少陰舌下。又云：舌下兩脈者，廉泉也。此總係任經穴，而實為腎經脈氣所發。

It does not produce a substantial amount [of fluids] because it is not water from an external source; rather, it is formed by the channels and network-vessels of the whole body. For those who practise self-cultivation, the water[526] they swallow is precisely water from this Quán (Spring), thus it is called Lián Quán (Ridge Spring). Also, *the Nèijīng* states, "The foot shàoyīn is below the tongue."[527] It also states, "The

---

[524] I.e., needle it obliquely upwards.

[525] For this entire statement, *the Sùzhù* actually states, "刺可入同身寸之三分，留三呼，若灸者，可灸三壯。With needling, one can insert 3 fēn of body-inch, retain for 3 respirations; for moxibustion, one can moxa 3 cones."

[526] I.e., the spittle.

[527] From *Sùwèn* Chapter 59.

two vessels below the tongue are Lián Quán (Ridge Spring)."[528] Even though it is classified as a rèn channel point, it is in fact where the vessel qì of the kidney channel effuses.

任之肺病：咳嗽上氣，喘息嘔沫。

Lung diseases of the rèn: cough with qì ascent, panting with vomiting of foam.

注：此皆肺之有餘也，泄此穴以降肺有餘之氣。

Explanation: these are both due to superabundance of the lung, drain this point in order to descend the superabundance of lung qì.

任之心病：舌下腫難言，舌根縮急不食，舌縱涎出口瘡。

Heart diseases of the rèn: swelling below the tongue with difficulty speaking, retraction and tension of the tongue with no desire to eat, protracted tongue with drooling and mouth sores.

注：以上皆心之熱也，泄此穴以退心之熱。

Explanation: all of the above are due to heat of the heart, drain this point in order to abate the heat of the heart.

Twenty-Fourth Point of the Rèn Channel
Chéng Jiāng – Sauce Receptacle (REN-24)
任經第二十四穴承漿

穴在脣稜下陷中，開口取之。大腸脈、胃脈、督脈、任脈四脈相會之所。《素》注：鍼二分，留五呼，灸三壯。《銅人》：灸七壯至七七壯。《明堂》：鍼三分，得氣即泄，留三呼，徐徐引氣而出，日灸七壯，過七七壯，停四、五日，復灸七七壯。若一嚮不灸，恐足陽明脈斷，其病不愈，停息復灸，令血脈宣通，其病立愈。

This point is located in the depression below the edge of the [lower] lip, open the mouth to locate it. It is the meeting place of the four vessels, the large intestine vessel, stomach vessel, dū vessel, and rèn vessel. *The Sùzhù states,* **"Needle 2 fēn, retain for 5 respirations, and moxa 3 cones."** *The Tóngrén states,* **"Moxa 7 to 49 cones."**

The Míngtáng states, **"Needle 3 fēn, obtain qì then promptly drain, retain for 3 respirations, slowly direct the qì to exit, and moxa 7 cones daily; after 49 cones [in total], stop after 4 or 5 days, and then moxa up to 49 cones again. If**

---

[528] From *Sùwèn* Chapter 36.

one never performs moxa [at this point], there is a danger that the foot yángmíng vessel will be severed;[529] as a result, the disease will not be relieved. After resting, one should resume performing moxa, this will perfuse the blood vessels; as such, the disease will be immediately cured."

注：穴名承漿者，口中飲食所餘，而在外者，此穴其承之之地，故曰承漿。乃胃、大腸、督、任四脈相會之所，治病之要穴也。

Explanation: regarding the point name Chéng Jiāng (Sauce Receptacle), when residuals of food and drink linger outside of the mouth [while eating], this point is the place that Chéng (Receives) it, thus it is called Chéng Jiāng (Sauce Receptacle). As it is the meeting place of the four vessels, the stomach, large intestine, dū, and rèn [vessels], it is an essential point for treating diseases.

任之胃病：偏風半身不遂，口眼喎斜，面腫消渴，口齒疳蝕生瘡，暴瘖不能言。

Stomach diseases of the rèn: hemilateral wind and hemiplegia, deviated eyes and mouth, swollen face with dispersion-thirst, gān-erosion and sores of the mouth and teeth, and sudden loss of voice.

注：口眼喎斜，乃受風也。面腫消渴，胃有熱也。口齒疳蝕，亦胃有熱也。暴瘖不能言，熱結於舌也。以上俱宜泄此穴，以此穴爲手、足陽明、督、任脈相會之地。多灸更妙。

Explanation: deviated eyes and mouth is due to contraction of wind. Swollen face with dispersion-thirst is due to the presence of heat in the stomach. Gān-erosion of the mouth and teeth is also due to the presence of heat in the stomach. Sudden loss of voice is due to heat binding the tongue. For all of the above, it is appropriate to drain this point, as this point is the meeting place of the hand and foot yángmíng, dū and rèn vessels. Frequently utilising moxa [on this point] is even more miraculous.

---

[529] For this problematic sentence, *the Shènghuì Fāng* (992 CE), *the Zīshēng* (1220 CE), and even the usually unreliable *Zhēnjiǔ Jùyīng* (1526 CE) all have a completely different line, "若一面灸，恐足陽明脈斷。If one continues to moxa, there is a danger that the foot yángmíng vessel will be severed." While the original message seems more fitting, as it explains the rationale for why one should rest for 4-5 days before performing moxa again, the line from this current manuscript does not seem to make complete sense. This scribal error seems to have appeared when *the Dàchéng* was compiled in 1601 CE, which was inherited to this writing by Yuè Hánzhēn.

Extra Points Associated with the Rèn Channel
任經奇穴

Goat Faeces[530] (UEX-LE 1)
Yáng Shǐ – 羊矢

在會陰旁三寸，股內橫紋中，皮肉間有核如羊矢。可刺三分，灸七壯。一傳治婦
人產後昏迷，不省人事。

**This point is 3 cùn to the side of Huì Yīn (REN-1); on the transverse crease on
the inner thigh, between the flesh and skin, there is a node that resembles a
piece of Yáng Shǐ (Goat Faeces). One can pierce it 3 fēn, and moxa 7 cones. One
transmitted source states that it treats postpartum fainting and loss of
consciousness.**

Intestine's Bequeathal (UEX-CA 43)
Cháng Yí – 腸遺

挾中極旁，相去二寸半。《千金》云：治大便難，灸隨年壯。

This point clasps the sides of Zhōng Jí (REN-8), 2 and a half cùn apart from it.
The Qiānjīn **states, "To treat difficult defecation, moxa cones according to one's
age."**

Uterine Gate (UEX-CA 39)
Bāo Mén – 胞門

子户、氣門

[Alternate names:] Zǐ Hù (Infant's Door), Qì Mén (Qì Gate)

《千金》云：子臟門塞不受精，妊娠不成。若墮胎腹痛，漏胞見赤，灸胞門五十
壯，關元左邊二寸是也。右邊名子户。若胞衣不出，及子死腹中，或腹中積聚，
皆鍼入胞門一寸。

The Qiānjīn **states, "When the gate of the infant's viscus[531] is blocked, one will
not be able to receive the essence; as such, pregnancy will not occur. In case of
a threatened miscarriage with abdominal pain, foetal spotting with**

---

530 *Grasping the Wind* names it "Goat Arrow."
531 I.e., the uterus.

observable bleeding, moxa 50 cones on Bāo Mén (Uterine Gate), which is 2 cùn to the left side of Guān Yuán (REN-4); on the right side, it is named Zǐ Hù (Infant's Door). If there is retention of placenta, death in utero, or accumulations and gatherings in the abdomen, for all cases, needle Bāo Mén (Uterine Gate) to a depth of 1 cùn."

又云：胎孕不成，灸氣門穴，在關元旁三寸，各五十壯。又：漏胎下血不禁，灸百壯。

It also states, "For inability to conceive, moxa the point Qì Mén (Qì Gate), which is located 3 cùn to the side of Guān Yuán (REN-4); moxa 50 cones on each [side]."[532] In addition, "For unrestrained leaking of blood during pregnancy, moxa 100 cones."

Body Intersection (UEX-CA 42)
Shēn Jiāo – 身交

在小腹下橫紋中。《千金翼》云：白崩中，灸小腹橫紋當臍孔直下一百壯。及治胞落癲，灸身交五十壯，三報之。又治大小便不通，又治溺床者，可灸七壯。

This point is located on the transverse crease below the lower abdomen. *The Qiānjīn Yì* states, "For white flooding, moxa 100 cones on the traverse crease on the lower abdomen that is directly below the umbilicus. Also, to treat uterine prolapse and downfall, moxa 50 cones on Shēn Jiāo (Body Intersection), repeat 3 times. In addition, to treat stoppage of defecation and urination, also to treat bed wetting, one can moxa 7 cones."

Dragon's Chin (UEX-CA 3)
Lóng Hàn – 龍頷

在鳩尾上寸半。《千金翼》云：主心痛冷氣，止灸百壯，勿鍼。

This point is located 1 cùn and a half above Jiū Wěi (REN-15). *The Qiānjīn Yì* states, "To govern heart pain with cold qì, moxa up to 100 cones; needling is prohibited."

---

[532] "50 cones" in *the Qiānjīn* is actually "100 cones."

Sea Source (EX-HN 11)
Hǎi Quán – 海泉

在舌下中央脈上，主治消渴，鍼出血。

This point is located on the centre vessel below the tongue; to govern the treatment of dispersion-thirst, bleed it.

Golden Liquid [on the] Right (EX-HN 12)
& Jade Humour [on the] Left (EX-HN 13)
Zuǒ Jīn Jīn Yòu Yù Yè – 左金津右玉液

在舌下兩旁紫脈上，主治消渴、口瘡、舌腫、喉痺，宜用三棱鍼出血。

These two points are on the purple vessels on the two sides below the tongue. They govern the treatment of dispersion-thirst, mouth sores, swollen tongue, and throat impediment, it is appropriate to utilise the three-edged needle to bleed them.

Ghost Seal (UEX-HN 33)
Guǐ Fēng – 鬼封

《千金》云：第十三次下鍼，在舌頭當舌中下縫，刺貫出舌上。仍以一板橫口吻，安鍼頭，勿令舌動，名鬼封。

***The Qiānjīn* states, "It is the thirteenth point to be needled in sequence;[533] it is located at the crevice below the centre of the tongue. Peirce through the tongue and emerge it above, place a small wooden plate horizontally at the lips to stabilize the tip of the needle and prevent the tongue from moving.[534] It is named Guǐ Fēng (Ghost Seal).**

---

[533] Referring to the Thirteen Ghost Points needling sequence.

[534] One needs to pull the patient's tongue out to needle this point properly; after the needle pierces through the tongue, a slender wooden plate is likely placed behind the needle (deeper into the mouth) but pressing against the two corners of the lips, forming a cross shape with the needle. The placement of the wooden plate would then prevent the person from withdrawing the tongue, as the shaft of the needle would likely be pressing against the upper lip, while the needle handle would be pressing against the wooden plate.

The Point Inside of the Lip (UEX HN 29)
Chún Lǐ Xué – 唇裏穴

《千金翼》云：唇裏正當承漿邊各一寸，鍼三鋥，主治馬黄黄疸。此名鬼市，百邪癲狂，當在第八次下鍼。

The Qiānjīn Yì states, "This point is inside the lip, exactly 1 cùn on each side [on the inside of] Chéng Jiāng (REN-24), pierce with a fire needle 3 times,[535] it governs the treatment of jaundice that is the colour of a yellow horse." This point is named Guǐ Shì (Ghost Market), [it treats] the hundred evils causing epilepsy and mania, it should be the eighth point to be needled in sequence.

---

[535] It is uncertain what "zēng 鋥 (fire needling)" really is. In the relevant passage in *the Qiānjīn Yì*, the Sòng imperial editors themselves mentioned that they did not understand what this character meant and simply kept the character as it was. We have adopted the interpretation of Huáng Lóngxiáng et al. from their authoritative work of *Zhōngguó Zhēnjiǔ Cìjiǔfǎ Tōngjiàn* 中国针灸刺灸法通鉴 (*Comprehensive Reflection on Methodologies of Chinese Acupuncture and Moxibustion*, 2004 CE), which establishes that this term "zēng 鋥" often appears as the verb for the subject "火针 fire needle" – thus, it likely means fire needling. On a further note, according to Sūn Sīmiǎo's description, "火針亦用鋒針，以油火燒之，務在猛熱，不熱即有損於人也。For fire needling, a lancing needle is also utilized; burn it with grease fire and ensure that it is fiercely hot; if it is not hot enough, it will injure the person." In modern clinic, tungsten three-edged needles or specialty fire needles made with heat-resistant alloys should be utilized for such a technique; otherwise, as regular stainless-steel needles may soften upon heating, it may become difficult to insert or prone to breaking for such an application.

The Dū Channel & Points

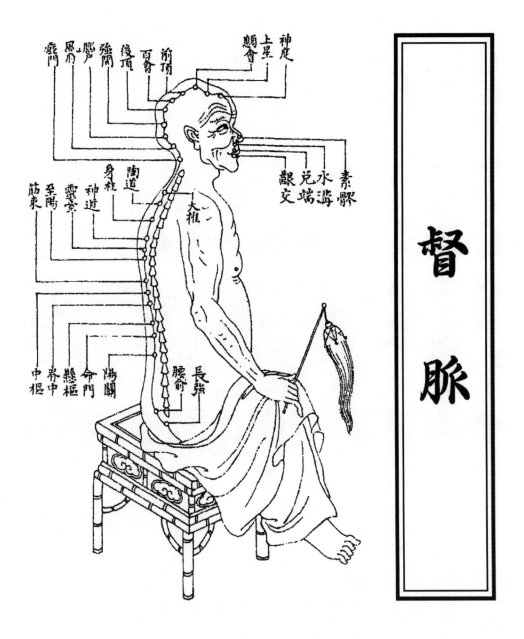

督脈

The Dū Channel & Points
督經

Overview of the Dū Channel
督經總論

思蓮子曰：督行人身之背，所以統一身之陽，任行人身之腹，所以統一身之陰，
人身之有任督，猶天地之有子午也。督統一身之陽，所以爲陽脈之海。而人身陽
最大者，莫大於足太陽。人之太陽挾背而下行，督行於太陽之中而上行，其脈起
於腎下胞中，至於小腹，乃却行於腰橫骨圍之中央，系溺孔之端，男子循莖下仍
行於篡，女子絡陰器，合篡間，俱繞篡屏翳穴，即前陰後陰之間會陰穴也。

**Master Sīlián says, the dū [vessel] travels on the back of the human body, that
is why it commands the yáng of the whole body; the rèn [vessel] travels on the
abdomen of the human body, that is why it commands the yīn of the whole
body; the rèn and dū [vessels] of the human body resemble zǐ and wǔ[536] of the
heaven and earth.**

**The dū [vessel] commands the yáng of the whole body, that is why it is the sea
of the yáng vessels. Yet, for the greatest yáng in the human body, none is
greater than the foot tàiyáng. While the tàiyáng [channel] of a person clasps
the back as it descends, the dū [vessel] travels between the tàiyáng [pathways]
as it ascends. The [dū] vessel commences in the womb below the kidneys and
arrives at the lower abdomen; thereupon, it returns to surround the centre of
the transverse bone and connects with the tip of the urethra;[537] in males, it
follows the bottom of the penis and travels to the perineum;[538] in females, it
networks with the genitals[539] and unites at the perineum. In both [genders], it**

---

[536] Zǐ 子 is the first earthly branch; in daily hours, it denotes the time between 11 pm to 1 am,
the peak of yīn, when the yáng is engendered; whereas wǔ 午 is the seventh earthly
branch; in daily hours, it denotes the time between 11 am to 1 pm, the peak of yáng, when
the yīn is engendered.

[537] Lit. urine hole.

[538] This seems to be a scribal error in the manuscript. While the manuscript has zuǎn 纂
(compile, edit), it should be another similarly looking character, cuàn 篡 (perineum),
instead in lieu of the context.

[539] Lit. yīn organs.

encircles Píng Yì (REN-1),[540] which is precisely Huì Yīn (REN-1), which is located between the anterior yīn and posterior yīn.[541]

別繞臀，至少陰與太陽中絡者，合少陰上股內廉，由陰尾尻骨兩旁，足太陽經之會陽穴，遂貫脊與足少陰會於本經絡穴，在骶骨端之長強穴，遂並脊裏上行，歷二十一椎下之腰腧穴，十六椎下之陽關穴，十四椎下之命門穴，十三椎下之懸樞穴，十一椎下之脊中穴，

It diverges to encircle the buttocks, where it reaches the network-vessel between the shàoyīn and tàiyáng [channels], and it then unites with the shàoyīn [channel] at the inner aspect of the upper thigh. From Huì Yáng (BL-35) of the tàiyáng channel on the two sides of the yīn sacrum and coccyx bones, thereupon, it pierces the spine and meets with the foot shàoyīn at the network point of this channel, Cháng Qiáng (DU-1), which is located at the tip of the sacrum.

Thereupon, it ascends in the interior of the spine to pass through Yāo Shù (DU-2) below the twenty-first vertebra, Yáng Guān (DU-3) below the sixteenth vertebra, Mìng Mén (DU-4) below the fourteenth vertebra, Xuán Shū (DU-5) below the thirteenth vertebra, Jǐ Zhōng (DU-6) below the eleventh vertebra,

十椎下之中樞穴，九椎下之筋縮穴，七椎下之至陽穴，六椎下之靈臺穴，五椎下之神道穴，三椎下之身柱穴，大椎下之陶道穴，而與足太陽會，

Zhōng Shū (DU-7)[542] below the tenth vertebra, Jīn Suō (DU-8) below the nineth vertebra, Zhì Yáng (DU-9) below the seventh vertebra, Líng Tái (DU-10) below the sixth vertebra, Shén Dào (DU-11) below the fifth vertebra, Shēn Zhù (DU-12) below the third vertebra, and Táo Dào (DU-13) below Dà Zhuī (DU-14) to meet with the foot tàiyáng [channel].

又上歷大椎上之大椎穴，而與手太陽、足太陽、手少陽、足少陽、足陽明會合，

It continues to ascend and passes through Dà Zhuī (DU-14) above the great vertebra[543] to meet and unite with the hand tàiyáng, foot tàiyáng, hand shàoyáng, foot shàoyáng, and foot yángmíng [channels].

---

[540] This is an alternate name for REN-1 (Huì Yīn, 會陰).

[541] I.e., the exterior genitals and the anus.

[542] While Yuè Hánzhēn mentions DU-7 in this section discussing the pathway, he does not seem to regard it as a channel point for the dū channel, however, it is included as an extra point instead. For a more thorough discussion, see the entry for Zhōng Shū (Central Pivot) in the associated extra points.

[543] I.e., first thoracic vertebra. See footnote in DU-14.

遂離背而入項，至於本經之啞門穴，又會陽維入系舌本，上行至本經之風府穴，又會足太陽、陽維，同入腦中，循枕骨上行本經之腦戶穴，又上歷本經百會穴後三寸之強間穴，

Thereupon, it departs the upper back to enter the nape, arrives at Yǎ Mén (DU-15) of this channel, where it meets with the yángwéi [vessel] to enter and connect with the base of the tongue. It ascends to reach Fēng Fǔ (DU-16) of this channel, where it meets with the foot tàiyáng [channel] and yángwéi [vessel]; thereupon, they enter the brain together. It continues to ascend by following the pillow bone to Nǎo Hù (DU-17) of this channel. It continues to traverse upwards to Qiáng Jiān (DU-18) of this channel, at 3 cùn behind Bǎi Huì (DU-20).

又上歷本經百會穴後寸半之後頂穴，遂上巔歷本經之在百會穴，百會穴前寸半之前頂穴，百會前三寸之顖會穴，

It continues upwards to Hòu Dǐng (DU-19) of this channel, at 1 cùn and a half behind Bǎi Huì (DU-20). Thereupon, it ascends to Bǎi Huì (DU-20) of this channel at the vertex, and [passes through] Qián Dǐng (DU-21) at 1 cùn and a half in front of Bǎi Huì (DU-20), and Xìn Huì (DU-22) at 3 cùn in front of Bǎi Huì (DU-20).

又前行過顖會前一寸之上星穴，又前行至顖會前二寸，直鼻上入髮際五分之神庭穴，至此穴又爲足太陽、督脈之會，循額中至鼻柱，經鼻準頭本經之素髎穴，下循人中本經之水溝穴，與手陽明大腸經、足陽明胃經會，

It continues to move forward and traverse Shàng Xīng (DU-23) at 1 cùn in front of Xìn Huì (DU-22). It again moves forwards to arrive at Shén Tíng (DU-24), which is at 2 cùn in front of Xìn Huì (DU-22), directly above the nose, and 5 fēn into the hairline; as it arrives at this point, it also serves as the meeting between the foot tàiyáng [channel] and dū vessel.

It follows the centre of the forehead to arrive at the nose beam.[544] It passes by Sù Liáo (DU-25) of this channel at the tip of the nose. It descends to Shuǐ Gōu (DU-26) of this channel by following the human centre,[545] where it meets with the hand yángmíng large intestine channel and the foot yángmíng stomach channel.

至本經之直唇上端之兌端穴，又下唇入上齒縫中，而至本經之齦交穴，與任脈、足陽明經交會而終；

It arrives at Duì Duān (DU-27) of this channel directly above the edge of the [upper] lip. It continues to descend the lip to enter into the cleft of the upper

---

[544] The stem of the nose.
[545] I.e., the philtrum, but also an alternate name for DU-26.

teeth, and arrives at Yín Jiāo (DU-28) of this channel, where it meets and intersects with the rèn vessel and foot yángmíng channel, where it then terminates.

而督又有別絡自長強走任脈者，前行由少腹直上貫臍之中央，上貫心入喉，上頤環唇，上行系兩目之中央，下會足太陽於目內眥睛明穴，

The dū [channel] has a network-vessel that diverges from Cháng Qiáng (DU-1) towards the rèn vessel; its pathway in front ascends vertically to pierce the centre of the umbilicus, ascends to pierce the heart and enter the throat, ascends to the chin to encircle the lips, ascends to connect with the centre between the two eyes, and descends to meet with the foot tàiyáng at Jīng Míng (BL-1) located at the inner canthus.

又上額與足厥陰會於巔，入絡於腦，又別自腦下項，循肩胛，與手、足太陽、少陽會於大杼，第一椎下兩旁，去脊中一寸五分陷中，挾脊抵腰中，入循膂絡腎。

It ascends the forehead to meet with the foot juéyīn [channel] at the vertex, and enters to network with the brain. A divergence descends from the brain to the nape, follows the scapula to meet with the hand and foot tàiyáng and shàoyáng [channels] at Dà Zhù (BL-11), which is below and beside the first vertebra on each side, in the depression 1 cùn 5 fēn on each side of the spine. It continues and clasps the spine to reach the lumbus, where it enters to network with the kidneys by following the paravertebral sinews.

按督脈自會陰同任、衝分行而後，督之正脈既自下而上行於背，衝、任自會陰而前上行於腹，而督又有別絡，自長強由前行，由任脈而上行於腹，貫心入喉上頤，

From my observation, at Huì Yīn (REN-1), the dū vessel parts with the rèn and chōng [vessels] and travels to the rear. Whereas the principal vessel of the dū ascends from below on the back, the chōng and rèn [vessels] travel to the front from Huì Yīn (REN-1) and ascend to the abdomen. Moreover, the dū [vessel] also has a divergent network-vessel that travels to the front from Cháng Qiáng (DU-1); it follows the rèn vessel to ascend the abdomen, pierces the heart, enters the throat, and ascends to the chin,

遂分兩歧而環唇，分系兩目，分會兩足太陽於兩目上睛明穴，上額與厥陰會於巔，入腦，又自腦下項，循肩胛與手、足太陽會於大椎，在第一椎下兩旁，去挾脊中各一寸五分陷中，分兩歧挾脊抵腰中，入循膂絡腎。

Thereupon, it divides into two forking paths to encircle the lips, it divides [again] to connect with both eyes, where it divides to meet with the foot tàiyáng [channel] at Jīng Míng (BL-1) above both eyes. It ascends the forehead, meets with the foot juéyīn [vessel] at the vertex, and enters the brain. It continues to descend from the brain to the nape, following the shoulder to meet with the hand and foot tàiyáng [channels] at Dà Zhuī (DU-14),[546] which is below and beside the first vertebra on each side, in the depression 1 cùn 5 fēn on each side of the spine. Thereupon, it divides into two [pathways], clasps the spine [as it descends], and arrives at the lumbus, where it enters to network with the kidneys by following the paravertebral sinews.

人之身雖有陰陽之分，而陽常有餘抱乎陰，即以督任而言，督雖主乎背，任雖主乎腹，而督之絡，又自腹而分行抱任至巔，又抱督脈上行，在背督之正脈，下挾脊而入腰，

Although the body is divided into yīn and yáng, the yáng is always superabundant and it embraces the yīn; likewise, regarding the dū and rèn [vessels], although the dū [vessel] governs the back, and although the rèn [vessel] governs the abdomen, a network-vessel of the dū [vessel] diverges from the abdomen to embrace the rèn [vessel] as it [ascends to] arrive at the vertex; in addition, it further embraces the upper pathway of the dū vessel, which is the principal vessel of the dū [channel] located on the upper back; it clasps the spine as it descends and enters the lumbus.

雖督任兩經，在人身猶天地之有子午，而實則督抱乎任，陽抱乎陰，猶天抱乎地，而地在天中之象焉。至任之別絡名尾翳者，不過自鳩尾而反下行，散於腹。實則腹皮痛，虛則癢搔而已。

Although the two channels of dū and rèn in the human body resemble zǐ and wǔ[547] of the heaven and earth, yet in actuality, it is the dū [vessel] that embraces the rèn [vessel]; [likewise], it is the yáng that embraces the yīn, which resembles an image of the heavens embracing earth, with the earth situated within the heavens.

As for the divergent network-vessel of the rèn [vessel] that is called Wěi Yì (REN-15),[548] it simply turns around to descend from turtledove tail[549] and spreads into the abdomen. When it is replete, there will be pain of the abdominal skin; when it is vacuous, there will be itching and scratching;[550] and that is all.

---

[546] Based on the location description, this is possibly a scribal error for Dà Zhù (BL-11).

[547] Regarding earthly branches "zǐ and wǔ," see footnote 536.

[548] Tail Screen, this is an alternate name for REN-15 (Turtledove Tail) and refers to the xiphoid process.

[549] Also the name of REN-15.

[550] These two preceding lines are referring to the rèn divergent network vessel, and are from *Língshū* Chapter 10.

不能如督之周環於身之前後如輪，抱結任脈在內也。所以人之身，陽常有餘，陰常不足，觀於督任而益明矣。

[The rèn vessel] cannot compare with the dū [vessel], which encircles the front and rear of the body like a wheel, embracing and binding the rèn vessel within it. That is why in the human body, yáng is always superabundant and yīn is always insufficient; one only needs to observe the dū and rèn [vessels] and it will become increasingly clear.

但分之以見陰陽之各有攸司，合之以見陰陽之渾淪無間，一而二，二而一也。

When they are differentiated, one may observe that each of yīn and yáng has their own command; when they are united together, one may observe that yīn and yáng appear hazy and indistinguishable; as such, one is divided into two, and two are united into one.

至督脈所生之病，則從小腹上衝心而痛，不得前後，爲衝疝，女子爲不孕，癃閉遺溺，嗌乾，治在任經之腰橫骨上毛際中央之曲骨穴，甚者治任經之臍下一寸之陰交穴。

For diseases that the dū vessel engenders, there is surging into the heart from the lower abdomen with pain, inability to move forwards and backwards, surging mounting, infertility in females, dribbling urinary block with enuresis, and dry throat; these are treated by Qū Gǔ (REN-2) of the rèn channel, which is located at the centre of the pubic hair region above the pubic bone on the waist. If [the disease] is severe, treat Yīn Jiāo (REN-7) of the rèn channel, which is 1 cùn below the umbilicus.

王啓玄曰：此乃任衝二脈之病，不知何以屬之督脈。李瀕湖則正之曰：督脈雖行於背，而督之別絡自長強走任脈者，則由小腹直上貫臍中，上貫心入喉中，上頤環唇，而分入於目之內眥，故有此症，啓玄蓋未深考也。

Wáng Qǐxuán[551] says, "These are surely diseases of the two vessels, the rèn and chōng, but I do not know why they belong to the dū vessel."[552] Lǐ Bīnhú[553] remedied this by saying, "Although the dū vessel travels on the back, for the divergent network-vessel of the dū that goes to the rèn vessel from Cháng Qiáng (DU-1), it ascends vertically from the lower abdomen to pierce the centre of the umbilicus, ascends to pierce the heart and enter the centre of the throat, ascends the chin to encircle the lips, divides into two [pathways] and

---

[551] I.e., the self-styled name of Wáng Bīng.
[552] From Wáng Bīng's commentary on *Sùwèn* Chapter 60.
[553] I.e., the self-styled name of Lǐ Shízhēn.

enters the inter canthus; thus, [the dū vessel] has these signs. [Wáng] Qǐxuán has undoubtedly failed to investigate this thoroughly."[554]

至督之正經行於背者爲病，則《素問》有曰：督脈實則脊強反折，虛則頭重高搖，挾脊之有過者，取之所別也。而《難經》又曰：督脈爲病，脊強而厥。

As for the diseases of the principal channel of the dū that travels on the back, the *Sùwèn* also states, "When the dū vessel is replete, there will be stiffness of the spine and arching backwards; when it is vacuous, there will be heavy-headedness and swaying at the top [of the body]; on [the pathway] that clasps the spine and traverses these [regions], choose the place where it diverges."[555]

Moreover, *the Nánjīng* also states, "When the dū vessel is diseased, there will be stiffness of the spine with reversal."[556]

《金匱》曰：脊強者，五痓之總名，其症卒暴口噤而背反強，而瘈瘲，藥之不已，可灸身柱、大椎、陶道穴。其所取之穴，則皆督脈正行於背之穴也。

The Jīnguì states, "Stiffness of the spine is the general name for the five types of tetany, the signs are sudden clenching of the jaw, stiffness of the back with backwards arching, as well as tugging and slackening. When medicinals are ineffective, one can moxa Shēn Zhù (DU-12), Dà Zhuī (DU-14), and Táo Dào (DU-13)."[557] For the points chosen, these are all points of the principal pathway of the dū vessel on the upper back.

由是觀之，督之正經爲病，則宜取背之穴，督之別絡爲病，則宜取在腹之穴，亦督抱乎任之義也。

By observing these, when the principal channel of the dū is diseased, it is appropriate to choose points on the upper back; when the divergent network-vessel of the dū is diseased, it is appropriate to choose points on the abdomen; as such, this also portrays the meaning of the dū [vessel] embracing the rèn [vessel].

至督之脈有病而見乎寸口者，王氏《脈經》曰：尺寸俱浮，直上直下，此爲督脈，主腰脊強痛，不得俯仰，大人癲病，小兒風癎疾。

As for what can be observed at the cùnkǒu [pulse] when there is a disease in the dū vessel, Mister Wáng [Shúhé] says in *the Màijīng*, "When both the chǐ and

---

[554] From Diseases of the Dū Vessel in *the Qíjīng Bāmài Kǎo* 奇經八脈考 (*An Investigation of the Eight Extraordinary Channels*, 1578 CE).

[555] From *Língshū* Chapter 10 instead of the *Sùwèn* as indicated, though the first line can be found in *Sùwèn* Chapter 60.

[556] From *Nánjīng* Difficulty 29.

[557] From Vol. 2, Chapter 1 of *the Jīnguì Yùhán Jīng* 金匱玉函經 (*the Canon of the Golden Cabinet and Jade Sheath*), a lesser-known work by Zhāng Zhòngjǐng.

cùn [positions] are floating, with [the three positions] going up and down together, this is the [pulse]of the dū vessel; it governs stiffness and pain of the lumbus and spine, inability to move forwards and backwards, epileptic disease in adults, and wind-epilepsy in children."[558]

又曰：脈來中央浮，直上直下痛者，督脈也，動苦腰背膝寒，大人癲，小兒癇，宜灸頂上三壯。蓋督之百會穴也。又《金匱》曰：痓家脈築築而弦，直上下行。蓋痓乃督脈之症也。

He also says, "For an arriving pulse that is floating in the centre, when there is pain above and below, this is the [pulse] of dū vessel. There is discomfort in the lumbus and upper-back upon movement, cold [sensation] in the knees,[559] epilepsy in adults, and episodic epilepsy in children, it is appropriate to moxa 3 cones at the upper vertex."[560] Undoubtedly, this is referring to Bǎi Huì (DU-20) of the dū [channel].

Moreover, *the Jīnguì* states, "For those with tetany, the pulse is string-like as though it is pounding with a pestle, with [the three positions] going up and down together."[561] Surely, this is because tetany is a disease sign of the dū vessel.

《素問》曰：風氣循風府而上，則爲腦風，風入系頭，則爲目風眼寒。亦督脈之症也。

The Sùwèn states, "When wind qì follows Fēng Fǔ (DU-16) as it ascends, it will become brain wind;[562] when wind enters to connect with the head, this will become eye wind and cold sensation in the eyes."[563] These are also disease signs of the dū vessel.

王氏曰：腦戶乃督脈、足太陽之會。太陽挾督脈而下行，統在乎背，故督與太陽之症，恒相近也。蓋督爲一身陽經之海，而總統十二經，其病脈一見於寸口，則十二經不復朝焉。

---

[558] From *Màijīng* Vol. 2, Chapter 4.

[559] The primary manuscript has "cold [sensation] in the umbilicus" instead. The editors of this manuscript, Zhāng and Zhà, have amended to "cold [sensation] in the knees" according to *the Màijīng*. Nevertheless, as Yuè Hánzhēn relied heavily on the channel pathway to explain channel indications, there is a distinct possibility that he intentionally edited this part and made it "cold [sensation] in the umbilicus," as the dū vessel pathway passes by the umbilicus but not the knees.

[560] Also from *Màijīng* Vol. 2, Chapter 4.

[561] Also from Vol. 2, Chap. 1 of *the Jīnguì Yùhán Jīng* 金匱玉函經 (*the Canon of the Golden Cabinet and Jade Sheath*).

[562] *The Practical Dictionary* defines brain wind as "a disease similar to head wind.... characterised by aversion to cold on the nape and extreme cold of DU-17 area with unbearable pain."

[563] From *Sùwèn* Chapter 42.

Mister Wáng [Bīng] commentates, "Nǎo Hù (DU-17) is the meeting of the dū vessel and foot tàiyáng [channel]."[564] As the tàiyáng [channel] clasps the dū vessel and descends, it commands the back; thus, the disease signs of the dū [vessel] and tàiyáng [channel] are usually identical. Undoubtedly, the dū [vessel] is the sea of the yáng of the entire body, it has the overall command of the twelve channels; hence, when the diseases pulse [of the dū vessel] appears at the cùnkǒu [position], the twelve channels are no longer present at the court.[565]

而一身之氣血，總爲督脈所用，故直上直下，三部如一，則知爲督脈受病，而不復責十二經之症矣。

For the qì and blood of the entire body, they are as a whole commanded by the dū vessel, that is why [the dū pulse] goes up and down together, as though the three [pulse] positions were one single entity; as such, one knows that when the dū vessel has contracted a disease, one no longer seeks the disease signs of the twelve channels.

共穴二十七。背上穴，脊中下五穴，脊中上七穴，並脊中共十三穴。自頭至額共穴十，百會前四穴，後六穴。鼻至唇共四穴，隨穴所在，而治症焉。凡取脊間督脈諸穴，當於骨節突處取之，但驗於魚，爲可知也。若取於節下，必不見效。

There are in total twenty-seven points [of the dū vessel].

For the points on the back, there are five points below Jǐ Zhòng (DU-6) and seven points above Jǐ Zhòng (DU-6); including Jǐ Zhòng (DU-6), there are thirteen points in total. From the head to the forehead, there are ten points in total; there are four points in front of Bǎi Huì (DU-20), as well as six points behind. From the nose to the [upper] lip, there are four points in total.

Based on where these points are located, they treat their respective disease signs. In general, when choosing the various points of the dū vessel on the spine, one should find the protrusion of the bone joint to locate it. This can be demonstrated by simply examining a fish's [skeleton]. If one locates [the point] below the joint, it will certainly be ineffective.

---

[564] From Wáng Bīng's commentary on *Sùwèn* Chapter 42

[565] I.e., the pulse. Note: with a disease in the dū vessel, all three pulse positions would go up and down together, thus superseding any individual pulse indicators in all twelve pulse positions. As such, the twelve channels cannot be diagnosed in this case.

First Point of the Dū Channel
Cháng Qiáng – Long and Strong (DU-1)
督脈第一穴長強

一名氣之陰郄
Alternate name: Yīn Cleft of Qì

一名撅骨
Alternate name: Peg Bone

一名窮骨
Alternate name: End Bone

一名骨骶
Alternate name: Sacral Bone

穴在脊骶端，鍼三分，伏地取之，足少陰腎經、足少陽膽經之會，爲督脈之絡，
別走任脈。《銅人》：鍼三分，轉鍼以大痛爲度，灸不及鍼，日灸三十壯，止二
百壯，此乃痔之根。《甲乙》：鍼二分，留七呼。《明堂》：灸五壯，治下漏五
痔，疳蝕下部，刺三分，伏地取之，以大痛爲度，灸亦良，日三十壯，至七日
止，但不及鍼。

**This point is located at the end of the sacral spine, needle 3 fēn, lie prostrate to
locate it. It is the meeting of the foot shàoyīn kidney channel and foot
shàoyáng gallbladder channel. It is the network point of the dū vessel, which
diverges to go to the rèn vessel.** *The Tóngrén* **states, "Needle 3 fēn, rotate the
needle**[566] **until one experiences great pain; moxa is inferior to needling, and
moxa 30 to 200 cones daily, as this [point] is where haemorrhoids [take] root."**
The Jiǎyǐ **states, "Needle 2 fēn, and retain for seven respirations."** *The
Míngtáng* **states, "Moxa 5 cones to treat the five types of leaking haemorrhoids
and gān-erosion in the lower body; pierce 3 fēn, lie prostrate to needle it until
one experiences great pain; moxa is also favourable, moxa 30 cones daily, stop
after 7 days, but [this treatment] is inferior to needling."**

注：身長之骨，莫長於脊骨，故曰長，而此穴正當其下之最銳處，故曰
強。又爲足少陰腎、足少陽膽會督脈之處，生痔之根，在於此穴。凡灸鍼此穴者，
須慎冷食房勞，以防再發。

Explanation: among the Cháng (Long) bones of the body, there is none
Cháng (Longer) than the backbone, thus it is called Cháng (Long); furthermore, as
this point is located exactly at the sharpest point of the lower [backbone], thus it is
called Qiáng (Strong). In addition, as this place is where the dū vessel meets with the

---

[566] For "轉鍼 rotate the needle," *the Tóngrén* actually has "抽鍼 tug/pull the needle."

foot shàoyīn kidney and foot shàoyáng gallbladder [channels], this point is where the root of haemorrhoids is engendered. In general, for those who have moxibustion or needling performed at this point, they must avoid cold drinks and food and sexual taxation, so as to avoid a reoccurrence.

督之本病：腰脊痛，驚癇瘛瘲，狂病，小兒顖陷，頭重。

Principal diseases of the dū: pain in the lumbar spine, fright epilepsy with tugging and slackening, manic disease, depressed fontanels in infants, and heavy-headedness.

注：督之上行部分，皆在腰脊，故穴之在脊者，治腰脊病居多。如此穴而上如腰腧，如命門，如懸樞，如脊中，如筋縮，如至陽，如身柱，如陶道，如啞門，計十六穴，皆治腰脊病。

Explanation: the ascending pathway of the dū [vessel] is located entirely at the lumbus and spine; thus, points located on the spine predominantly treat diseases of the lumbar spine. For example, this point and those above such as Yāo Shù (DU-2), Mìng Mén (DU-4), Xuán Shū (DU-5), Jǐ Zhōng (DU-6), Jīn Suō (DU-8), Zhì Yáng (DU-9), Shēn Zhù (DU-12), Táo Dào (DU-13), and Yǎ Mén (DU-15), these sixteen points in total, they all treat diseases of the lumbar spine.

無非以此經自下上行，或風寒濕氣勞閟，一有逆於其間，而腰脊之病作。應相其上下而酌用之，實則泄之，虛則補之，急痛者爲實，悠悠痛者爲虛也。

This is simply because as this channel ascends from below, whether [one contracts] wind cold, damp qì, taxation, or inhibited [faecal passing], once any of them manifests as counterflow within this space, a disease of the lumbar spine will occur. One ought to deliberate the selection [of points] based on whether [the pain] is located above or below; when there is repletion, drain it; when there is vacuity, supplement it.; while urgent pain indicates repletion, unabating pain indicates vacuity.

督脈統一身之陽，驚癇瘛瘲，乃本經所司也，故此症而取此經之穴者凡十三穴，乃長強、命門、脊中、筋縮、神道、身柱、陶道、啞門、後頂、百會、前頂、神庭、水溝也。此穴乃督脈發生之上原，故必取之。

As the dū vessel commands the yáng of the whole body, fright epilepsy with tugging and slackening is surely what this channel controls; thus for this sign, thirteen points from this channel in total can be chosen, Cháng Qiáng (DU-1), Mìng Mén (DU-4), Jǐ Zhōng (DU-6), Jīn Suō (DU-8), Shén Dào (DU-11), Shēn Zhù (DU-12), Táo Dào (DU-13), Yǎ Mén (DU-15), Hòu Dǐng (DU-19), Bǎi Huì (DU-20), Qián Dǐng (DU-21), Shén Tíng (DU-24), and Shuǐ Gōu (DU-26). Yet, as this point is the upper source where the dū vessel engenders and emerges, it must be chosen.

狂病屬陽，督乃陽也，取在下之穴，以泄上有餘之陽。顖會乃本經在頂之穴，陷則本經之陽氣衰矣，宜補此穴，而復灸之以昇其陽。頭重乃火上昇也，泄在下之穴以降上逆之火。

Manic disease belongs to yáng, as the dū [vessel] is surely yáng, choose this point that is located below in order to drain the superabundant yáng that is above. Xìn Huì (DU-22) is a point of this channel that is located on the vertex, when the [fontanel] is depressed, the yáng qì of this channel has become debilitated, it is appropriate to supplement this point; one should further moxa in order to raise the yáng. Heavy-headedness is due to ascending fire, drain this point that is located below in order to descend the counterflow ascent of fire.

督之腎病：大小便難，五淋，疳蝕下部，驚恐失精，傷風下血，久痔漏。

Kidney diseases of the dū: difficult urination and defecation, five stranguries, gān-erosion in the lower body,[567] fright and fear with seminal loss, wind damage with bloody stool, and chronic haemorrhoids and fistulae.

注：腎司二便，此穴既會足少陰腎經而上行，腎之氣滯，所以有二便俱難之症，宜泄此穴以調腎氣之鬱。五淋，皆腎火有餘也，泄此穴以散腎火。

Explanation: the kidneys control the urine and stool; furthermore, since [the dū vessel] meets with the foot shàoyīn kidney channel at this point as it ascends, when there is qì stagnation of the kidneys, there will be the sign of difficult [passing] in both defecation and urination, it is appropriate to drain this point in order to regulate the depression of kidney qì. All of the five stranguries are superabundance of kidney fire, drain this point in order to disperse the kidney fire.

疳蝕下部，火盛極矣，泄此穴以散下部之火。驚恐傷腎而失精，此穴近精出之路，宜補之以收其脫。此穴正在穀道之後，本經自會陰後行，繞穀道會於此穴，痔病下血，雖為大腸有餘之症，然下垂而結於此處，故為痔之根本，宜鍼灸兼施，而毒始去。

Gān-erosion in the lower body is indicative of the extreme exuberance of fire, drain this point in order to disperse the fire in the lower body. When fear and fright damage the kidneys, this will lead to seminal loss; as this point is nearby the pathway where essence is discharged, it is appropriate to supplement this [point] in order to contract the desertion [of essence].

---

[567] *The Practical Dictionary* defines gān diseases as "a disease of infancy of childhood characterised by emaciation, dry hair, heat effusion of varying degree, abdominal distension with visible superficial veins, yellow face and emaciated flesh, and loss of essence-spirit vitality."

This point is located exactly below the anus.[568] From Huì Yīn (REN-1), the [dū] channel travels to the rear, encircles the anus and meets at this point. Although haemorrhoids with bloody stool is a sign of superabundance in the large intestine, yet, as this is the place where [haemorrhoids] sag and form, thus [this point] is where the haemorrhoids takes root; it is appropriate to use both needling and moxa, so that the toxin will be eliminated.

督之脾病：洞泄嘔血。

Spleen disease of the dū: throughflux diarrhoea and retching of blood.

注：洞泄乃陽氣之下脫也，宜補此穴以收下脫之氣。嘔血乃胃病也，氣逆而上，乃有此症，宜泄此穴以降上逆之氣。

Explanation: throughflux diarrhoea is due to sunken and deserted yáng qì, it is appropriate to supplement this point in order to contract the sunken and deserted qì. Retching of blood is a stomach disease, when there is qì counterflow ascent, there will be this sign, it is appropriate to drain this point in order to descend the ascending counterflow of qì.

督之肝病：瞻視不正。

Liver disease of Dū: crooked gaze.

注：督之絡，入面而過目系，絡有邪焉，而後有瞻視不正之症，故宜泄此穴以降其邪。

Explanation: the network-vessel of the dū enters the face and traverses the eye connector, when there is a presence of evil in the network-vessel, it will lead to the sign of crooked gaze, thus it is appropriate to drain this point in order to descend the evil.

Second Point of the Dū Channel
Yāo Shù – Lumbar Transport Point (DU-2)
督經第二穴腰腧

一名背解
Alternate name: Back's Resolution

一名髓孔
Alternate name: Marrow Hole

---

[568] Lit. pathway of grain.

一名腰柱
Alternate name: Lumbar Pillar

一名腰户
Alternate name: Lumbar Door

穴在二十一椎下宛宛中，挺身伏地舒身，兩手相重支額，縱四體後，乃數脊之椎分明而取此穴。《銅人》：鍼八分，留三呼，泄五吸，灸七壯至七七壯，灸後必慎房勞、舉重強力等事，將養之。《明堂》：灸三壯。《千金》云：腰卒痛，去窮骨上一寸，灸七壯者即此。

This point is located in the depression below the twenty-first vertebra; [have the patient] lie prostrate, straighten and relax the body, place one hand on top of the other [under] the forehead to prop it up; after the four limbs are relaxed, count the precise number of vertebrae to locate this point.

The Tóngrén **states, "Needle 8 fēn, retain for 3 respirations, and drain for 5 exhalations; moxa 7 to 49 cones; after moxa, be careful of activities such as sexual taxation, lifting heavy objects, or exertion of excessive force, they must recuperate."** *The Míngtáng* **states, "Moxa 3 cones." This is precisely what is stated by** *the Qiānjīn*, **"For sudden lumbar pain, moxa 7 cones at 1 cùn above Qióng Gǔ (DU-1)."**[569]

　　注：穴名腰腧者，腰中至要之穴也，再合其四名之義而思之，則此穴更可知也。

Explanation: this point is named Yāo Shù (Lumbar Transport Point) because it is the most important point in the centre of the Yāo (Lumbus); by further incorporating and contemplating the meaning of its four [alternate] names, one can come to an even deeper understanding of [the name of] this point.

　　二十一椎之下，椎盡矣，背解者，脊之上通於背者至此而盡，故曰背解。腦為髓海，而脊通之，至此而下輸，故曰髓孔。此椎下接於橫骨，猶柱之立於壁也，故曰腰柱。風寒濕由此穴而入，遂成腰痛之症，故曰腰户。而圖以腰腧名之，盡概上四名之義，故曰至要之穴也。

Below the twenty-first vertebra, [this is where] the vertebrae end; thus, for Bèi Jiě (Back's Resolution), as the spine above goes through the back to arrive here and terminates, thus it is called Bèi Jiě (Back's Resolution).

The brain is the sea of marrow, and the spine connects with it. As [the spine] arrives here and transports downwards, thus it is called Suǐ Kǒng (Marrow Hole).

---

[569] Lit. "End Bone," which is an alternate name for DU-1.

In the below, this vertebra joins with the transverse bone;[570] as such, it resembles a Zhù (Pillar) that is upbearing a wall, thus it is called Yāo Zhù (Lumbar Pillar).

When wind, cold, or damp enters this point, consequently, there will be the sign of pain in the Yāo (Lumbus), thus it is called Yāo Hù (Lumbar Door).

From my conjecture, [this point] is named as Yāo Shù (Lumbar Transport Point), because it completely encapsulates the meaning of the four [alternate] names; therefore, it is said to be the most important point [on the lumbus].

督之本病：腰胯痛不得俯仰，婦人月水閉，溺赤，足痹不仁。

Principal diseases of the dū: pain in the lumbus and hip with inability to bend forwards and backwards, blockage of monthly water, red urine, and foot impediment with insensitivity.

注：腰腧正腰中至要之處，一爲風寒濕所中，則痛而不得俯仰，宜鍼以散其氣，灸以溫其寒與濕。此穴之內，與胞近矣，婦人月水閉，乃氣滯也，宜鍼以通其氣，氣通則血行矣。溺赤者，乃熱也，宜取此穴以散其熱。足痹不仁，則陽氣不行於上矣，宜取此穴以通下行之陽氣。

Explanation: Yāo Shù (DU-2) is located precisely at the most important place at the centre of the lumbus; once it is struck by wind, cold, or damp, there will be pain with inability to bend forwards and backwards; it is appropriate to needle in order to disperse the qì, moxa in order to warm the combined cold and damp. On the interior of this point, it is nearby the womb; as blockage of monthly water is due to qì stagnation, it is appropriate to needle in order to free the qì; once the qì is freed, the blood will begin to flow.

Red urine is due to heat, it is appropriate to choose this point in order to disperse the heat. When there is foot impediment with insensitivity, the yáng qì will fail to travel to the above, it is appropriate to choose this point in order to free the yáng qì that is traveling to the below.

督之脾病：溫瘧汗不出。

Spleen disease of the dū: warm malaria with absence of sweating.

注：有熱而無寒者，謂之溫瘧，若此與熱病何異？但發熱有時，不若熱病之恒熱也。汗不出，則一身之陽氣全閉而不通，故取此穴，以通一身之陽，陽氣通則汗出矣，汗出而熱即解。

Explanation: When there is fever but absence of chills, this is warm malaria; for this [type of malaria], how does one distinguish it from febrile diseases? Simply,

---

[570] I.e., the pelvic bone.

there are periodic fevers [in warm malaria], which is dissimilar to the constant fevers of those with febrile disease. When there is absence of sweating, throughout the entire body, the yáng qì is completely blocked and not flowing freely, thus choose this point in order to free the yáng of the whole body; once the yáng qì is free, there will be sweating; once there is sweating, the heat will immediately be resolved.

督之腎病：傷寒，四肢熱不已。

Kidney diseases of the dū: cold damage and incessant heat in the four limbs.

注：此乃陽鬱於內，不得宣通之症，取此穴以通督脈之陽，督之陽通，而一身之陽全通，而熱遂汗解矣。

Explanation: for these signs, yáng is depressed in the interior and unable to perfuse to flow freely, choose this point in order to free the yáng of the dū vessel; once the yáng of the dū [vessel] flows freely, the entirety of the yáng of the whole body will flow freely; consequently, as sweating occurs, the heat will cease.

Third Point of the Dū Channel
Yáng Guān – Yáng Pass (DU-3)
督經第三穴陽關

穴在十六椎下，坐而取之。《銅人》：鍼五分，灸三壯。

This point is located below the sixteenth vertebra, sit to locate it. *The Tóngrén* states, "Needle 5 fēn, and moxa 3 cones."

注：陽關者，督經之陽氣，自腰腧而上行者，已六椎而至此穴，有關之象焉，故曰陽關。

Explanation: regarding Yáng Guān (Yáng Pass), the yáng qì of the dū channel has already ascended six vertebrae from Yāo Shù (DU-2) to arrive at this point, it has the image of a Guān (Pass), thus it is called Yáng Guān (Yáng Pass).

督之肝病：膝外不可屈伸，風痺不仁，筋攣不行。

Liver diseases of Dū: inability to bend and stretch the outside of the knees, wind impediment with insensitivity, and hypertonicity of the sinews with inability to walk.

注：膝之外，乃足少陽部分也，督之經爲風寒濕所侵，膝動則牽乎脊而不可屈伸矣，取此穴於上，督之邪去，則膝能屈伸矣。

Explanation: the outside of the knee is the area of the foot shàoyáng [channel]; when the channel of the dū is invaded by wind, cold, or damp, as any movement of the knee involves the spine, there will be an inability to bend and stretch [the knee]. Choose this point that is above to eliminate the evil of the dū [channel], then the knee will be able to bend and stretch.

Fourth Point of the Dū Channel
Mìng Mén – Life Gate (DU-4)
督經第四穴命門

一名屬累
Alternate name: Adjoining Connector[571]

穴在十四椎下，伏而取之。《銅人》：鍼五分，灸三壯。一云：平臍用綫牽而取之。一曰：刺三分，灸二十七壯。《神農經》：治腰痛，可灸七壯。

This point is located below the fourteenth vertebra, lie prostate to locate it. *The Tóngrén* states, "Needle 5 fēn, and moxa 3 cones." Another source states, "It is level with the umbilicus, draw a string to locate it." Another source states, "Pierce 3 fēn, and moxa 27 cones." *The Shénnóng Jīng* states, "One can moxa 7 cones to treat lumbar pain."

注：此穴與臍對，正在內兩腎之中間，而足太陽兩腎腧穴之內，乃人至命之地，故曰命門。年二十以上者，灸恐絕嗣。

Explanation: this point is the counterpart to the umbilicus, it is located exactly in centre of the space between the two kidneys inside; as it is on the inside of the two Shèn Shù (BL-23) points of the foot tàiyáng [channel], it is surely the place of supreme [importance] to a person's Mìng (Life), thus it is called Mìng Mén (Life Gate). For those twenty years and older, do not moxa due to the risk of severing their descendants.[572]

督之本病：腰腹相引，小兒發癇，張口搖頭，身反折角弓，骨蒸五臟熱，頭痛如破，身熱如火，汗不出。

一云：治腎虛腰痛，赤白帶下，男子泄精，耳鳴，手足冷，痺攣疝，驚恐，頭眩瘂瘲，急腹痛。

Principal diseases of the dū: radiating [pain] between the lumbus and abdomen, onset of epilepsy in children, gaping mouth with shaking of the head, backwards arched-stiffness of the body, steaming bone and heat of the

---

[571] *Grasping the Wind* names it "Connected."
[572] I.e., causing infertility.

five zàng-viscera, splitting headache, fire-like body heat, and absence of sweating.

Another source states: it treats kidney vacuity lumbar pain, red and white vaginal discharge, seminal discharge in males, tinnitus, cold hands and feet, impediment with hypertonicity and mounting, fright and fear, dizzy head with tugging and slackening, and tense abdominal pain.

注：此穴前與臍乎，故有腰腹相引之症，乃氣之滯而不行也，宜泄此穴以通其鬱。癇之爲病，火自命門，鼓痰而上膈，遂昏迷不省人事，角弓反張，皆督經之本症，宜泄此穴，而降其上逆之火。命門者，相火之本，此火一發，五臟之火俱熾而熱，故宜泄此穴以降火，火降則汗出矣。

Explanation: this point is the counterpart to the umbilicus in front, thus there is the sign of radiating [pain] between the lumbus and abdomen, which is due to stagnation of qì that is no longer flowing, it is appropriate to drain this point in order to free the depression.

For the disease of epilepsy, the fire from Mìng Mén (DU-4) arouses the phlegm to ascend the diaphragm; as a result, it causes the person to lose consciousness and have backwards arched-back rigidity, all of which are principal signs of the dū channel, it is appropriate to drain this point in order to descend the counterflow ascent of fire.

Mìng Mén (DU-4) is the foundation of ministerial fire; once this fire effuses, the fire of the five zàng-viscera will become intense and hot, thus it is appropriate to drain this point in order to descend the fire; when the fire descends, sweating will occur.

督之脾病：寒熱痎瘧。

Spleen disease of the dū: chills and fever with intervallic malaria.

注：邪自風府而入爲瘧，日下一椎，過脊中而至命門，則邪愈深矣，急取此穴而截下行之邪，使勿入陰分。

Explanation: when evil enters Fēng Fǔ (DU-16), it will manifest as malaria and descend one vertebra each day; if it traverses Jǐ Zhōng (DU-6)[573] to arrive at Mìng Mén (DU-4), the evil is moving deeper, urgently choose this point to intercept the evil that is descending, do not let it enter the yīn aspect.

---

[573] This could also mean centre of the spine or mid-spine.

Fifth Point of the Dū Channel
Xuán Shū – Suspended Pivot (DU-5)
督經第五穴懸樞

穴在十三椎下，伏而取之。《銅人》：鍼三分，灸三壯。

This point is located below the thirteenth vertebra, lie prostrate to locate it. *The Tóngrén* states, "Needle 3 fēn, and moxa 3 cones.

注：脊中之穴，平分二十一椎之中，而此穴乃在其下。樞者，所以司開合之軸也。脊中司俯仰曲伸，亦猶門之闔，在於樞也，此穴在脊中之下，有樞之象焉。曰懸者，以其橫懸爲俯仰之樞，而非若門之樞，立而司開合者也。

Explanation: the point Jǐ Zhōng (DU-6) is located exactly at the midpoint of the twenty-one vertebrae, and this point (DU-5) is located below it.

Shū (Pivot) refers to the axis that controls opening and closing. The Shū (Pivot) is what allows Jǐ Zhōng (DU-6) to command the [the movement of] leaning forwards and backwards, as well as bending and stretching, as though it is the closing of a gate; as this point (DU-5) is located below Jǐ Zhōng (DU-6), it also has the image of a Shū (Pivot).

Speaking of Xuán (Suspended), it is because this [point] is horizontally Xuán (Suspended) to serve as a Shū (Pivot) for bending forwards and backwards, rather than a vertical Shū (Pivot) of a gate that controls opening and closing.

督之本病：腰脊强，不能屈伸。

Principal disease of the dū: stiffness of the lumbar spine with inability to bend and stretch.

注：此穴有邪入之，則痛而腰脊强不能屈伸，而樞之用廢，故急泄之，以散其邪。

Explanation: when evil enters this point, there will be pain that leads to stiffness of the lumbar spine with inability to bend and stretch; as such, the function of the pivot has become disabled, thus urgently drain it in order to disperse the evil.

督之脾病：積氣上下行，水穀不化，下利，痰留腹中。

Spleen diseases of the dū: qì accumulations that move up and down, indigestion of water and grain, diarrhoea, and phlegm that lodges in the abdomen.

注：樞所以司上下者，邪留之亦上下行，而水穀不爲之化，乃寒邪客之也，宜鍼以散之，灸以溫之。腹中有留痰，十四椎與臍平，則十三椎正值腹之中微上矣，痰留者，乃邪客而滯留者也，宜取此穴，灸之溫之，鍼之散之。

Explanation: the pivot is what controls [the movement] above and below, thus, when the evil lodges at the [pivot], it will also travel up and down. As for the failure of water and grain to be transformed, this is due to cold evil that lodges at [this point], it is appropriate to needle in order to disperse it and to moxa in order to warm it.

Regarding the phlegm that lodges in the abdomen, as the fourteenth vertebra is level with the umbilicus, precisely, the thirteenth vertebra is slightly above the centre of the abdomen; for the lodged phlegm, it is the visiting evil that has stagnated and lodged; hence, it is appropriate to choose this point and moxa it in order to warm it and needle it in order to disperse it.

Sixth Point of the Dū Channel
Jǐ Zhōng – Middle of the Spine[574] (DU-6)
督經第六穴脊中

一名神宗
Alternate name: Spirit Gathering

一名脊腧
Alternate name: Spine Transport Point

穴在十一椎下，伏而取之。《銅人》：鍼五分，得氣即泄，禁灸，灸之令人腰傴僂。

This point is located below the eleventh vertebra, lie prostate to locate it. *The Tóngrén* states, "Needle 5 fēn, obtain qì then promptly drain, and moxibustion is contraindicated, as moxa will make the person become hunchbacked.

注：脊共二十一椎，上十椎，下十椎，此穴在十一椎之下，區處其中，故爲脊中。禁灸者，火入脊中，督之上下氣脈中絕，腰之所以傴僂也。

Explanation: the Jǐ (Spine) has twenty-one vertebrae in total; above [this point], there are ten vertebrae, and below it, there are also ten vertebrae; this point is located below the eleventh vertebra and situated in the Zhōng (Middle) [of the spine], thus it is the Jǐ Zhōng (Middle of the Spine). Regarding the contraindicated use of moxa, when fire enters the Jǐ Zhōng (Middle of the Spine), the upper and

---

[574] *Grasping the Wind* names it "Spinal Centre."

lower portions of the qì vessel of the dū will be severed in the Zhōng (Middle); as a result, the back will become stooped.

督之本病：風癎癲邪，五痔便血。

Principal diseases of the dū: wind epilepsy with epileptic evil, and five [types of] haemorrhoids with bloody stool.

注：風癎癲邪，乃督之本病也，解見前。五痔便血，亦督經本病也，下臨長强，治脊中上下之氣，氣通而毒散矣。

Explanation: wind epilepsy with epileptic evil is a principal disease of the dū [channel], see the previous explanations. The five [types of] haemorrhoids with bloody stool are also principal diseases of the dū channel; [as the dū channel] arrives at Cháng Qiáng (DU-1) below, by treating the ascending and descending qì at Jǐ Zhōng (DU-6), the [flow of] qì will become free; as a result, the toxin will dissipate.

督之脾病：黄疸，腹滿不嗜食，積聚下利，小兒脱肛。

Spleen diseases of the dū: jaundice, abdominal fullness with no pleasure in eating, accumulations and gatherings with diarrhoea, and prolapse of the rectum in children.

注：此穴正在足太陽經兩脾腧之中，脾有濕熱，而成黄疸，而腹爲之滿不嗜食，旁治脾腧，中治脊中，皆去此病之根也。脾腧治積聚者也，兩脾腧所挾之脊中，治積聚則亦宜取之。下利脱肛，乃大腸之氣脱也，督經環肛門而上，上脊之中，乃攝下十椎者也，脱肛之症，故責之。

Explanation: this point is located exactly in the middle between the two Pí Shù (BL-20) points of the foot tàiyáng channel; when there is a presence of damp heat in the spleen, it will manifest as jaundice; as a result, there will be fullness in the abdomen with no pleasure in eating; hence, by either treating with Pí Shù (BL-20) on the sides or by treating with Jǐ Zhōng (DU-6) in the middle, both will eliminate the root of the evil.

As Pí Shù (BL-20) treats accumulations and gatherings, thus for Jǐ Zhōng (DU-6) that is clasped between the two Pí Shù (BL-20) points, it should also be chosen for the treatment of accumulations and gatherings. Diarrhoea and prolapse of the rectum are due to qì desertion of the large intestine; dū channel ascends after encircling the anus, and it ascends to the middle of the spine; thus, it administers the lower eleven vertebrae; therefore, for the sign of prolapse of the rectum, one should seek this point.

督之肺病：溫病。

Lung disease of the dū: warm disease.

注：寒中人久而成溫，督統一身之陽，而脊中又爲二十一椎之中，脊中氣通，則上下之氣悉通而汗出矣。

Explanation: after cold strikes a person, if it remains [untreated] for an extended period of time, it will be become a warm [disease]; as the dū [vessel] commands the yáng of the entire body, and Jǐ Zhōng (DU-6) is situated exactly in the middle of the twenty-one vertebrae, once the qì flows freely at Jǐ Zhōng (DU-6), all qì above and below will flow freely; as a result, sweating will occur.

Seventh Point of the Dū Channel
Jīn Suō – Sinew Contraction (DU-8)[575]
督經第七穴筋縮

穴在九椎下，伏而取之。《銅人》：鍼五分，灸三壯。《明堂》：灸七壯。

This point is located below the nineth vertebra, lie prostrate to locate it. *The Tóngrén* states, "Needle 5 fēn, and moxa 3 cones." *The Míngtáng* states, "Moxa 7 cones."

注：人之俯仰，在乎脊筋之伸縮，伸而不縮，則脊強矣，縮而不伸，則傴僂矣，此穴正在脊中之上，當脊筋伸縮之際，故曰筋縮。

Explanation: for a person's movement of bending forwards and backwards, it relies on the stretching and Suō (Contracting) of the spinal Jīn (Sinews). When one can stretch but not Suō (Contract), the spine will become stiff; when one can Suō (Contract) but not stretch, one will become hunched. As this point is located just above Jǐ Zhōng (DU-6), it is exactly at the juncture where the spinal Jīn (Sinews) stretches and Suō (Contracts), therefore it is called Jīn Suō (Sinew Contraction).

督之本病：脊急強，目轉反戴上視，目瞪，癇病多言，癲疾狂走，心痛。

Principal diseases of the dū: tension and stiffness of the spine, eyes spinning and rolling backwards, upwards gazing eyes, staring eyes, epilepsy diseases with excessive speaking, epileptic disease and manic walking, and heart pain.

注：本經受邪，則脊爲之強，而筋不能伸縮矣，目反戴上視者，督之絡入系於目，本經有病，既中於筋，目系亦筋也，所以有反戴上視之症矣，宜取此穴。

Explanation: when this channel contracts evil, the spine will become stiff, and the sinews will be unable to stretch and contract; for eyes rolling backwards and gazing upward, the network-vessel of the dū enters to connect with the eyes;

---

[575] Note: Zhōng Shū (DU-7) is listed as an associated extra point at the end of the chapter.

when this channel has a disease, it will precisely strike the sinews; in addition, the eye connector is also a sinew, this is why there is the sign of eyes rolling backwards and gazing upward; therefore, it is appropriate to choose this point.

癇病多言，肝之病爲怒，此多言，亦肝之有餘也，以九椎之兩旁爲肝腧，則癇病多言亦責之。癲疾狂走，皆筋病也，故亦責此穴。肝氣逆於心而痛作焉，治此穴者，泄肝氣也。

Regarding epilepsy disease with excessive speaking, in liver diseases, anger will manifest; for this [sign of] excessive speaking, it is also due to the superabundance of the liver; as Gān Shù (BL-18) is located on the two sides of the nineth vertebra, thus for epilepsy disease with excessive speaking, also seek this [point]. Epileptic disease and manic walking are both sinew diseases, thus also seek this point. When there is counterflow liver qì affecting the heart, it will cause pain in [the heart], thus treat this point to drain the liver qì.

Eighth Point of the Dū Channel
Zhì Yáng – Arrival at the Yáng[576] (DU-9)
督經第八穴至陽

穴在七椎下，俯而取之。《銅人》：鍼五分，灸三壯。《明堂》：灸五壯。

This point is located below the seventh vertebra, bow one's head to locate it. *The Tóngrén* states, "Needle 5 fēn, and moxa 3 cones." *The Míngtáng* states, "Moxa 5 cones."

注：此穴之旁，爲足太陽之膈腧穴，膈之上乃純氣之府，血爲陰，氣爲陽，故曰至陽。言督經自下而上行者，至此則入於陽分也。

Explanation: beside this point (DU-9) is Gé Shù (BL-17) of the foot tàiyáng [channel]; above the diaphragm, it is surely the mansion of pure qì; as blood is yīn and qì is Yáng (Yáng), thus it is called Zhì Yáng (Arrival at Yáng). This is to say the pathway of the dū channel ascends from the below to Zhì (Arrive) here, where it enters the Yáng (Yáng) aspect.

督之本病：腰脊痛，背中氣上下行，腹中鳴。

Principal diseases of the dū: pain in the lumbar spine, qì that moves up and down the middle of the back, and rumbling in the abdomen.

---

[576] *Grasping the Wind* names it "Extremity of Yáng."

注：氣之自下而上行者，有滯於入膈之所，則不能上行，而腰脊痛作，宜泄此穴以降之。背之中，正督經所行之地，氣不能上膈，遂覺上而復下，氣逆於腹，而腹爲之鳴，亦宜泄此穴以散之。

Explanation: for the qì that ascends from below, if it becomes stagnated at the location where it enters the diaphragm, it will no longer be able to ascend; as a result, there will be pain in the lumbar spine, it is appropriate to choose this point in order to descend it.

The middle of the back is precisely the place where the dū channel travels; when the qì is unable to ascend to the diaphragm, consequently, one will feel [the qì] first moving upwards before it moves downwards; as a result, there will be qì counterflow in the abdomen, which leads to rumbling in the abdomen, it is appropriate to drain this point in order to disperse it.

督之脾病：胃中氣寒不能食，四肢腫痛，少氣難言，寒熱解㑊，淫濼脛痠。

Spleen diseases of the dū: cold qì in the stomach with inability to eat, swelling and pain in the four limbs, scantness of breath with difficulty speaking, chills and fever with lethargy and fatigue, pain and weakness in the lower legs.

注：此穴正在前胃脘上之所，膈腧所治病，有膈胃寒痠、飲食不下之症，故此穴亦治胃寒不食。脾主四肢，督統一身之陽，指氣而言也。陽氣不暢於四肢，遂有腫痛、少氣難言之症，宜補此穴以助其氣。寒熱解㑊、淫濼脛痠，皆陰有餘而陽不足之症也，宜補此穴以助其陽。

Explanation: this point is located exactly above where the stomach duct is; as the diseases treated by Gé Shù (BL-17) are cold and aching in the diaphragm and stomach, as well as inability to get food and drink down, this point also treats stomach cold and inability to eat.

The spleen governs the four limbs; [when it is said that] the dū [vessel] commands the yáng of the whole body, this is referring to the qì. When yáng qì is impeded in the four limbs, consequently, there will be signs of swelling and pain, scantness of breath with difficulty speaking, it is appropriate to supplement this point in order to assist the qì. Chills and fever with lethargy and fatigue, pain and weakness in the lower legs, all these are signs of superabundance of yīn with insufficiency of yáng, it is appropriate to supplement this point in order to assist the yáng.

督之肺病：卒痓忤，攻心胸，胸肋支滿，身羸瘦。

Lung diseases of the dū: sudden infixation and hostility[577] attacking the heart and chest, propping fullness of the chest and rib-sides, and generalised marked weakness and emaciation.

注：膈之上乃心肺之府也，氣虛而邪始侵之，宜補此穴以助其陽。氣滯於胸及脇，而身爲之瘦，氣滯之病也，宜泄此穴以散其滯。

Explanation: above the diaphragm is the repository of the heart and lung, when there is qì vacuity, evil will begin to invade them, it is appropriate to supplement this point in order to assist the yáng. When qì stagnates at the chest and rib-sides, yet the body is emaciated, this is a disease of qì stagnation, it is appropriate to drain this point in order to disperse the stagnation.

Ninth Point of the Dū Channel
Líng Tái – Divine Terrace[578] (DU-10)
督經第九穴靈臺

穴在六椎下，俯而取之。《銅人》缺治病，禁鍼，此穴見《素問》。

This point is located below the sixth vertebra, bow one's head to locate it. Its [indications of] disease treatment are absent in *the Tóngrén*. It is forbidden to needle. For this point, see *the Sùwèn*.[579]

注：督經自下而上，至陽之穴，既過膈矣。膈之上有空虛之處，任脈爲膻中，膻中，虛空之象也，

Explanation: as the dū channel ascends from below to the point of Zhì Yáng (DU-9), it has traversed past the diaphragm. Above the diaphragm, there is a place of hollowness, which is Dàn Zhōng (REN-17) on the rèn vessel; as such, Dàn Zhōng (REN-17) has an image of the hollow space.

---

[577] Note: while we have translated zhùwǔ 痓忤 literally as "infixation and hostility," it should be understood as "zhòng è 中惡 (malignity strike)," which *Practical Dictionary* defines as, "A disease attributed in ancient times to the malign work of demons... are due to catching some unright qì and are characterized by sudden counterflow cold of the limbs, goose pimples, blackish green-blue head and face, essence-spirit failing to confine itself, deranged raving, clenched jaw, spinning head and collapse, and clouding unconsciousness. They are observed in vehement reversal, visiting hostility... or after attending funerals or going into temples or graveyards.'"

[578] *Grasping the Wind* names it "Divine Tower."

[579] We believe this is referring to commentary on *Sùwèn* Chapter 59 by Wáng Bīng, as DU-11 is not mentioned in the primary text.

在督經既過膈，五臟皆系於背，心爲人身至靈之官在上，穴在其下，有臺之象，狀脊之內載其心之象也。治病缺者，心不受邪，不宜干之也，所以禁鍼。

[This point] is located on the dū channel after it has traversed past the diaphragm. All five zàng-viscera connect with the back; the heart is the utmost Líng (Divine) official in the human body, while it is located above, this point is located below it; thus, [this point] has the image of a Tái (Terrace), which depicts the image of how the heart is held up on the inside of the spine. As for the reason why its [indications] of disease treatment are absent, the heart does not contract evil,[580] thus, it is not appropriate for one to interfere with it, that is why [this point] is contraindicated for needling.

督之肺病：氣喘不能臥。

Lung disease of the dū: panting with inability to lie down.

注：俗灸之以治氣喘不能臥，火到便愈。氣滯於肺而喘作，灸以通之，滯散而喘息。

Explanation: it is a common practise to moxa it in order to treat panting with inability to lie down; as soon as the fire arrives, they will recover. When there is qì stagnation in the lung, panting will occur, moxa it in order to free it; when the stagnation disperses, the panting will cease.

Tenth Point of the Dū Channel
Shén Dào – Spirit Path (DU-11)
督經第十穴神道

穴在五椎下，俯而取之。《銅人》：灸七七壯，止百壯，禁鍼。《明堂》：灸三壯，鍼五分。《千金》：灸五壯。

This point is located below the fifth vertebra, bow one's head to locate it. *The Tóngrén* states, "Moxa 49 to 100 cones, and needling is contraindicated." *The Míngtáng* states, "Moxa 3 cones, and needle 5 fēn." *The Qiānjīn* states, "Moxa 5 cones."

---

[580] Note: this seems to allude to the statement from *Língshū* Chapter 71, "諸邪之在於心者，皆在於心之包絡。 For the various types of evil in the heart, they are all located within the pericardiac network of the heart."

注：此穴在足太陽經兩心腧之中，正在心之後，心爲主宰之官，神明出
焉，故曰神道。《銅人》禁鍼，亦不宜輕干之意也。雖《明堂》有鍼五分之文，還
從《銅人》爲是。

Explanation: this point is located in the middle between the two Xīn Shù (BL-15) of the foot tàiyáng channel. It is located exactly behind the heart; as the heart is the official of governing and dictating, the bright Shén (Spirit) emanates from it, thus it is called Shén Dào (Spirit Path).

When *the Tóngrén* states, "needling is contraindicated," this also conveys the concept that it is not appropriate for one to carelessly interfere with [the heart]. Although it is written in *the Míngtáng* that [it can be] "needled 5 fēn," one should still follow *the Tóngrén* instead.

督之本病：小兒風癇，可灸七壯

Principal disease of the dū: one can moxa 7 cones for wind epilepsy in children.

注：若痰、若火逆，而上行過膈，而使心神爲之昏，乃癇症也，灸以散其
痰與火，乃從治之法也。

Explanation: when phlegm or counterflow of fire ascends to traverse past the diaphragm, this will cloud the heart spirit, which is a sign of epilepsy; moxa it in order to disperse the phlegm and fire, which is a method of co-acting treatment.[581]

督之心病：恍惚悲愁，健忘驚悸。

Heart diseases of the dū: abstraction with sorrow and anxiety, and forgetfulness with fright palpitations.

注：前症皆心氣不足所致，宜灸此穴以温之。

Explanation: all of the above signs are a result of insufficient heart qì, it is appropriate to moxa this point in order to warm it.

督之肺病：傷寒，發熱頭痛，進退往來，痎瘧。

Lung diseases of the dū: cold damage, fevers with headache that comes and goes with varying severity, and intervallic malaria.

注：頭痛者，督經之症也，而發熱、進退往來，則邪干於神之所致，故宜
取此穴。督經之風府受邪，日下一椎，故心亦有瘧。

---

[581] According to the *Practical Dictionary*, the co-acting treatment is "The nonroutine principle of treating false signs with medicinals of opposite nature, e.g., treating heat with heat, cold with cold, the stopped by stopping, and flow by promoting flow."

Explanation: headache is a sign of the dū channel; fevers that come and go with varying severity is a result of evil invading the spirit, thus it is appropriate to choose this point. When the dū channel contracts an evil at Fēng Fǔ (DU-16), [the evil] will descend one vertebra each day, thus there can also be malaria in the heart.

《內經》云：心瘧，令人煩心，甚欲得清水，反寒多，不甚熱。注云：唯其多熱，所以寒多，蓋熱極生寒也，寒既久，則火少衰，所以不能熱，此心瘧也。《內經》取乎少陰經穴神門治之，瘧症如此者，亦宜取督經神道穴治之也。

The Nèijīng states, "For heart malaria, it will cause the person to have vexation of the heart; when it is severe, [the patient] will desire cool water, yet, there will be predominantly chills instead with infrequent fevers."[582] The [Nèijīng] Zhù states, "Precisely, owing to the intense heat, as a result there are predominantly chills; undoubtedly, when heat reaches the extreme, it will engender cold; when cold remains for an extended period of time, fire will become scant and debilitated, that is why there are no fevers; this is heart malaria."[583] The Nèijīng selects the shàoyīn channel point, Shén Mén (HE-7), to treat it. For malaria signs like this, it is also appropriate to choose Shén Dào (DU-11) of the dū channel to treat it.

督之腎病：失欠，牙車磋，張口不合。

Kidney diseases of the dū: yawning, teeth grinding, and gaping mouth with inability to close it.

注：《內經》云：熱病，氣穴在四椎下間主膈中熱，五椎下間主肺熱。注云：四椎下間無穴，五椎下間乃神道穴也。

Explanation:[584] the Nèijīng states, "For febrile disease, whereas the qì hole[585] that is located in the space below the fourth vertebra governs heat in the diaphragm, [the qì hole] in the space below the fifth vertebra governs heat in the lung."[586] The [Nèijīng] Zhù states, "While there is no point in the space below the fourth vertebra, Shén Dào (DU-11) is the point in the space below the fifth vertebra."[587]

---

582 From Sùwèn Chapter 36, where it further states "刺手少陰 pierce the shàoyīn."

583 This comes from the commentary for Sùwèn Chapter 36 by Mǎ Shì 馬蒔.

584 We believe this explanation to be misplaced, as it seems to continue the discussion of the lung diseases from the previous section and has little to do with kidney diseases; however, we have left it in place according to the arrangement of the manuscript.

585 Lit. point.

586 From Sùwèn Chapter 32.

587 This is commentary from Chapter 32 of the Sùwèn by Mǎ Shì 馬蒔.

Eleventh Point of the Dū Channel
Shēn Zhù – Pillar of the Body[588] (DU-12)
督經第十一穴身柱

穴在第三椎下，俯而取之。《銅人》：鍼五分，灸七七壯，止百壯。《明堂》：灸五壯。《下經》：灸三壯。《神農》：治咳嗽，可灸十四壯。

This point is located below the third vertebra, bow one's head to locate it. *The Tóngrén* states, "Needle 5 fēn, and moxa 49 to 100 cones." *The Míngtáng* states, "Moxa 5 cones." *The Xiàjīng* states, "Moxa 3 cones." *The Shénnóng* states, "One can moxa 14 cones to treat cough."

注：人之肩所以能負重者，以有身柱也，脊骨爲人一身之柱，而此穴近上，猶其用力負重之所，故曰身柱。

Explanation: what enables a person's shoulders to carry weight, it is because of Shēn Zhù (Pillar of the Body). The spine is the Zhù (Pillar) of the whole Shēn (Body); as this point is near the top [of the spine], it is the place where one exerts force and carries weight; therefore, it is called Shēn Zhù (Pillar of the Body).

督之本病：癲病狂走，瘈瘲，怒欲殺人，身熱狂言見鬼，小兒驚癇，腰脊痛。

Principal diseases of the dū: withdrawal disease with manic walking, tugging and slackening, anger with desire to kill people, generalised heat with manic raving and visions of ghosts, fright epilepsy in children, and pain in the lumbar spine.

注：《難經》云：治長洪伏三脈，風癇惡人與火，灸三椎、九椎。九椎者，筋縮也。瘈瘲之病，癲狂病，皆督經本症也。洪長伏三脈，亦必左右寸關尺上下如一，則知眞爲督經受病，十二經不朝寸口之脈，則單取督經爲宜也。腰脊痛，在下而取之上，以散其鬱。

Explanation: *the Nànjīng*[589] states "To treat the three pulses of long, surging, and hidden, as well as wind epilepsy with aversion to people and fire, moxa [below] the third and nineth vertebrae." [The point below] the nineth vertebra is Jīn Suō (DU-8). Both the diseases of tugging with slackening and withdrawal with mania are principal signs of the dū channel.

---

588 *Grasping the Wind* names it "Body Pillar."

589 This citation does not come from the *Nànjīng* 難經, but from *Cǐshì Nánzhī* 此事難知 (*Difficult Subjects to Understand*, 1308 CE) by Wáng Hàogǔ instead. This exact paraphrase first appeared in *the Zhēnjiǔ Jùyīng* 針灸聚英 (*Gathered Blooms of Acupuncture and Moxibustion*, 1529 CE), and was likely miscopied during the compilation of *Zhēnjiǔ Dàchéng*.

For the three pulses of surging, long, and hidden, the entire left and right cùn, guān and chǐ [positions] must go up and down together as though they are one entity; as such, one knows that it is truly a contraction of disease in the dū channel, when all twelve channels do not assemble at the cùnkǒu pulse [positions].[590] For this, it is appropriate to seek the dū channel alone. For pain in the lumbar spine, while [the pain] is located below, [a point] above is chosen in order to disperse the depression.

Twelfth Point of the Dū Channel
Táo Dào – Kiln Path (DU-13)
督經第十二穴陶道

穴在一椎下，俯而取之，足太陽、督脈之會。《銅人》：鍼五分，灸五壯。

This point is located below the first vertebra, bow one's head to locate it. It is the meeting of the foot tàiyáng [channel] and dū vessel. *The Tóngrén* states, "Needle 5 fēn, and moxa 5 cones."

注：陶者，窑也，中虛而能容物之象也。胸與腹在下與前而中虛，此穴在其上之最高處，有陶之象焉，故曰陶道。

Explanation: Táo (Kiln) is a ceramic oven; it has the image of being empty in its centre and able to store objects within. The chest in front and the abdomen below are both empty in their centre; as this point is located above them at the most elevated place, it has the image [that resembles the solid top of] a Táo (Kiln), thus it is called Táo Dào (Kiln Path).

督之本病：脊强，煩滿汗不出，頭重目瞑，瘈瘲，恍惚不樂，痎瘧，寒熱洒淅。

Principal diseases of the dū: stiffness of the spine, vexation with fullness and absence of sweating, heavy-headedness with heavy eyes, tugging and slackening, abstraction with unhappiness, intervallic malaria, chills and fever as though after a soaking.

注：督之初受風寒之邪，自風府而入，日下一節，而爲痎瘧，宜於初得時，入風府尚未久，其邪尚未深，早取此穴以截之。脊强、煩滿汗不出，亦初受天寒也，急灸此穴，出汗甚易。頭重目瞑、瘈瘲、恍惚不樂，乃癇病之輕者，督之本病，宜首治此穴。

Explanation: when the dū [vessel] initially contracts the evil of wind and cold, [the evil] enters through Fēng Fǔ (DU-16); each day, it will descend one

---

[vertebral] joint, manifesting as intervallic malaria; at the time of onset when [the evil] enters Fēng Fǔ (DU-16), when the evil has not remained for long and not yet penetrated deeper, it is appropriate to use this point early in order to intercept [the evil].

For stiffness of the spine, vexation and fullness with absence of sweating, these are also the onset of contracting the cold of the heavens,[591] urgently moxa this point and it should easily cause sweating. As for heavy-headedness with heavy eyes, tugging and slackening, and abstraction with unhappiness, these are all mild forms of epilepsy, which are principal diseases of the dū [vessel], it is appropriate to treat this point first.

Thirteenth Point of the Dū Channel
Dà Zhuī – Great Vertebra[592] (DU-14)
督經第十三穴大椎

一名百勞
Alternate name: Hundred Taxations

穴在大椎上陷者宛宛中，手、足三陽、督脈之會。鍼五分，留三呼，泄五吸，灸以年為壯。

This point is located in the depression above the great vertebra.[593] It is the meeting of the three hand and foot yáng [channels] and dū vessel. Needle 5 fēn, retain for 3 respirations, drain for 5 exhalations, and moxa the number of cones in accordance with one's age.

注：按鍼灸各書，載督脈大椎為手、足三陽經、督脈之會，

Explanation: according to various books of acupuncture and moxibustion, they all record Dà Zhuī (Great Vertebra) of the dū vessel as the meeting of the three hand and feet yáng channels and dū vessel. Hence, I have meticulously investigated [these meetings].

---

[591] I.e., external cold.
[592] *Grasping the Wind* names it "Great Hammer." Note: when this character, 椎, is read as chuí, it means the hammer (noun) or to hammer down (verb); whereas, when it is read as zhuī, it means the vertebra/vertebrae (noun). As this name is typically read as Dà Zhuī, which literally means "great/protruding vertebra" in Chinese, which we think is a more fitting interpretation in the context of this point.
[593] I.e., the first thoracic vertebra.

今細考手陽明大腸經，循巨骨穴上出天柱之會，上會於大椎。手太陽小腸經，由肩外腧、肩中腧諸穴，上會大椎。手少陽三焦經，其支行者，從膻中而上出缺盆之外，上項，過大椎，是手陽明、太陽、少陽俱有會大椎之可據矣。

The hand yángmíng large intestine channel follows Jù Gǔ (LI-16) to ascend, emerges to meet with Tiān Zhù (BL-10), and further ascends to meet with Dà Zhuī (Great Vertebra).

The hand tàiyáng small intestine channel follows the points, Jiān Wài Shù (SI-14) and Jiān Zhōng Shù (SI-15), and ascends to meet with Dà Zhuī (Great Vertebra).

For the hand shàoyáng sānjiāo channel, a branch pathway follows Dàn Zhōng (REN-17), ascends to emerge at the outside of Quē Pén (ST-12), and further ascends the neck to traverse Dà Zhuī (Great Vertebra).

As such, the meetings of all hand yángmíng, tàiyáng, and shàoyáng [channels] with Dà Zhuī (Great Vertebra) can be verified.

至足三陽則有可議者，足少陽膽經，過天牖，行手少陽之脈前，下至肩上，至肩井，卻左右交出手少陽之後，過大椎，是足少陽會督於大椎也。

As for the three leg yáng [channels], these are debatable.

The foot shàoyáng gallbladder channel traverses Tiān Yǒu (SJ-16), travels in front of the vessel of the hand shàoyáng, descends to the top of the shoulder, and arrives at Jiān Jǐng (GB-21); thereupon, the left and right [pathways] pull back to intersect behind the hand shàoyáng [channel] and traverse Dà Zhuī (Great Vertebra). This is the meeting of the foot shàoyáng [channel] with Dà Zhuī (Great Vertebra).

足太陽脈直行者，由通天、絡卻、玉枕入絡腦，復出下項，抵天柱而下過，從膊過督之陶道穴前，陶道爲督與足太陽之會，即此也，然陶道在大椎之下，大椎在陶道之上，僅隔一脊節，既下過陶道，未有不上大椎者，此可言會也。

The vertical pathway of the foot tàiyáng vessel follows Tōng Tiān (BL-7), Luò Què (BL-8), and Yù Zhěn (BL-9) to enter and network with the brain; it returns to emerge and descend the nape, and arrives at Tiān Zhù (BL-10); thereupon, it further descends after traversing [Tiān Zhù (BL-10)], follows the shoulder, and traverses in front of Táo Dào (DU-13) of the dū vessel. Thus, Táo Dào (DU-13) is [said to be] the meeting of the foot tàiyáng [channel] and the dū vessel, and this is exactly the reason for it. In addition, since Táo Dào (DU-13) is located below Dà Zhuī (Great Vertebra) and Dà Zhuī (Great Vertebra) is located above Táo Dào (DU-13), there is only one vertebra that separates them; as [the foot tàiyáng vessel] descends to traverse Táo Dào (DU-13), it is implausible that it does not ascend to Dà Zhuī (Great Vertebra). therefore, for this [meeting], it can be inferred from these statements.

若足陽明胃經，則純行面之前，自接手陽明之交，起於鼻之兩旁迎香穴，左右相交於頞中，過足太陽之睛明穴，遂下循鼻外，雖有上下曲折支別之行，而實無下後項大椎之絡，是會督脈之大椎者，止手、足五陽，而無足陽明也。概手、足三陽，尚未細考故耳。

As for the foot yángmíng stomach channel, it only travels on the front of the face. It commences at Yíng Xiāng (LI-20) at the two sides of the nose, which is the intersection where it receives from the hand yángmíng [channel]; subsequently, the left and right [pathways] intersect with each other at the bridge of the nose; it then traverses Jīng Míng (BL-1) of the foot tàiyáng [channel]; thereupon, it descends following outside of the nose. Although it has pathways that ascend, descend, bend, twist, branch out, and diverge, there is in fact no network-vessel that descends to Dà Zhuī (Great Vertebra) at the rear of the nape.

Therefore, only the five yáng [channels] of the hand and feet meet with Dà Zhuī (Great Vertebra) of the dū vessel, while the foot yángmíng [channel] does not [meet with it]. Undoubtedly, regarding [the claim that this point is the meeting with] "the three yáng of the hand and foot," it has not been examined in detail.

督之本病：骨蒸，前板齒燥，溫瘧，痎瘧。

Principal diseases of the dū: steaming bone, dryness of the front teeth, warm malaria, and intervallic malaria.

注：脊為一身骨之主，而大椎又為脊骨之主，骨熱宜取此穴，以去其熱。齦交既為本經所止之穴，則前齒自為督經之所主，大椎為脊骨之主於項後，板齒為督經之首於唇前，有前後相應之義，故取此穴以治之。板齒燥乃熱极也，泄大椎以去其熱，而燥解矣。

Explanation: the spine is the governor of the bones of the whole body, and Dà Zhuī (DU-14) further serves as the governor of the spine, thus for steaming bone, it is appropriate to choose this point in order to eliminate the heat.

Yín Jiāo (DU-28) is the point where this channel terminates, hence, the front teeth are governed by the dū channel; since Dà Zhuī (DU-14) is the governor of the spine located in the rear on the nape, and the front teeth is the frontmost aspect of the dū channel located in the front by the [upper] lip, they demonstrate the meaning of mutual correspondence between the front and rear, thus choose this point in order to treat [the front teeth]. When the front teeth are dry, this is due to extreme heat; drain Dà Zhuī (DU-14) in order to eliminate the heat, then the dryness will resolve.

張仲景曰：太陽與少陽並病，頸項強痛，或眩冒，時如結胸，心下痞硬者，當刺大椎第一間。蓋以此穴爲二經相會之地，故二經病並取之也。

Zhāng Zhòngjǐng said, "For tàiyáng and shàoyáng dragover disease, stiffness in the neck and nape, possibly with veiling dizziness, periodic binding in the chest, and hard glomus below the heart, one should pierce Dà Zhuī (DU-14) in the first space."[594] Undoubtedly, this point is the place where these two channels meet with each other,[595] thus for a disease of these two channels, choose it.

督經受邪，日下一節而爲瘧。溫瘧，有熱而無寒也；痎瘧，寒熱交作也。責大椎治其始也。

When the dū channel contracts evil, every day, [the evil] will progress down one [vertebral] joint and manifest as malaria. In warm malaria, there is a presence of fevers but absence of chills; in intervallic malaria, there is alternating chills and fever; [in both cases], seek Dà Zhuī (DU-14) to treat it at the onset.

督之肺病：肺脹脇滿，嘔吐上氣，五勞七傷乏力，風勞食氣，氣注背膊拘急，頸項強不得回顧。

Lung diseases of the dū: distension of the lung with fullness of the rib-sides, retching and vomiting with qì ascent, five taxations and seven damages with lack of strength, wind taxation with food qì, qì infixation with hypertonicity of the upper-back and arms, and stiffness in the neck and nape with inability to look behind.

注：此穴在肺之上，故所治多肺病。肺脹乃鬱於肺中也，嘔吐上氣，皆氣逆於胸胃之間也，取此穴以散其滯。

Explanation: as this point is situated above the lung, thus what it treats are predominantly lung diseases. Distension of the lung is due to depression within the lung; for retching and vomiting with qì ascent, all of them are caused by counterflow qì in the space of the chest and stomach; choose this point in order to disperse the stagnation.

五勞七傷，陰不足以匹陽之症也，久之而陽亦弱，而力乏矣，取此穴以泄陽之有餘。風勞者，因風症久而成勞也；食氣者，氣爲食滯而不舒也。故灸此穴以

---

[594] From Line 142 of the *Shānghán Lùn*, the quote continues "肺腧、肝腧，慎不可發汗，發汗則讝語。脈弦，五六日，讝語不止，當刺期門 [Pierce] Fèi Shù (BL-13), Gān Shù (BL-18), be cautious as to not cause sweating, if there is sweating delirious speech will follow. When the pulse is string-like, after 5 to 6 days the delirious speech has not ceased, one should pierce Qī Mén (LR-14)."

[595] I.e., the dū channel and foot tàiyáng channel.

去風，灸此穴以散氣。氣注背膊拘急、不得回顧，乃風寒之邪入客此穴，而上行於項也，急多灸以溫之。

Regarding the five taxations and seven damages, these are signs of yīn insufficiency that is unable to match the yáng, which over an extended period of time leads to weakness of the yáng as well; as a result, there will be a lack of strength, choose this point in order to drain the superabundance of yáng. Wind taxation is because chronic wind signs have progressed to taxation [disease]; food qì is constrained qì caused by food stagnation. Therefore, moxa this point in order to eliminate the wind, and moxa this point in order to disperse the qì.

For qì infixation with hypertonicity of the upper-back and arms, as well as inability to look behind, this is because wind and cold evils have ascended the nape after having entered and lodged at this point, urgently use moxa a great number [of cones] in order to warm it.

Fourteenth Point of the Dū Channel
Yǎ Mén – Mute's Gate (DU-15)
督經第十四穴啞門

一名舌厭
Alternate name: Tongue Repression

一名舌橫
Alternate name: Tongue's Horizontal

一名瘖門
Alternate name: Loss of Voice Gate

穴在項後入髮際五分，項中央宛宛中，俯頭取之，督脈、陽維之會，入系舌本。《素》注：鍼四分。《銅人》：鍼二分。可繞鍼八分，留三呼，泄五吸，泄盡更留鍼取之，禁灸，灸之令人啞。

This point is located on the nape, 5 fēn into the posterior hairline, in the depression at the centre of the nape, bow one's head to locate it. It is the meeting of the dū vessel and yángwéi [vessel], it enters to connect with the root of the tongue. _The Sùzhù_ states, "Needle 4 fēn." _The Tóngrén_ states, "Needle 2 fēn; surround-needling[596] can also be performed with 8 fēn [insertion], retain for 3 respirations, drain for 5 exhalations; further retain the

---

[596] See explanation section.

needle after draining is finished;[597] moxibustion is contraindicated, if moxibustion is performed, it will make the person mute.

注：此督經自下而上，離背而入項第一穴也，與陽維會而入系舌本，故不宜深鍼，從《銅人》鍼二分爲宜。其言繞鍼八分者，蓋既鍼二分之後，遂卧其鍼，而旁入八分，以泄之也。啞門之名，著戒垂後，誤灸之，則必啞也。

Explanation: as the dū channel ascends from below, this is the first point to enter the nape after [the channel] departs the upper back. Since it meets with the yángwéi [vessel] and enters to connect with the root of the tongue, thus it is inappropriate to needle deeply; hence, it is appropriate to follow [the instruction of] *the Tóngrén* to "needle 2 fēn."

As for the statement that "surrounding needling can also be performed with 8 fēn [insertion]," undoubtedly, after needling it 2 fēn [deep], one then lays down the needle and further insert 8 fēn to the side in order to drain it. Regarding the name of Yǎ Mén (Mute's Gate), this is an issued warning bequeathed to the later generations; if one mistakenly moxa [this point], it will certainly cause one to become Yǎ (Mute).

督之本病：脊强反折，瘛瘲癲疾，頭重風汗不出。

Principal diseases of the dū: arched-back rigidity, tugging and slackening with withdrawal disease, heavy-headedness and [head] wind with absence of sweating.

注：脊强反折等疾，乃督之本病也，取此穴以泄在上之邪。頭重風汗不出，風入督經而頭爲之重，以督脈行於頭上也，邪入之而頭遂重，取此穴以散其風，而汗自出矣。

Explanation: for various diseases like arched-back rigidity, all of them are principal diseases of the dū [vessel], choose this point in order to drain the evil from above. For heavy-headedness and [head] wind with absence of sweating, when wind enters the dū channel, the head will become heavy, because the dū vessel travels to the top of the head; when the head becomes heavy after evil enters [the dū vessel], choose this point in order to disperse the wind, and sweating will naturally occur.

督之心病：舌急不語，重舌。

Heart diseases of the dū: tension of the tongue with inability to speak, and double tongue.[598]

---

[597] I.e., retain the needle after 5 respirations.

[598] While this is called double tongue, it is referring to an enlargement below the tongue that has the resemblance of the tongue, it is attributed to accumulated heat of the heart and spleen surging upwards.

注：舌者，心之竅也，此穴在舌之後，鍼以泄其火，而舌急重舌之病自愈矣。

Explanation: the tongue is the orifice of the heart; as this point is located at the rear of the tongue, needle it in order to drain the fire, and the diseases of tension of the tongue and double tongue will naturally recover.

督之腎病：諸陽熱氣盛，衄血不止，寒熱風啞。

Kidney diseases of the dū:[599] all types of yáng heat with qì exuberance, incessant nosebleeds, and chills and fevers with wind muteness.

注：一身之陽，俱逆而炎上於肺，鼻者，肺之竅也，火載血而血溢出焉，督脈統諸陽，陽維維諸陽，既俱會於此穴，一鍼而諸陽之火散，則衄止。風傷肺而寒熱作，久之成啞，鍼此穴以散其風，而降其火。

Explanation: when there is counterflow of all yáng in the entire body, it will blaze upwards towards the lung; as the nose is the orifice of lung, when the blood is carried by fire, the blood will spill out; while dū vessel commands all yáng, the yángwéi [vessel] links together all the yáng; as both [vessels] meet at this point, once it is needled, the fire of all yáng will be dispersed and the [nose]bleeds will cease.

When wind damages the lung, there will be onsets of chills and fevers; if it remains for an extended period of time, [the person] will become mute, needle this point in order to disperse the wind and descend the fire.

Fifteenth Point of the Dū Channel
Fēng Fǔ – Wind Mansion (DU-16)
督經第十五穴風府

一名舌本
Alternate name: Root of the Tongue

穴在項後入髮際一寸，大筋宛宛中，疾言其肉立起，言休立止，足太陰、督脈、陽維之會。《銅人》：鍼三分，禁灸，灸之令人失音。《明堂》：鍼四分，留三呼。《素》注：鍼四分。一云：主泄腦中之熱，與大杼、缺盆、中府同。

This point is located on the nape, 1 cùn into the posterior hairline, in the depression between the great sinews. When one speaks quickly, the flesh will protrude; when one stops talking, [the protruding flesh] will flatten. It is the

---

[599] We speculate that kidney diseases may be an error for lung diseases, as the kidneys are not mentioned in the explanation.

meeting of the foot tàiyīn, dū vessel, and yángwéi [vessel]. *The Tóngrén* states, "Needle 3 fēn, and moxibustion is contraindicated as it will cause loss of voice." *The Míngtáng* states, "Needle 4 fēn, retain for 3 respirations." *The Sùzhù* states, "Needle 4 fēn." Another source states, "It governs the draining of heat in the brain, [its therapeutic effect] is the same as Dà Zhù (BL-11), Quē Pén (ST-12), and Zhōng Fǔ (LU-1)."

注：風自後來者，此穴先受之，故曰風府。凡一切風寒之邪，俱由此穴入，而後及於周身，故有風府之稱。

Explanation: when Fēng (Wind) sweeps through [a person] from behind, this point will first contract [the wind evil], thus it is called Fēng Fǔ (Wind Mansion). In general, for all evils of cold and Fēng (Wind), they all enter through this point and subsequently reach the whole body, thus is it designated as Fēng Fǔ (Wind Mansion).

風者陽邪，宜自陽穴中入，經曰：邪客於風府，循膂而下，衛氣一日夜大會於風府，明日日下一節，故其作晏，每至於風府，則腠理開，腠理開則邪氣入，邪氣入則病作，以此日作稍晏也，其出於風府，日下一節，二十五日下至骶骨，二十六日入於脊內，故日作益晏也。

As Fēng (Wind) is a yáng evil, it is fitting that it enters through a yáng point, as *the Canon* states, "When the evil lodges at Fēng Fǔ (Wind Mansion), it descends by following the paravertebral sinews. During each [cycle of] day and night, the wèi-defensive qì has a great assembly at Fēng Fǔ (Wind Mansion); in addition, on every subsequent day, [the lodged evil] descends one [vertebral] joint; this is the reason why [the malaria disease] manifests progressively later on each passing day. Thus, whenever [the wèi-defensive qì] reaches Fēng Fǔ (Wind Mansion), the interstices will open; when the interstices open, evil qì will enter; when evil qì enters, the [malaria] disease will occur; hence, [the malaria disease] will manifest slightly later on every subsequent day. Once [the evil] emerges from Fēng Fǔ (Wind Mansion), every day, it descends one [vertebral] joint; after twenty-five days, it will reach the sacrum; and after twenty six days, it will enter the inside of the spine; thus, on every subsequent day, [the malaria disease] manifests progressively later."[600]

督之本病：頭痛項急，不得回顧，頭中百病，振寒汗出，頭重惡寒，傷寒狂走，欲自殺，目盲視。

---

[600] This is a paraphrase from *Sùwèn* Chapter 35 and *Língshū* Chapter 79. Note: This is quite a difficult passage to translate as a few key subjects are missing in crucial lines. Even classical annotators themselves disagree on what these subjects should be, e.g., after the great assembly of wèi-defensive qì, what goes down the vertebrae? (wèi-defensive qì or latent evil?) Also, what opens the interstices? (wèi-defensive qì or latent evil?) As we noticed that Yuè Hánzhēn's interpretation of *the Nèijīng* seems to align closer to Mǎ Shì's annotation, we have thus translated according to the latter's interpretation.

Principal diseases of the dū: headache with tension of the nape and inability to look behind, the hundred diseases of the head,[601] quivering with cold while sweating, heavy-headedness and aversion to cold, cold damage with manic walking, desire to kill oneself, and blindness.

注：風府，風邪客之，頭爲之痛，項爲之急，宜泄此穴以去風府之風。頭中百病，俱從風府而邪入之，故治頭痛，不可捨此穴。振寒而汗不出，則爲傷寒，汗出者則爲傷風，風必由風府而入，故此穴宜必取之也。風，陽邪也，邪中人者深，遂有狂走欲自殺之症，先從風府以去在上之邪。目盲視者，邪由督絡入於目也，當泄後之穴。

Explanation: When wind evil lodges in Fēng Fǔ (DU-16), the head will become painful, and the nape will become tense, it is appropriate to drain this point in order to eliminate the wind at Fēng Fǔ (DU-16). Regarding the hundred diseases of the head, they all begin from an evil entering Fēng Fǔ (DU-16), thus, to treat headache, one must not forgo this point.

Quivering with cold and absence of sweat is due to cold damage; when there is sweating instead, it is due to wind damage; as wind must enter through Fēng Fǔ (DU-16), thus it is most appropriate for this point to be chosen. As wind is a yáng evil, when the evil strikes a person, it penetrates deeply, consequently, there will be signs of manic walking with desire to kill oneself; one should first utilise Fēng Fǔ (DU-16) in order to eliminate the evil that is above.

For blindness, the evil enters the eyes through the dū network-vessel, one should drain from the point that is behind [the eyes].

督之肝病：偏風，半身不遂。

Liver diseases of Dū: hemilateral wind and hemiplegia.

注：陽氣不至之處而邪客之，遂有不遂之症，治風府之總穴，以去其風而補其陽。

Explanation: when the evil lodges in the place where the yáng qì fails to reach, there will be signs of paralysis; Fēng Fǔ (DU-16) is the command point to treat this, as it eliminates the wind and supplements the yáng.

督之脾病：馬黃，黃疸。

Spleen diseases of the dū: [jaundice that is] the colour of a yellow horse, and jaundice.

---

[601] "The hundred diseases" is a euphemism for all kinds of diseases.

注：二症皆脾胃有濕熱所致，乃取此穴，蓋督之絡，由下而上行，故取此穴。

Explanation: both of these two signs are caused by damp heat in the stomach and spleen, yet why should one choose this point? Undoubtedly, since the network-vessel of the dū [vessel] ascends from below, thus choose this point.

督之心病：中風，舌緩不語。

Heart diseases of the dū: wind strike, and slack tongue with inability to speak.

注：舌者，心之竅也。舌緩者，風中於舌，急泄舌上之本穴。

Explanation: the tongue is the orifice of the heart; in addition, slack tongue is due to wind strike at the tongue, urgently drain the root point that is above the tongue.[602]

Sixteenth Point of the Dū Channel
Nǎo Hù – Brain's Door (DU-17)
督經第十六穴腦戶

一名匝風
Alternate name: Circumference Wind

一名會額
Alternate name: Meeting of the Forehead

一名合顱
Alternate name: Skull Union

穴骨枕上，本經強間穴後一寸半，足太陽、督脈之會。《銅人》：禁灸，灸之令人啞。《明堂》：鍼三分。《素》注：鍼四分。《素問》：刺腦戶，刺入立死。又云：此穴鍼灸俱不宜。

This point is located above the pillow bone, 1 cùn and a half behind Qiáng Jiān (DU-18) of this channel. It is the meeting of the foot tàiyáng [channel] and dū vessel. *The Tóngrén* states, "Moxibustion is contraindicated, as moxa will make the person mute."[603] *The Míngtáng* states, "Needle 3 fēn." *The Sùzhù* states, "Needle 4 fēn." *The Sùwèn* states, "When piercing Nǎo Hù (DU-17), if the needle

---

602 Note: The secondary manuscript has, "急泄舌本之上穴 urgently drain the point that is above the root of the tongue."

603 *The Tóngrén* actually states, "禁鍼，灸之令人鍼 needling is contraindicated, as needling will make the person mute."

enters [deeply], there will be immediate death."[604] Another source states, "For this point, both needling and moxa are inappropriate."[605]

注：此穴細按之，真有小孔陷中，其云鍼灸俱不宜，此言真當。而又有所主治之病何也？還以他穴代之為是。

Explanation: by carefully palpating this point, there is truly a small opening inside a depression. As for the statement that "both piercing and moxa are inappropriate," this should be regarded as true. Yet, why are there diseases that [this point] governs the treatment of? Still, it is better to use other points as a substitute for [this point].

主病：面赤目黄，面痛，頭重腫痛，瘦瘤。

Governed diseases: red face with yellowing of the eyes, facial pain, heavy-headedness with swelling and pain, and goitre.[606]

Seventeenth Point of the Dū Channel
Qiáng Jiān – Unyielding Space (DU-18)
督經第十七穴強間

一名大羽
Alternate name: Great Feather

穴在後頂後一寸半。《銅人》：鍼二分，灸七壯。《明堂》：灸五壯。

This point is located 1 cùn and a half behind Hòu Dǐng (DU-19). *The Tóngrén* states, "Needle 2 fēn, and moxa 7 cones." *The Míngtáng* states, "Moxa 5 cones."

注：穴在腦戶之上，後頂之下，最堅固之所，故曰強間，鍼二分者，不宜深入也。

Explanation: as this point is located above Nǎo Hù (DU-17) and below Hòu Dǐng (DU-19), it is in the place that is most firm and solid, thus it is called Qiáng Jiān (Unyielding Space); only needle 2 fēn, as it is inappropriate to needle deeply.

---

[604] From *Sùwèn* Chapter 52, which actually states, "刺頭中腦戶，入腦立死 when piercing Nǎo Hù (DU-17) on the head, if it enters the brain, there will be immediate death."

[605] We are unable to locate the exact source of this quote; however, the phrase "禁刺灸 piercing and moxibustion are contraindicated" appears in *the Lèijīng Túyì* 類經圖翼 (*the Illustrated Wings of the Classified Canon*, 1624 CE).

[606] Translator's note: no explanation given for these diseases.

督之本病：頭痛目眩，腦旋煩心，嘔吐涎沫，項強不得回顧，狂走不臥。

Principal diseases of the dū: headache with dizzy vision, spinning brain with vexation of the heart, retching and vomiting of foamy drool, stiffness of the nape with inability to look behind, and manic walking with inability to lie down.

注：此症乃命門之火，載痰而上衝，過膈而至巔，遂有頭痛目眩，頭旋煩心，嘔吐涎沫之症，泄此穴以散其上逆之火。項強不得回顧，項受風也，泄之以散其風。狂走不臥，純陽無陰之症也，泄之以散火而弱陽。

Explanation: these are signs of the fire of mìngmén, which surges upwards carrying phlegm; as it traverses the diaphragm to reach the vertex, consequently, there will be signs of headache and dizzy vision, spinning brain and vexation of the heart, retching and vomiting of foamy drool; drain this point in order to disperse the counterflow ascent of fire.

Stiffness of the nape with inability to look behind is due to the nape contracting wind, drain this [point] in order to disperse the wind. Manic walking with inability to lie down is a sign of pure yáng in the absence of yīn, drain this [point] in order to disperse the fire and weaken the yáng.

Eighteenth Point of the Dū Channel
Hòu Dǐng – Behind the Vertex (DU-19)
督經第十八穴後頂

一名交衝
Alternate name: Intersection Hub

穴在百會後一寸半，枕骨上。《銅人》：鍼二分，灸五壯。《明堂》：鍼四分。《素》注：鍼三分。

This point is located 1 and a half cùn behind Bǎi Huì (DU-20), above the pillow bone.[607] The Tóngrén states, "Needle 2 fēn,[608] and moxa 5 cones." The Míngtáng states, "Needle 4 fēn." The Sùzhù states, "Needle 3 fēn."[609]

注：穴在百會之後，百會爲頂也，故曰後頂。一名交衝者，足太陽兩脈，既左右交於頂之百會而下，此穴正當左右交衝之中，故曰交衝。

---

607 I.e., the occipital bone.
608 For "2 fēn," the Tóngrén actually states "3 fēn."
609 For "3 fēn," the Sùzhù actually states "4 fēn."

Explanation: this point is located Hòu (Behind) Bǎi Huì (DU-20); as Bǎi Huì (DU-20) is on the Dǐng (Vertex), thus this point is called Hòu Dǐng (Behind the Vertex). An alternate name is Jiāo Chōng (Intersection Hub), because as the left and right vessels of the foot tàiyáng descend after having intersected at Bǎi Huì (DU-20) on the Dǐng (Vertex), this point is exactly located at the Chōng (Hub) where the left and right [pathways] Jiāo (Intersect), thus it is called Jiāo Chōng (Intersection Hub).

督之本病：頸項強急，惡風寒，風眩目眈眈，額顱上痛，狂走癲疾不臥，瘛發瘲瘲，頭偏痛，歷節汗出。

Principal diseases of the dū: stiffness and tension of the neck and nape, aversion to wind and cold, wind dizziness with blurred vision, skull pain above the forehead, manic walking with withdrawal disease and inability to lie down, tugging and slackening at the onset of epilepsy, hemilateral headache, and joint-running wind with sweating.

注：前症俱爲督經至頭之本病，故取此穴，以散其邪。歷節痛而有汗，則亦風邪中之也，取此穴以散風止汗。

Explanation: all of the above signs are principal diseases of the dū channel, which arrives at the head, thus choose this point in order to disperse the evils. For joint-running wind pain with sweating, this is also because of a strike by wind evil, drain this point in order to disperse the wind and cease the sweating.

Nineteenth Point of the Dū Channel
Bǎi Huì – Hundred Meetings[610] (DU-20)
督經第十九穴百會

一名五會
Alternate name: Fivefold Meeting[611]

一名巔上
Alternate name: Mountain Top

一名天橫
Alternate name: Celestial Horizon[612]

---

[610] *Grasping the Wind* names it "Hundred Convergences."

[611] *Grasping the Wind* names it "Fivefold Confluence."

[612] I.e., the milky way, or sometimes more specifically as five stars (19, φ, 14, σ, and μ) of the Auriga constellation. In *the Zhēnjiǔ Dàchéng*, this alternate name is listed as Tiān Mǎn 天滿 (Celestial Fullness) instead.

穴在前頂後一寸五分，頂中央旋毛中，可容豆，直兩耳尖，手、足三陽、督脈之會。《素》注：鍼二分。《銅人》：灸七壯，止七七壯。凡灸頭頂，不得過七七壯，緣頭皮薄，灸不宜多，鍼二分，得氣即泄。

This point is located 1 cùn 5 fēn behind Qián Dǐng (DU-21), at the vertex, in the centre of the hair whorl, where it can hold a small bean; it is directly above the apex of both ears. It is the meeting of the three hand and foot yáng [channels] and the dū vessel. *The Sùzhù* states, "Needle 2 fēn."[613] The *Tóngrén* states, "Moxa 7 to 49 cones. For all applications of moxa on the vertex of the head, one should not exceed 49 cones, because the scalp skin is thin, so it is not appropriate to apply large amounts of moxa; needle 2 fēn, obtain qì, then promptly drain."

又《素》注：鍼四分。《神農經》云：治頭風，可灸三壯，小兒脫肛，可灸三壯至五壯，艾炷如小麥大。

The Sùzhù also states, "Needle 4 fēn." *The Shénnóng Jīng* states, "One can moxa 3 cones to treat head wind; one can moxa 3 to 5 cones to treat prolapse of the rectum in children; the cones should be the size of a wheat grain."

注：此穴云在旋毛中，如遇旋毛偏者，何以定之？雙旋者何以定之？還以東西兩耳尖，南北完督之中，十字相直處，再退些子是穴。《性理》北溪陳氏曰：此穴猶天之極星居北之意也。

Explanation: this point is said to be in the centre of the hair whorl, but if the hair whorl is situated to the side, how does one locate it then? Or what if there are two whorls, how does one locate it then? One should still locate the centre between the two ears on the east and west, as well as the entire dū vessel along south and north; this point is slightly behind [the centre] where the [two axes] cross each other perpendicularly. Mister Chén of Běixī[614] says in *the Xìnglǐ*,[615] "The imagery of this point is so that it resembles the heavenly pole star which dwells in the north."[616]

如云手足三陽、督脈之會，今考手三陽經，無至百會之絡。足少陽雖行於頭，乃足太陽有絡此穴，從巔至百會，抵耳上角，過足少陽之率谷、浮白、竅陰穴，而少陽膽經，則未有至百會之絡也。

---

[613] For "2 fēn," *the Sùzhù* actually states "3 fēn."

[614] I.e., Chén Chún 陳淳 (1159 – 1223 CE), a student of the influential Neo-Confucian Zhū Xī. As he lived on the shore of the Běixī 北溪 (Northern Stream) of the Lóngjiāng 龍江 (Dragon River) in the Fújiàn Province, he came to be known as Master of Běixī 北溪 (Northern Stream).

[615] From *Sìshū Xìnglǐ Zìyì* 四書性理字義 (*Nature, Principles, and Meaning of Characters in the Four Classics*, c. early 13th century CE).

[616] I.e., the north star.

Regarding the statement that it is the meeting of the three hand and foot yáng [channels] and the dū vessel, from my current investigations, the three hand yáng channels do not have any network-vessels that arrive at Bǎi Huì (Hundred Meetings).

Although the foot shàoyáng travels on the head, it is the foot tàiyáng that networks with this point; [such a network-vessel] follows the vertex to arrive at Bǎi Huì (Hundred Meetings), reaches the corner of the ears, and traverses Lǜ Gǔ (GB-8), Fú Bái (GB-10), and [Tóu] Qiào Yīn (GB-11) of the foot shàoyáng; however, as for the shàoyáng gallbladder channel itself, in fact, it does not have any network-vessels that reach Bǎi Huì (Hundred Meetings).

若足陽明胃經，則所行在面之前部分，而並無上巔會百會之絡。若足太陽之經，起自內眥睛明穴，上額循攢竹，過神庭，歷曲差、五處、承光、通天，乃自通天斜行，左右交於頂上督經於百會耳。

As for the foot yángmíng stomach channel, the area where it travels is on the front of the face; as such, it does not have any network-vessels that ascend to the vertex and Huì (Meet) with Bǎi Huì (Hundred Meetings).

As for the channel of foot tàiyáng, it commences from Jīng Míng (BL-1) at the inner canthus, ascends following Zǎn Zhú (BL-2), traverses Shén Tíng (DU-24), and passes through Qū Chà (BL-4), Wǔ Chù (BL-5), Chéng Guāng (BL-6), and Tōng Tiān (BL-7); thereupon, it travels obliquely from Tōng Tiān (BL-7), with the left and right pathways intersecting at Bǎi Huì (Hundred Meetings) on the vertex on the dū channel.

所謂手、足三陽會於此穴者，乃以足太陽爲一身之巨陽，其行於周身，皆通於手、足三陽相會之絡，太陽既會百會，即有手、足三陽統會相通之義。

When it is said that the three hand and foot yáng [channels] Huì (Meet) at this point, this is because the foot tàiyáng is the great yáng of the whole body; as it travels around the entire body, it connects and Huì (Meets) with all network-vessels of three hand and foot yáng channels; since the tàiyáng [channel] Huì (Meets) with Bǎi Huì (Hundred Meetings), thus, there is the notion that all three hand and foot yáng [channels] Huì (Meet) with one another [at this point].

若手、足三陽真有絡有經，有別至於此穴，則古經末載也。又按督脈既通一身之陽，而此穴又爲督脈聚陽之所，凡頭上之病，無所不治，而氣病獨爲要穴。

Even if the three hand and foot yáng [channels] truly have a network-vessel, channel, or divergence that arrives at this point, it is not recorded in the ancient canons. In addition, from my observation, since the dū vessel connects with yáng of the entire body, and this point is further the place where the yáng accumulates on the dū vessel, thus, for all diseases on the head, there is none that it fails to treat; as such, for qì diseases, it is alone as the most important point.

督之本病：頭風，中風語言蹇澀，口噤不開，偏風半身不遂，心煩悶，驚悸健忘，忘前失後，心神恍惚，無心力，瘀癧，脫肛，風癇，青風心風，角弓反張，羊鳴多哭，語言不擇，登時即死，吐沫，汗出而嘔，飲酒面赤，腦重目眩，食無味。

Principal diseases of the dū: head wind, wind strike with difficult sluggish speech, clenched jaw with inability to open it, hemilateral wind with hemiplegia, vexation and fullness of the heart, fright palpitations with forgetfulness, forgetting what occurs prior and losing what occurs later, abstraction of the heart spirit, feeble heart, intervallic malaria, prolapse of the rectum, wind epilepsy, blue-green wind[617] with heart wind, arched-back rigidity, excessive crying that sounds like the bleating of goats, unfiltered speech, abrupt death-like appearance, vomiting of foam, sweating with retching, red face after drinking liquor, heavy-brain with dizzy vision, and inability to perceive flavour in food.

　　注：以上如心神恍惚、無心力，此心經症也，何以責督脈？蓋心爲身之中，督亦爲身之中，此穴爲頭之中，乃氣有餘而血不足之症，取此穴以散氣，而配不足之血。餘俱督經本症，應責此穴。

　　Explanation: for above signs such as abstraction of the heart and feeble heart, these are signs of the heart channel, so why should one seek the dū vessel? Because while the heart is the centre of body, the dū is also on the centre of the body; likewise, this point is in the centre of the head; thus, for signs of superabundance of qì and insufficiency of blood, choose this point in order to disperse the qì, and match it [with a point to treat] insufficiency of the blood. For the remaining [signs], they are all principal dū channel signs, one ought to seek this point.

---

617 This may refer to the disease green-blue wind internal obstruction, which according to the *Practical Dictionary* is "A disease of the eye in which the pupil takes on a green-blue colour and is sometimes dilated, accompanied by a faint red areola surrounding the black wheel (ciliary congestion). Green-blue wind internal obstruction is accompanied by mild distension in the head, mild aversion to light and tearing, and gradual decrease in visual acuity."

Twentieth Point of the Dū Channel
Qián Dǐng – Front of the Vertex[618] (DU-21)
督經第二十穴前頂

穴在顖會後一寸半骨間陷中。《銅人》：鍼一分，灸三壯至七壯。《素》注：鍼
四分。《神農》：治小兒急慢驚風，可灸三壯，炷如小麥。

This point is located in the depression between the bones, 1 cùn and a half behind Xìn Huì (DU-22). *The Tóngrén* **states, "Needle 1 fēn, and moxa 3 to 7 cones."** *The Sùzhù* **states, "Needle 4 fēn."** *The Shénnóng* **states, "One can moxa 3 cones to treat both urgent and chronic fright wind in children, [the cones should] resemble the size of a wheat grain."**

注：百會爲頂，此穴在百會之前，故曰前頂。

Explanation: Bǎi Huì (DU-20) is located on the Dǐng (Vertex); as this point is located in Qián (Front) of Bǎi Huì (DU-20), thus it is called Qián Dǐng (Front of the Vertex).

督之本病：小兒驚癇瘈瘲，發即無時，頭風目眩，鼻多清涕，頂腫痛，面赤腫。

Principal diseases of the dū: fright epilepsy in children with tugging and slackening, with no fixed time of onset, head wind with dizzy vision, copious clear snivel, swelling and pain on the vertex, and redness and swelling on the face.

注：以上皆督經之症也，取此穴宜也。

Explanation: all of the above are signs of the dū channel, it is appropriate to choose this point.

督之脾病：水腫。

Spleen disease of the dū: water swelling.

注：水腫而責此穴者，孔開於上，而水泄於下之義。

Explanation: for water swelling, one can also seek this point, as it exemplifies the concept of opening a hole above [to allow] the water to drain below.

---

[618] *Grasping the Wind* names it "Before the Vertex."

Twenty-First Point of the Dū Channel
Xìn Huì – Fontanel Meeting (DU-22)
督經第二十一穴顖會

穴在上星後一寸陷中，《銅人》：灸二七壯，初灸不痛，病去即痛，痛乃止灸。
若是鼻塞，灸至四日漸退，七日頓愈。鍼二分，留三呼，得氣即瀉，八歲以下不
可鍼，緣顖門未合，恐傷其骨，令人失音。《素》注：鍼四分。《神農》：治頭
風疼痛，可灸三壯，小兒急慢驚風，灸三壯，炷如小麥。

This point is located in the depression 1 cùn behind Shàng Xīng (DU-23). *The Tóngrén* states, "Moxa 14 cones;[619] at the beginning, the moxa should not cause pain; when the disease is eliminated, there will be pain; once there is pain, one should stop moxa. If there is nasal congestion, it will abate after 4 days of moxa, and it will suddenly recover after 7 days. Needle 2 fēn, retain for 3 respirations, obtain qì then promptly drain; those who are 8 years and younger cannot be needled here, because the fontanel gate has not yet joined together, there is a risk that [needling] will damage the bone and cause loss of voice."[620]

The Sùzhù states, "Needle 4 fēn." *The Shénnóng* states, "One can moxa 3 cones to treat head wind with pain; one can moxa 3 cones to treat both urgent and chronic fright wind in children, [the cones should] resemble the size of a wheat grain."

注：顖會者，乃人之顖門，以與督脈會，故曰顖會。鍼固不宜深，灸亦不
宜多，灸多恐火氣入腦也。

Explanation: regarding Xìn Huì (Fontanel Meeting), surely, since the Xìn (Fontanel) gate Huì (Meets) with the dū vessel, thus it is called Xìn Huì (Fontanel Meeting). Deep needling is entirely inappropriate; likewise, [using] a large amount of moxa is also inappropriate, for the risk that fire qì will enter the brain.

督之本病：腦虛冷，飲酒過多，腦痛如破，衄血面赤，暴腫，頭皮腫，生白屑
風，頭眩顏青，目眩，鼻塞不聞香臭，驚悸，目上戴不識人。

Principal diseases of the dū: vacuity cold in the brain, brain pain as if it is broken after drinking excessive amounts of liquor, nosebleeds with red face, fulminant swelling, swelling of the scalp skin, generation of white scaling-wind,[621] dizzy head with blue-green facial complexion, dizzy vision, nasal

---

[619] For "moxa 14 cones," *the Tóngrén* actually states "moxa 3 to 49 cones."

[620] For "cause loss of voice," *the Tóngrén* actually states "cause premature death."

[621] *The Practical Dictionary* defines this as "a scaling skin disease of the neck, which can spread over the face, nose, and ears."

congestion that inhibits the sense of smell, fright palpitations, and upward staring eyes with inability to recognise people.

注：前症皆督經本症，責此穴固宜。

Explanation: all of the above signs are principal signs of the dū channel, undoubtedly, it is appropriate to seek this point.

Twenty-Second Point of the Dū Channel
Shàng Xīng – Upper Star (DU-23)
督經第二十二穴上星

一名神堂
Alternate name: Spirit Hall

穴在神庭後入髮際一寸陷中，容豆。《素》注：鍼三分，留六呼，灸五壯。以細三稜鍼，宣泄諸陽熱氣，不令上衝頭目。

This point is located behind Shén Tíng (DU-24), in the depression 1 cùn into the hairline, where it can hold a small bean. *The Sùzhù* states, "Needle 3 fēn, retain for 6 respirations, and moxa 5 cones. Use a fine three-edged needle to diffuse and drain all types of yáng and heat qì, as to prevent it from surging into the head and eyes."

注：此穴在額之最高處陷中如豆大，如星以懸於天者然，故曰上星。不宜多灸，恐拔氣上，令目不明。

Explanation: this point is located at the highest place on the forehead, in the depression that resembles the size of a small bean; it is like a Xīng (Star) that is hang-ing in the heavens, thus it is called Shàng Xīng (Upper Star). It is not appropriate to use a large amount of moxa, for the risk of pulling the qì upwards, which will cause dim vision.

督之本病：面赤腫，頭風頭皮腫，面虛，鼻中瘜肉，鼻塞頭痛，目眩目睛痛，不能遠視，口鼻出血不止，痎瘧振寒，熱病汗不出。

Principal diseases of the dū: redness and swelling of the face, head wind with swelling of the scalp skin, vacuity [swelling] on the face,[622] polyps in the nose, nasal congestion with headache, dizzy vision with pain of the eyeball, near-

---

[622] Upon a brief research, there seems to be a scribal error that removed the character, 腫 (swelling), when this indication was copied from *the Zhēnjiǔ Zīshēng Jīng* 針灸資生經 (*the Classic of Support-ing Life with Acupuncture and Moxibustion*, 1220 CE) to *the Zhēnjiǔ Jùyīng* 針灸聚英 (*Gathered Blooms of Acupuncture and Moxibustion*, 1529 CE). So, the indication here should be restored as "面虛腫 vacuity swelling on the complexion."

sightedness, incessant bleeding from the mouth and nose, intervallic malaria and quivering with cold, and febrile disease with absence of sweating.

注：頭鼻面目諸病，皆督經本病也，應責此穴。痎瘧乃寒熱交作之症也，而振寒不已，取此穴以宣久鬱之陽。熱病汗不出，乃五十九刺之一也。

Explanation: for the various diseases of the head, nose, face, and eye, they are all principal diseases of the dū channel, one ought to seek this point.

Intervallic malaria presents with the sign of alternating chills and fever, as well as incessant quivering with cold, choose this point in order to diffuse the chronically depressed yáng. As for febrile disease with absence of sweating, [this point] is one of the fifty-nine piercings.[623]

Twenty-Third Point of the Dū Channel
Shén Tíng – Spirit Courtyard[624] (DU-24)
督經第二十三穴神庭

穴在直鼻上入髮際五分，足太陽、督脈之會。《素》注：灸三壯。《銅人》：灸二七壯，止七七壯。禁鍼，鍼則令人發狂，目失精。歧伯曰：凡欲療風，勿令灸多。緣風性輕，多即受傷，惟宜灸七壯，至三七壯止。張子和曰：目腫目臀，鍼神庭、上星、顖會、前頂，臀者可使立退，腫者可使立消。

This point is located 5 fēn into the hairline, directly above the nose. It is the meeting of the foot tàiyáng [channel] and dū vessel. *The Sùzhù* states, "Moxa 3 cones." *The Tóngrén* states, "Moxa 14 to 49 cones. Needling is contraindicated; if it is needled the person will become manic and their eyes will lose their essence.

Qì Bó says, "Should one desire to cure wind, one should avoid a large amount of moxa. Because the nature of wind is light, a large amount of moxa will cause damage [to the area], it is appropriate to only moxa 7 to 21 cones."[625]

---

[623] This refers to fifty-nine piercings (points) for the treatment of febrile diseases and malaria in *Sùwèn* Chapters 32, 36, 58, and 61, as well as *Língshū* Chapters 19 and 23.

[624] *Grasping the Wind* names it "Spirit Court."

[625] Note: This quote appears in *the Tóngrén*, which attributes it to Qì Bó, i.e., *the Nèijīng*; however, it cannot be found in any existing copy of *the Nèijīng*, nor is it found in any known surviving acupuncture literature dated prior to *the Tóngrén*.

Zhāng Zǐhé[626] says, "For swelling of the eyes and eye screens, needle Shén Tíng (DU-24), Shàng Xīng (DU-23), Xìn Huì (DU-22), and Qián Dǐng (DU-21), the eye screens will immediately abate, the swelling will immediately disperse."[627]

思蓮子議曰：神庭者，額之上乃人神所遊之所，而此穴乃其庭也。

Master Sīlián comments, "Regarding Shén Tíng (Spirit Courtyard), above the forehead is surely the place where the person's Shén (Spirit) wanders, and this point is surely [the place of] its Tíng (Courtyard)."

督之本病：登高而歌，棄衣而走，角弓反張，吐舌癲疾，風癇，目上視不識人，頭風目眩，鼻出清涕不止，驚悸不得安寢，嘔吐煩滿。

Principal diseases of the dū: climbing to high places and singing, casting off one's clothes and running around, arched-back rigidity, protrusion of the tongue with withdrawal disease, wind epilepsy, upward gazing eyes with inability to recognise people, head wind with dizzy vision, incessant discharge of clear snivel from the nose, fright palpitations with inability to sleep peacefully, retching and vomiting with vexation and fullness.

注：以上皆督經本症，應責此穴。

Explanation: all of the above are principal signs of the dū channel, one ought to seek this point.

Twenty-Fourth Point of the Dū Channel
Sù Liáo – White Bone-Hole (DU-25)
督經第二十四穴素髎

一名面正
Alternate name: Face Centre

穴在鼻柱上端準頭，此穴諸書缺治。《外臺》：鍼一分，不宜灸。《素》注：鍼三分。

This point is located at the tip of the nose above the nose beam. This point's [indications of] disease treatment are absent in various books. *The Wàitái* states, "Needle 1 fēn, and it is not appropriate to moxa." *The Sùzhù* states, "Needle 3 fēn."

---

[626] I.e., the courtesy name of Zhāng Cóngzhèng 張從正 (1156-1228 CE), founder of the Attack Evil School of Thought.

[627] From Chapter 8 of *Rúmén Shìqīn* 儒門事親 (*Confucian Filiality*, 1228 CE) by Zhāng Zǐhé.

注：素者，始也，順也，潔也。人之生也先鼻，有始之義焉，自山根而下，至此而止，有順之義也，穴在面中最高處，有潔之義焉，故曰素髎。

Explanation: Sù (White) is the beginning, the compliant, and the unsullied. When a person is born, the nose is the first [to emerge]; therefore, [this point] carries the meaning of the beginning. As [the dū channel] descends from the mountain root,[628] it stops upon arriving at this place, which bears the meaning of being compliant. In addition, as this point is located at the highest place at the centre of the face, it has the meaning of being unsullied; therefore, it is called Sù Liáo (White Bone-Hole).

督之本症：鼻中瘜肉不消，多涕生瘡，鼻窒喘息不利，鼻喎僻，鼽衄。

Principal diseases[629] of the dū: polyps in the nose that do not disperse [without intervention], excess snivel and generation of sores, nasal congestion with panting and inhibition [of breathing], deviated nose, and nosebleeds.

注：前症皆鼻病有餘之症，故宜取此穴以泄之。

Explanation: all of the above signs are signs of nasal diseases due to superabundance, thus it is appropriate to choose this point in order to drain it.

Twenty-Fifth Point of the Dū Channel
Shuǐ Gōu – Water Trough (DU-26)
督經第二十五穴水溝

一名人中
Alternate name: Human Centre

穴在鼻柱下溝中央，近鼻孔陷中，督脈、手、足陽明之會。《素》注：鍼三分，留六呼，灸三壯。《銅人》：鍼四分，留五呼，得氣即泄，灸不及鍼，日灸三壯。《明堂》：日灸三壯至二百壯。《下經》：灸五壯。

This point is located in the centre of the groove below the nose beam,[630] in the depression nearby the nostrils. It is the meeting of the dū vessel, and hand and

---

[628] According to the *Practical Dictionary*, this place is "the region between the two inner canthi of the eye; the root of the nose."

[629] While the primary manuscript has "脾病 spleen diseases" here, we have amended it to "本病 principal disease" according to the secondary manuscript, as we find it more fitting for the context.

[630] Also nose beam, according to the *Practical Dictionary,* "it is the region below the nose, [also] the stem of the nose.

foot yángmíng [channels]. *The Sùzhù* **states, "Needle 3 fēn, retain for 6 respira-tions, and moxa 3 cones."**

The Tóngrén **states, "Needle 4 fēn, retain for 5 respirations, obtain qì then prompt-ly drain; while moxa is inferior to needling it, one can still moxa 3 cones."** *The Míngtáng* **states, "Moxa 3 to 200 cones daily."** *The Xiàjīng* **states, "Moxa 5 cones."**

注：穴名水溝者，以其形有水溝之象，而治水病者，必取此穴以出水，故名水溝以誌之。

Explanation: this point is named Shuǐ Gōu (Water Trough), this is because its shape resembles a Shuǐ Gōu (Water Trough); moreover, whenever one treats Shuǐ (Water) diseases, one must choose this point in order to discharge Shuǐ (Water), thus it is named Shuǐ Gōu (Water Trough).

一名人中者，蓋人身之竅，三偶在此穴之上，三奇在此穴之下，合爲泰卦，而此穴在其中，故曰人中。

As for the alternate name Rén Zhōng (Human Centre), undoubtedly, because for the orifice of the human body, three of them are in pairs above this point,[631] and three of them are single below it;[632] together, they form the tài hexagram.[633] As this point is situated in the Zhōng (Centre),[634] thus it is called Rén Zhōng (Human Centre).

---

[631] I.e., eyes, ears, and nose; all three of these orifices have two openings.

[632] I.e., mouth, urethra, and anus; all three of these orifices have only one opening.

[633] Note: This should be regarded as imagery symbolism. Each orifice with two openings can be interpreted as the yīn line (--), whereas each orifice with one opening can be interpreted as the yáng line (—); as such, the orifices above DU-26 form the earth trigram (☷), while those below form the heavenly trigram (☰). With the heaven trigram above, earth trigram below, one receives tài 泰 hexagram (hexagram 11, "peace").

[634] I.e., DU-26 is situated in the strategic location between the upper and lower trigrams. Side Note: By conventional wisdom, one would want the heaven trigram above and the earth trigram below, as it would reflect the natural world; interestingly, by such arrangement, it actually-forms the pǐ 否 hexagram (hexagram 12, obstruction) in *the Yìjīng*. The reason is that, with the heaven trigram above and the earth trigram below, the heavenly yáng above will ascend further while the earthly yīn below will descend further, resulting in a separation and lack of interaction between the heavens and earth. On the other hand, in the case of tài 泰 hexagram (hexagram 11, "peace"), with the earth trigram above and the heaven trigram below, the earthly yīn above will descend while the heavenly yáng below will ascend, resulting in an interaction between the heavens and earth. DU-26 is situated precisely at this location where the interaction between the heavens and earth takes place. Moreover, in the study of "三才 Three Powers," humans are situated between the heavens and earth; therefore, by Rén (Human) in its alternate name, it is also indicative of the location of DU-26 between the heavens and earth.

足陽明胃自鼻上下行環唇者，交於此地，手陽明自下齒縫中，復出挾兩口吻上行，交於人中之內，而督脈自上下行者，從兩陽明相交之處而過之，故爲手、足陽明、督脈之會也。

After the foot yángmíng stomach [channel] descends from the nose above to encircle the lips, [its left and right pathways] intersect at this place. After the hand yángmíng [channel] re-emerges from the cleft in the lower teeth, it ascends while clasping the lips, and intersects [its left and right pathways] on the inside of Rén Zhōng (Human Centre). Furthermore, the dū vessel descends from the above to traverse this place, where the two yángmíng [channels] intersect; therefore, [this point] is the meeting of the hand and foot yángmíng [channels] and dū vessel.

督之本病：癲癇，語不識尊卑，乍哭乍笑，中風口噤，牙關不開，卒中惡鬼擊，喘渴，目不可視，口喎僻。

Principal diseases of the dū: withdrawal epilepsy, speaking without recognition of social status,[635] abrupt alternating between weeping and laughing, wind strike with clenched jaw with inability to open the jaw, sudden malignity stroke as though one is attacked by ghosts,[636] panting with thirst, inability to see, and deviated mouth.

注：諸風邪病，上取百會，下取人中，維俱督經之穴，而百會乃太陽會督之所，人中乃陽明會督之所，兩經皆血氣有餘之經，與督會則陽愈盛，故取此穴以泄之。

Explanation: for all the diseases of wind evil, choose Bǎi Huì (DU-20) above and choose Rén Zhōng (DU-26) below, as they link together all of the points of the dū channel; in addition, Bǎi Huì (DU-20) is where the tàiyáng [channel] meets with the dū [vessel], while Rén Zhōng (DU-26) is where the yángmíng [channels] meet with the dū [vessel]; as both of these channels are channels that are superabundant in blood and qì, when they meet with the dū [vessel], the yáng will become increasingly exuberant, thus choose this point in order to drain it.

督之脾病：消渴，飲水無度，水氣遍身腫，面腫唇動，狀如蟲行，黃疸，馬黃瘟疫，遍身黃。

---

[635] I.e., Lack of social etiquette when speaking.

[636] *The Practical Dictionary* notes, "Malignity stroke patterns are due to catching some unright (evil) qì and are characterized by sudden counterflow cold of the limbs, goose pimples, blackish green-blue head and face, essence-spirit failing to confine itself, deranged raving, clenched jaw, spinning head and collapse, and clouding unconsciousness. They are observed in vehement reversal, visiting hostility... or after attending funerals or going into temples or graveyards."

Spleen diseases of the dū: dispersion-thirst, drinking excessive amounts of water, water qì with swelling all over the body, swollen face with twitching lips as though insects were burrowing, jaundice that is the colour of a yellow horse, warm epidemic, and yellowing all over the body.

注：以上皆胃病也，脾弱不能運水下行膀胱，遂溢於四肢而上行及面，二陽明皆會此穴，故取此穴以泄水。灸三艾炷，如小雀矢大，灸不及鍼，水症面腫，鍼此穴，出水盡即愈。黃症皆由濕熱所致，泄此穴以去胃中之濕熱。瘟疫亦胃中有毒邪，泄此穴以解胃中之毒。

Explanation: all of the above are stomach diseases, when the spleen is weak, it will fail to transport water downwards into the bladder; consequently, it spills [water] to the four limbs and upwards to the face. Since both yángmíng [channels] meet at this point, thus choose this point in order to drain the water.

Moxa 3 cones, the cones should resemble the size of dropping from a small sparrow; however, moxa is inferior to needling. For water signs such as facial swelling, needle this point; once the water discharges completely, one will recover. Signs of yellowing are always a result of damp heat, drain this point in order to eliminate the damp heat in the stomach. Warm epidemic is also due to the presence of toxic evils in the stomach, drain this point in order to resolve the toxins within the stomach.

Twenty-Sixth Point of the Dū Channel
Duì Duān – Edge of the Opening[637] (DU-27)
督經第二十六穴兌端

穴在唇上端。《銅人》：鍼二分，灸三壯，炷如麥大。

This point is located at the upper edge of the [upper] lip. *The Tóngrén* states, "Needle 2 fēn, and moxa 3 cones, which resembles the size of a grain of wheat."

注：兌者，口也。穴在唇正中之端，故曰兌端。

Explanation: Duì (Opening) is the mouth.[638] This point is located exactly in the middle at the Duān (Edge) of the [upper] lip, thus it is called Duì Duān (Edge of the Opening).

---

[637] *Grasping the Wind* names it "Extremity of the Mouth."

[638] From Confucius's commentary in 易經說卦 *Book of Changes*: "Expounding the Hexagrams," "Qián (heaven trigram) is the head, kūn (earth trigram) the abdomen, zhèn (thunder trigram) the feet, xún (wind trigram) the thighs, kǎn (water trigram) the ears, gèn (mountain trigram) the hands, and duì 兌 (lake trigram) the mouth."

督之本病：癲疾吐沫，鼻塞痰涎，口噤鼓頷，唇吻强，齒齦痛，衄血不止。

Principal diseases of the dū: withdrawal disease with vomiting of foam, nasal congestion with phlegm-drool, clenched jaw with chattering of the chin, stiff lips, pain of the teeth and gums, and incessant nosebleed.

注：以上皆督經受邪之本症，宜泄此穴。

Explanation: all of the above are principal signs of the dū channel contracting evil, it is appropriate to drain this point.

督之心病：小便黄，舌乾消渴。

Heart diseases of the dū: yellow urine, and dry tongue with dispersion-thirst.

注：以上皆心火之熾也，唇爲脾經所司，乃泄其子，以衰其母之義。

Explanation: all of the above are due to the intense heat of heart fire, although the lips are what the spleen channel controls, this is the concept that one should drain the child in order to reduce the mother.

Twenty-Seventh Point of the Dū Channel
Yín Jiāo – Gum Intersection (DU-28)
督經第二十七穴齦交

穴在唇内齒上齦縫中，任經、督經、足陽明胃經之會。《銅人》：鍼三分，灸三壯。

This point is located in the cleft, in the centre of the gum above the teeth, on the inside of the lips. It is the meeting of the rèn channel, dū channel, and foot yángmíng stomach channel. *The Tóngrén* states, "Needle 3 fēn, and moxa 3 cones."

注：齦者，齒根也，爲三陽交會之所，故曰齦交。

Explanation: Yín (Gum) is the root of the teeth; in addition, as [this point] is the place where the three yáng Jiāo (Intersect) and meet, thus it is called Yín Jiāo (Gum Intersection).

督之本病：額頰中痛，頭項强，鼻中瘜肉蝕瘡，鼻塞不利。

Principal disease of the dū: pain in the forehead and bridge of the nose, stiffness of the neck and nape, polyps and eroding sores in the nose, and nasal congestion with inhibition [of breathing].

注：以上症皆督經之在此穴上者，取下穴以泄之，且爲督經之盡穴，一泄而督經之火盡泄。

Explanation: all of the above signs are located [in the areas of] the dū channel above this point, choose this point that is below to drain them; moreover, as it is the terminal point on the dū channel, once it is drained, the fire of the dū channel will be completely drained.

督之肝病：內眥赤癢痛，生白翳。

Liver diseases of Dū: itchiness and pain of the inner canthus, and generation of white eye screens.

注：此雖目病也，而足陽明經亦會於睛明，故取此穴泄之。

Explanation: although these are eye diseases, the foot yángmíng channel also meets at Jīng Míng (BL-1), thus choose this point in order to drain it.

督之胃病：牙疳腫痛，面赤心煩，馬黃黃疸，寒暑瘟疫，小兒面瘡，癬久不除，點烙亦佳。

Stomach diseases of the dū: gān of the teeth and gums with swelling and pain, red face with vexation of the heart, jaundice that is the colour of a yellow horse, warm epidemic in summer and winter, facial sores in children, and chronic lichens that do not heal, for which it is also adequate to [treat by] spot scolding.

注：以上皆胃經之症也。牙者，胃之經所行也，面亦胃經所行也。馬黃黃疸，皆胃有濕熱也；寒暑瘟疫，胃有毒也；小兒面瘡，胃經行於面，有風熱也，故取此穴。

Explanation: all of the above are signs of the stomach channel. While the teeth are where the stomach channel travels, the face is also where the stomach channel travels. For jaundice that is the colour of a yellow horse, it is because of the presence of damp heat in the stomach. For warm epidemic in summer and winter, it is because of the presence of toxin in the stomach. For facial sores in children, it is because of wind and heat in the stomach channel, which travels to the face, thus choose this point.

Extra Points Associated with the Dū Channel
督經奇穴

Five Points on the Spine and Upper Back (UEX-B 2)
Jǐ Bèi Wǔ Xué - 脊背五穴

《千金翼》云：治大人癲疾，小兒驚癇，灸背第二椎上，及下窮骨尖兩處，再以繩度量上下，中折復量至脊骨上點記之，共三處畢，復斷此繩，取其半者爲三折，而參合如乙字，以上角對中央一穴，下二角正挾脊兩邊，同灸之，凡五處也，各百壯。

The Qiānjīn Yì states, "**To treat withdrawal diseases in adults and fright epilepsy in children, moxa the two places: one above the second vertebra on the upper-back and another below the tip of the coccyx. Furthermore, use a rope to measure the distance between [these two points] above and below, fold the rope in half and mark [the midpoint] on the spine; as such, there are now three points in total. Cut off the rope [at its fold]; pick up [one rope] at half length, fold it into three segments of equal length, and join the ends together to form the shape of the character, 乙.[639] Place the upper angle on the middle point,[640] and the lower two angles will clasp the spine on the two sides. Moxa 100 cones on each of these five places.**

Circulating Qì (UEX-B 9)
Huí Qì - 迴氣

在脊窮骨上，赤白肉下，主五痔便血失屎，灸百壯。《千金翼》云：灸窮骨，惟多爲佳。又治赤白下痢，灸窮骨頭百壯，多多爲佳。又云：灸尾翠骨七壯，治脫肛，神良。《千金》作龜尾，即窮骨也。

This point is located on the coccyx, below the red and white flesh; moxa 100 cones to govern the five [types of] haemorrhoids, bloody stool, and faecal incontinence.

The Qiānjīn Yì states, "**Moxa on the coccyx, a greater amount [of moxa] is always better. Also, to treat red and white dysentery, moxa 100 cones on the head of the coccyx, it is better to have a higher and greater amount [of moxa].**"

---

639 In *the Qiānjīn Yì*, this character is actually ㄥ; as such, this means to fold the rope in half-length into an equilateral triangle.

640 I.e., the marked midpoint between the second vertebra and the tip of the coccyx.

It also states, "Moxa 7 cones on Wěi Cuì Gǔ (Tail Kingfisher Bone)[641] to treat prolapse of the rectum, it will be miraculously effective." *The Qiānjīn* refers to [this point] as Guī Wěi (Tortoise Tail),[642] which precisely indicates the coccyx.

《甲乙經》云：腰痛上寒，實則脊強，此穴主之。又云：癲疾發如狂者，面皮厚敦敦不治，虛則頭重，洞泄淋癃，大小便難，腰尻重難起，此穴主之。又云：小兒驚癇瘈瘲，脊強互相引，此穴主之。

The Jiǎyǐ Jīng states, "For lumbar pain with cold above, when it is replete, it will cause rigidity of the spine; this point governs it." It also states, "For withdrawal disease with [periodic] episodes of mania, thickening and firming of the facial skin that is untreatable; when it is vacuous, it will cause heavy-headedness, throughflux diarrhoea, strangury and dribbling urinary block, difficult urination and defecation, and heaviness of the lumbus with difficulty to stand up [from sitting]; this point governs these [signs]." It also states, "For fright epilepsy with tugging and slackening in children, as well as stiffness of the spine that radiates [between above and below], this point governs these [signs]."

Point [Below] the Seventeenth Vertebra (EX-B 8)
Shí Qī Zhuī Xué - 十七椎穴

《千金翼》云：轉胞腰痛，灸十七椎五十壯。

The Qiānjīn Yì states, "For shifted bladder and lumbar pain, moxa 50 cones [below] the seventeenth vertebra."

Lower Extreme Transport (EX-B 5)
Xià Jí Shù – 下極腧

《千金翼》云：十五椎名下極腧，主腹中疾，腰痛膀胱寒，澼飲注下，灸隨年壯。

The Qiānjīn Yì states, "It is [below] the fifteenth vertebra, and it is named Xià Jí Shù (Lower Extreme Transport); it governs the treatment of diseases within the abdomen, lumbar pain and cold in the bladder, afflux of liquids and downpour diarrhoea; moxa with the number of cones according to one's age."

---

[641] This is an alternate name for DU-1.
[642] This is also an alternate name for DU-1.

Central Pivot (DU-7)
Zhōng Shū - 中樞

此穴在第十椎節下間，俯而取之。此穴諸書皆失之，惟氣府論督脈下王氏注中有此穴。

This point is located in the space below the tenth vertebra, lie prostate to locate it. This point was omitted from all [previous] works, except for "the Treatise on the Qì Mansion,"[643] where this point appears in Mister Wáng's annotation after [the passage regarding] the dū vessel.

及考之《氣穴論》曰：背與心相控而痛，所治天突與十椎者，其穴即此。刺五分，禁灸，灸之令人腰痛傴僂。

In addition, upon investigating "the Treatise on the Qì Points,"[644] which states, "When there is a pain that radiates between the upper back and heart, that which treats [this pain] is Tiān Tū (REN-22) and [the point below] the tenth vertebra," that latter point precisely refers to this (DU-7). Pierce 5 fēn, and moxibustion is contraindicated; if one utilises moxa, it will cause lumbar pain with stooping."

Rear Alert Spirit (EX-HN 1)
Hòu Shén Cōng - 後神聰

去百會一寸，主治中風風癇，灸三壯。

This point is located 1 cùn from Bǎi Huì (DU-20); moxa 3 cones to govern the treatment of wind strike and wind epilepsy.

Front Alert Spirit (EX-HN 1)
Qián Shén Cōng -前神聰

去前頂五分，自神庭至此穴共四寸，主治中風風癇，灸三壯。

This point is 5 fēn from Qián Dǐng (DU-21). From Shén Tíng (DU-24) to this point, there is in total [a distance of] 4 cùn; moxa 3 cones to govern the treatment of wind strike and wind epilepsy.

---

643 *Sùwèn* Chapter 59.
644 *Sùwèn* Chapter 58.

Hall of Impression (EX-HN 3)

Yìn Táng - 印堂

在兩眉中間。《神農經》云：治小兒急慢驚風，可灸三壯，艾炷如小麥。

This point is located in the centre between the eyebrows. *The Shénnóng Jīng* **states, "One can moxa 3 cones to treat both urgent and chronic fright wind in children; the cones should resemble the size of a wheat grain."**

Junction of Nose and Forehead (UEX-HN 12)

Bí Jiāo È Zhōng - 鼻交頞中

《千金翼》云：主治癲風，角弓反張，羊鳴，大風青風，面風如蟲行，卒風多唾，健忘，心中憒憒，口噤，卒倒不識人，黃疸急黃，此穴皆主之。鍼入六分，得氣即泄，留三呼，泄五吸，亦宜灸，然不及鍼。慎忌酒、麵、生冷、醋、猪肉、魚、蒜、蕎麥、漿水。

The Qiānjīn Yì **states, "It governs the treatment of withdrawal wind, arched-back rigidity, bleating like a goat, great wind with blue-green wind, face wind as though the insects were burrowing, sudden wind with copious spittle, forgetfulness, restlessness in the heart, clenched jaw, sudden collapse with inability to recognise people, jaundice and acute yellowing; all of which are governed by this point. Insert the needle with 6 fēn, obtain qì then promptly drain, retain for 3 respirations, and drain for 5 exhalations; it is also appropriate to moxa, but it is inferior to needling. One should attentively avoid alcohol, flour-based foods, raw and cold food, vinegar, pork, fish, garlic, buckwheat, and sour millet water.**

《神農經》云：治小兒急慢驚風，可灸三壯，炷如小麥。《千金》云：此穴爲鬼市，治百邪癲狂。此當第一次下鍼，凡人中惡邪，先掐鼻下是也。鬼擊卒死者，須即灸之。

The Shénnóng Jīng **states, "One can moxa 3 cones to treat both urgent and chronic fright wind in children; the cones should resemble the size of a wheat grain."**

The Qiānjīn **states, "This point is Guǐ Shì (Ghost Market); it treats mania and withdrawal caused by hundred evils. This ought to be the first [point] to needle; whenever a person suffers a malignity stroke, first pinch below the nose. For a ghost attack that causes [a state that resembles] sudden death, one must immediately moxa it.**

393

The Yīnwéi Vessel

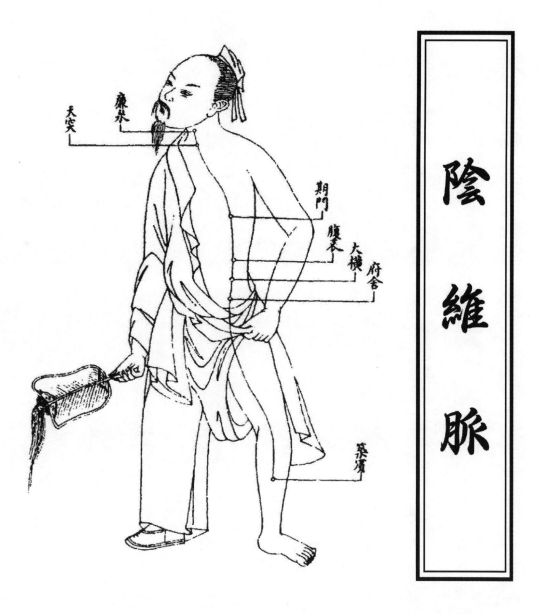

The Yīnwéi Vessel

陰維脈

思蓮子曰：陰維起於諸陰之交，其脈發於足少陰腎經築賓穴，在內踝上五寸腨肉之分中，爲陰維之郤。上循股內廉，上行入小腹，遂會足太陰脾經、足厥陰肝經、足少陰腎經、足陽明胃經於脾經之府舍穴。

Master Sīlián says, the yīnwéi [vessel] commences at the intersection of all yīn [channels]. This vessel emerges at Zhù Bīn (KI-9) of the foot shàoyīn kidney channel, the cleft [point] of the yīnwéi [vessel], which is located 5 cùn above the inner ankle [bone], in the centre of the calf muscle. It ascends following the inner ridge of the thigh, travelling to enter the lower abdomen; thereupon, it meets the foot tàiyīn spleen channel, the foot juéyīn liver channel, the foot shàoyīn kidney channel, and the foot yángmíng stomach channel at Fǔ Shè (SP-13) of the spleen channel.

此穴在脾經腹結穴下三寸，去腹中行四寸半，脾、肝、腎三經自下而上行，胃經自上而下行，陰維脈亦自下而上行，統會於此穴，入腹絡脾肝，結心肺，從脇上至肩。此穴爲太陰郤，三陰、陽明之別，既會此四經於此穴，又上腹會足太陰脾經於大橫穴，在腹哀下三寸六分。

This point (SP-13) is located 3 cùn below Fù Jié (SP-14) of the spleen channel, 4 and a half cùn from the midline; while the three channels, spleen, liver, and kidney, ascend from below, the stomach channel descends from above; likewise, the yīnwéi vessel ascends from below, meets with all [these channels] at this point (SP-13), where it enters the abdomen to network with the spleen and liver, binds with the heart and lung, and ascends to arrive at the shoulder from the rib-side. This point (SP-13) is the tàiyīn cleft [point] and the divergence of the three yīn and yángmíng [channels]; after meeting with these four channels at this point, [the yīnwéi vessel] continues to ascend the abdomen and meets the tàiyīn spleen channel at Dà Héng (SP-15), which is located 3 cùn 6 fēn[645] below Fù Āi (SP-16).

又上行會太陰脾經於腹哀穴，在膽經日月穴下一寸五分。二穴又並去中行四寸，遂循胸脇會足厥陰肝經於期門穴，乳下一寸五分，遂上胸膈挾咽，與任脈會於結喉下四寸半宛宛中之天突穴。又上行會任脈在結喉上二寸中央之廉泉穴。

---

645 For "3 cùn 6 fēn," the secondary manuscript has "3 cùn 5 fēn."

It continues to ascend to meet the tàiyīn spleen channel at Fù Āi (SP-16), which is located 1 cùn 5 fēn below Rì Yuè (GB-24) of the gallbladder channel; these two points are both 4 cùn from the midline. Thereupon, it follows the chest and rib-side to meet the juéyīn liver channel at Qī Mén (LR-14), which is located 1 cùn 5 fēn below the nipple.[646] Thereupon, it ascends the chest and diaphragm, clasps the pharynx, and meets with the rèn vessel at Tiān Tū (REN-22), which is located in the depression 4 and a half cùn below the laryngeal prominence. It continues to ascend and meets with the rèn vessel at Lián Quán (REN-23), which is located at the midline, 2 cùn above the laryngeal prominence.

其所經共七穴，一始腎之築賓，二會足三陰、足陽明於府舍，三會、四會，獨會足太陰之大橫、腹哀，五獨會足厥陰經於期門，六會、七會任經之天突、廉泉。

In total, it passes through seven points. The first is the beginning at Zhù Bīn (KI-9) of the kidney [channel]; the second is the meeting with the three foot yīn and foot yángmíng [channels] at Fǔ Shè (SP-13); the third and fourth meetings are only with the foot tàiyīn [channel] at Dà Héng (SP-15) and Fù Āi (SP-16); the fifth meeting is only with the juéyīn channel at Qī Mén (LR-14); the sixth and seventh meetings are with the rèn channel at Tiān Tū (REN-22) and Lián Quán (REN-23).

經之過，皆足三陰、任經之穴，起於腎，過於脾肝，而終於任脈。所行皆陰之營分也，故曰陰維維於陰，陰不能維於陰，則悵然失志，溶溶不能自收持。陰維爲病苦心痛，苦心痛者何也？營爲陰，陰維受邪，爲病在裏，故苦心痛。

All the traversing of this channel occurs at points of the three foot yīn and rèn channels; it commences at the kidney [channel], traverses the spleen and liver [channels], and terminates at the rèn vessel. Since it travels entirely in the yíng-nutritive aspect of the yīn, thus it is said that the yīnwéi [vessel] Wéi (Links)[647] the yīn together. When the [yīnwéi] fails to Wéi (Link) the yīn together, there will be disappointment, frustration, loss of will, and flaccidity with inability to support oneself. When the yīnwéi [vessel] is diseased, one will suffer from heart pain.[648] Why does one suffer heart pain? [Because] the yíng-nutritive is yīn; when the yīnwéi [vessel] contracts an evil, the disease will manifest in the interior, thus one will suffer from heart pain.

寸口脈，從少陰斜至厥陰者，是陰維脈部分，其陰不動則陰維無病，如其處脈動，苦癲癇，僵仆羊鳴。

---

[646] For "1 cùn 5 fēn below the nipple," the secondary manuscript has "4 cùn 5 fēn to the side of Jù Què (REN-14)."

[647] Note: while this "維 links" shares the same character as "wéi 維" of the "yīnwéi 陰維 vessel," it is used as a verb here to denote the function of the vessel.

[648] From *Nànjīng* Difficulty 29.

又苦僵仆失音，肌肉痺癢，應時自發，汗出惡風，身沉沉然也。取陽白、金門、
僕參。

At the cùnkǒu pulse, [the area] that extends obliquely from the shàoyīn to the juéyīn, this is the yīnwéi pulse area. When the yīn [aspect of the pulse] is not stirred, then there is no disease in the yīnwéi [vessel]. If the pulse at this position is stirred, one will suffer from withdrawal epilepsy, sudden collapse and bleating like a sheep.

When one suffers from sudden collapse and loss of voice, impediment and itchiness of the flesh that occurs spontaneously and periodically, and sweating with aversion to wind, with extreme heaviness of the body; in that case, choose Yáng Bái (GB-14), Jīn Mén (BL-63), and Pú Cān (BL-61).

陽白系膽經穴，在眉上一寸，直瞳子，手、足陽明、少陽、陽維五脈之會。金門
系膀胱經穴，在外踝下少後，丘墟後，申脈前，足太陽郄，陽維別屬。僕參亦系
膀胱經穴，在足跟骨下陷中，拱足取之，陽蹻之本。

Yáng Bái (GB-14) is by association a gallbladder channel point, it is located 1 cùn above the eyebrow, in line with the pupil; it is the meeting of five vessels, the hand and foot yángmíng and shàoyáng, as well as the yángwéi. Jīn Mén (BL-63) is by association a bladder channel point, it is located below and slightly behind the outer ankle [bone], behind Qiū Xū (BL-40), and in front of Shēn Mài (BL-62). It is the foot tàiyáng cleft [point], and the adjoint to the yángwéi divergence. Pú Cān (BL-61) is by association a bladder channel point, it is located in the depression of the heel bone, which is found by arching the foot; it is the root of the yángqiāo [vessel].

診得陰維脈沉大而實者，苦胸中痛，脅下支滿，心痛，其脈如貫珠者，男子兩脅
實，腰中痛，女子陰中痛，如有瘡狀。又陰維脈亦能使人腰痛。

In diagnosis, upon observing a yīnwéi pulse that is deep, large, and replete, one will suffer from pain in the chest, propping fullness under the rib-sides, and heart pain. If the pulse resembles a string of pearls, for males, there will be repletion in both rib-sides and pain in the lumbus; for females, there will be pain in the genitals, as though there is a physical manifestation of sores.[649] In addition, [a disease in] the yīnwéi vessel can also cause a person to have lumbar pain.

---

649 From *Màijīng* Vol. 2, Chapter 4.

經云：飛陽之脈，令人腰痛怫怫然，甚則悲以恐。

The Canon states, "[A disease in] the vessel of the flying yáng[650] will cause lumbar pain that makes the person anxious and depressed; when it is severe, there will be sadness accompanied by fear."[651]

王注曰：此陰維之脈也，去内踝上五寸腨肉分中，並足少陰經而上行者。刺飛揚之脈，在内踝上五寸，少陰之前，與陰維之會築賓也。此穴乃陰維發脈之始也。

Wáng [Bīng] commentates, "This is the vessel of the yīnwéi; it is 5 cùn above the inner ankle [bone] and in the centre of the flesh divide of the calf; it ascends together with the foot shàoyīn channel. To pierce the vessel of the flying yáng, do so at 5 cùn above the inner ankle [bone], in front of the shàoyīn, and where it meets with the yīnwéi [vessel],"[652] which is namely Zhù Bīn (KI-9). This point is the beginning of where the yīnwéi vessel emerges.

---

[650] According to the *Sùwèn* passage, this vessel occurs at "five cùn above the inner ankle and in front of the shàoyīn [channel]." Side note: Flying Yáng is very similar to the name of Fēi Yáng 飛揚 (BL-58 Taking Flight).

[651] From *Sùwèn* Chapter 41.

[652] From *Sùwèn* Chapter 41 commentary by Wáng Bīng.

The Yángwéi Vessel

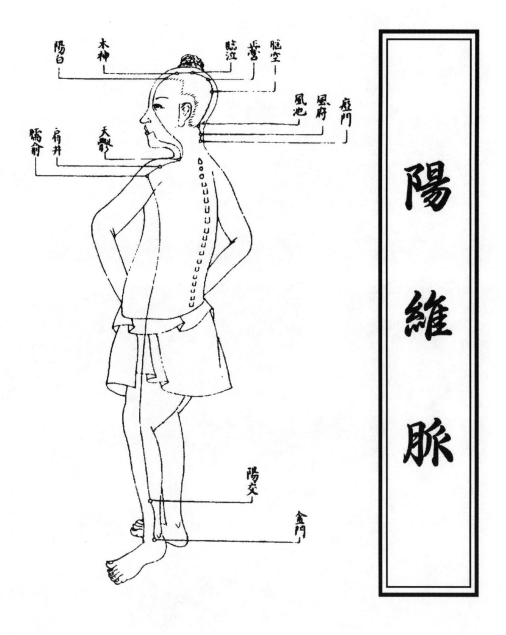

陽維脈

The Yángwéi Vessel

陽維脈

思蓮子曰：陽維起於諸陽之會，其脈發於足太陽外踝下、丘墟後、申脈前，足太
陽郄，陽維別屬於金門穴，遂上外踝七寸，會足少陽於斜屬太陽、陽明二陽之間
陽交穴，乃循膝外廉，上髀厭之環跳穴，而與足太陽、足少陽會，

**Master Sīlián says, the yángwéi [vessel] commences at the meeting of all yáng
[channels]. This vessel effuses below the outer ankle [bone] at Jīn Mén (BL-63)
of the foot tàiyáng, which is located behind Qiū Xū (GB-40) and in front of Shēn
Mài (BL-62); it is the foot tàiyáng cleft point and the adjoint to the yángwéi
divergence.**

**Thereupon, it ascends 7 cùn above the outer ankle [bone] to Yáng Jiāo (GB-
35), where it meets with the foot shàoyáng [channel] and obliquely adjoins to
the space between the two yáng [channels], the tàiyáng and yángmíng. It
continues to follow the outer face of the thigh and ascend to Huán Tiào (GB-
30) on the hip joint, where it meets with the foot tàiyáng and shàoyáng
[channels].**

遂抵小腹之側，而又會足少陽於章門下八寸，監骨上陷中之居髎穴，遂循脅肋斜
上於肘上，會於手陽明大腸經、手太陽小腸經，足太陽膀胱經於肘上七寸兩筋罅
陷中，在肩髃穴下一寸之臂臑穴，乃過肩之前，與手少陽會於在肩前去肩端三寸
之宛宛中臑會穴，及缺盆中上毖骨際陷中央之天髎穴，

**Thereupon, it reaches the side of the lower abdomen and further meets with
the foot shàoyáng [channel] at Jū Liáo (GB-29), which is located in the
depression above the haunch bone, 8 cùn below Zhāng Mén (LR-13).**

**Thereupon, it follows the rib-side, ascends obliquely to Bì Nào (LI-14) above
the elbow, which is located 7 cùn above the elbow, in the depression between
the two sinews, and 1 cùn below Jiān Yú (LI-15), where it meets with the hand
yángmíng large intestine channel, hand tàiyáng small intestine channel, and
foot tàiyáng bladder channel.**

**Then it traverses the front of the shoulder to meet the hand shàoyáng
[channel] at Nào Huì (SJ-13), which is located in the depression 3 cùn from the
edge of the shoulder, as well as Tiān Liáo (SJ-15), which is directly above the**

centre of Quē Pén (ST-12) and at the centre of the depression at the border of the hidden bone.[653]

却向後上行上肩，會手少陽三焦經、足少陽膽經、足陽明胃經於肩上陷中，大骨前寸半之肩井穴，遂却行向後入肩之後，會手太陽小腸經、陽蹻於肩後大骨下，胛上廉陷中之臑腧穴，

It turns back towards the rear and ascends over the shoulder to meet with the hand shàoyáng sānjiāo channel, foot shàoyáng gallbladder channel, and foot yángmíng stomach channel at Jiān Jǐng (GB-21), which is located in the depression above the shoulder, 1 cùn and a half in front of the great bone.

Thereupon, it [again] turns back towards the rear, enters the rear of the shoulder, where it meets with the hand tàiyáng small intestine channel and yángqiāo [vessel] at Nào Shù (SI-10), which is located in the depression on the upper ridge of the scapula, below the great bone behind the shoulder.

遂上頸循耳後，會手少陽三焦經、足少陽膽經於耳後髮際陷中之風池穴，

Thereupon, it ascends the neck to behind the ear, where it meets with the hand shàoyáng sānjiāo channel and foot shàoyáng gallbladder channel at Fēng Chí (GB-20), which is in the depression at the hairline behind the ear.

遂上頸之後，遂會足少陽膽經在頸之正行五穴，先會膽經於承靈後寸半，挾玉枕骨下陷中央之腦空穴，

Thereupon, it ascends the rear of the neck, where it meets with the five points on the principal pathway of the shàoyáng gallbladder channel on the neck [and head]: firstly, it meets with the gallbladder channel at Nǎo Kōng (GB-19), which is 1 cùn and half behind Chéng Líng (GB-18), in the centre of the depression that clasps the jade [pillow] bone.

次上會膽經正營穴後寸半之承靈穴，次上會膽經於目窗穴後寸半之正營穴，次上會膽經之臨泣穴後寸半之目窗穴，次上會膽經於在瞳人直上入髮際五分陷中之臨泣穴，

Next, it ascends to meet with the gallbladder [channel] at Chéng Líng (GB-18), which is 1 and a half cùn behind Zhèng Yíng (GB-17); then it ascends [again] to meet with the gallbladder [channel] at Zhèng Yíng (GB-17), which is 1 and a half cùn behind Mù Chuāng (GB-16);

Next, it ascends to meet with the gallbladder at Mù Chuāng (GB-16), which is 1 and a half cùn behind [Tóu] Lín Qì (GB-15); then, it ascends to meet with the

---

[653] I.e., the superior angle of the scapula.

gallbladder channel at [Tóu] Lín Qì (GB-15), which is in the depression 5 fēn into the hairline and directly above the pupil.

遂下頰與手少陽三焦經、足少陽膽經、手陽明大腸經、足陽明胃經並本經俱會於眉上一寸之直瞳人相對之陽白穴，循頸入耳，又出耳上，至直耳上入髮際之本神穴而終。

Thereupon, it descends the forehead; the hand shàoyáng sānjiāo channel, foot shàoyáng gallbladder channel, hand yángmíng large intestine channel, foot yángmíng stomach channel, and this channel then meet together at Yáng Bái (GB-14), which is 1 cùn above the eyebrow, in line with the pupil.

It follows the neck to enter the ear, then emerges at the top of the ear to arrive and terminate at Běn Shén (GB-13), which is into the hairline and directly above the ear.

維者，溢蓄不能環流灌溉諸經者也。

Regarding the wéi [vessels], by amassing what overflows and what fails to circulate, they irrigate all channels.[654]

其所歷共十六穴，一始發足太陽之金門穴、二會足少陽於足少陽之陽交，三會足少陽於足少陽之居髎穴，四上肘會手陽明、手太陽、足太陽於臂臑，五會上肩前會手少陽於少陽臑會、天髎，六會却會手、足少陽、足陽明於肩井，

It passes through a total of sixteen points: the first begins by emerging at Jīn Mén (BL-63) of the foot tàiyáng [channel]; the second is the meeting with the shàoyáng [channel] at Yáng Jiāo (GB-35) of the foot shàoyáng [channel]; the third is the meeting with the foot shàoyáng [channel] at Jū Liáo (GB-29) of the foot shàoyáng [channel];

The fourth is the meeting above the elbow with the hand yángmíng, hand tàiyáng, and foot tàiyáng [channels] at Bì Nào (LI-14); the fifth meeting occurs in front and above the shoulder, where it meets with the hand shàoyáng at Nào Huì (SJ-13) and Tiān Liáo (SJ-15) of the [hand] shàoyáng [channel]; the sixth meeting occurs as it pulls back to meet with the hand and foot shàoyáng and foot yángmíng [channels] at Jiān Jǐng (GB-21);

七會入肩後會手太陽、陽蹻於手太陽之臑腧，八會耳後會手、足少陽於足少陽之風池，九會遂上足少陽在頭之腦空、承靈、正營、目窗、臨泣五穴，足少陽由五穴而向後行，陽維由五穴而向前行，十會下頰與手少陽、足少陽、手陽明、足陽明會於足少陽之陽白，十一循頸入耳，與足少陽會於手少陽之本神。

---

[654] From *Nànjīng* Difficulty 28.

The seventh meeting occurs as it enters the rear shoulder, where it meets with the hand tàiyáng [channel] and yángqiāo [vessel] at Nào Shù (SI-10) of the hand tàiyáng [channel]; the eighth meeting occurs behind the ear, where it meets with the hand and foot shàoyáng [channels] at Fēng Chí (GB-21) of the foot shàoyáng [channel];

At the ninth meeting, it ascends through the five points of the foot shàoyáng [channel] on the head, which are Nǎo Kōng (GB-19), Chéng Líng (GB-18), Zhèng Yíng (GB-17), Mù Chuāng (GB-16), and [Tóu] Lín Qì (GB-15); while the foot shàoyáng [channel] follows these five points to travel towards the rear, the yángwéi [vessel] follows these five points to travel towards the front;

The tenth meeting occurs after it descends the forehead, where it meets with the hand shàoyáng, foot shàoyáng, hand yángmíng, and foot yángmíng [channels] at Yáng Bái (GB-14) of the foot shàoyáng [channel]; the eleventh [meeting] occurs after it follows the neck to enter the ear, where it meets with the foot shàoyáng [channel] at Běn Shén (GB-13) of the foot shàoyáng [channel].[655]

以上凡手之三陽經，足之三陽經，並陽蹻經，無不周環會合，所謂陽維起於諸陽之會，而維諸陽者此也。

At these aforementioned [meetings], all of the three yáng channels of the hand, the three yáng channels of the foot, as well as the yángqiāo channel, without exception, they all circulate, meet, and unite [with the yángwéi vessel]; that is why the yángwéi [vessel] is said to commence at the meeting of all yáng [channels] and further Wéi (Link) all yáng [channels] together.

如陽不能維於陽，則亦陰維之不能維於陰，亦悵然失志，溶溶不能自收持者也。陽維爲病，則苦寒熱。衛爲陽主表，陽維受邪，爲病在表，故苦寒熱。

If the [yángwéi vessel] fails to Wéi (Link) the yáng together, it is just like when the yīnwéi [vessel] fails to Wéi (Link) the yīn together, there will be disappointment and frustration, loss of will, and flaccidity with inability to support oneself.

When the yángwéi [vessel] is diseased, one will suffer from chills and fevers.[656] As the wèi-defensive qì is the yáng that governs the exterior, when the yángwéi [vessel] contracts evil, the disease is located in the exterior, thus there are chills and fever.

---

[655] "Běn Shén (GB-13) of the foot shàoyáng [channel]" is originally "Běn Shén (GB-13) of the hand shàoyáng [channel]" in the manuscript; we have changed it in accordance with the point listed.

[656] From Nànjīng Difficulty 29.

從少陽斜至太陽者，是陽維脈也。不動則陽維無病，如其部分脈動，則苦肌肉痺癢，皮膚痛下部不仁，汗出而寒。又苦癲仆羊鳴，手足相引，甚者失音不能言，宜取膽經之客主人。穴在耳前起骨有孔，乃手、足少陽、陽明四經相會之處。

[The wrist pulse] that extends obliquely from the shàoyáng to the tàiyáng, this is the yángwéi pulse. When it is not stirred, there is no disease in the yángwéi [vessel]. If the pulse at this position is stirred, one will suffer from impediment and itchiness of the muscles and flesh, skin pain, insensitivity of the lower body, sweating and chills. Also, one will suffer from epilepsy [that causes the person to] collapse and bleat like a sheep, and contraction of the hands and feet; when it is severe, there will be loss of voice with inability to speak, it is appropriate to choose Kè Zhǔ Rén (GB-3) of the gallbladder channel. This point is located in the hollow by the prominent bone in front of the ear, it is the meeting place of the four channels, the hand and foot shàoyáng and yángmíng [channels].

李氏曰：王氏以癲癇屬陽維、陰維，而《靈樞》以癲癇屬陽蹻、陰蹻，二說義理相同。王氏曰：診得陽維脈浮者，暫起目眩。陽盛實者，苦肩息，洒洒如寒。陽維之脈，亦令人腰痛。

Mister Lǐ [Shízhēn] says, "Mister Wáng [Shūhé] believes that withdrawal epilepsy pertains to the yángwéi and yīnwéi [vessels]; however, according to the Língshū, withdrawal epilepsy belongs to the yángqiāo and yīnqiāo [vessels]; these two theories agree with each other in their principles and reasoning."[657]

Mister Wáng [Shūhé] says, "When one is diagnosed with a yángwéi pulse that is floating, there will be dizzy vision upon standing up abruptly; for those with repletion of exuberant yáng, they will suffer from raised-shoulder breathing and continuous shivering with feeling of cold."[658] In addition, [a disease in] the yángwéi vessel can also cause a person to have lumbar pain.

經曰：陽維腰痛，痛上怫然腫，刺陽維之脈與太陽合腨間，去地一尺。王氏曰：陽維起於陽，則太陽之所生，並行而上至腨下，復與太陽合而上也。去地一尺，乃承山穴也，在銳腨腸分肉陷中，可刺七分。

The Canon states, "For lumbar pain of the yángwéi [vessel], the pain will ascend and [makes the person] anxious and depressed with the appearance of swelling; pierce the space on the calf, where the vessel of the yángwéi and the tàiyáng [channel] unite, 1 chǐ from the ground."[659]

---

[657] From the Qíjīng Bāmài Kǎo 奇經八脈考 (An Investigation of the Eight Extraordinary Channels, 1578 CE).

[658] From Màijīng Vol. 2, Chapter 4.

[659] From Sùwèn Chapter 41.

Mister Wáng [Bīng] says, "As the yángwéi [vessel] commences from the yáng, it is engendered by the tàiyáng [channel]; it travels parallel with [the tàiyáng channel] and ascends to arrive below the calf, where it further unites with the tàiyáng [channel] and ascends together. Regarding '1 chǐ from the ground,' this is referring to Chéng Shān (BL-57), which is located in the depression below the edges of the calf intestine; one can pierce 7 fēn into it."[660]

又云：肉里之脈，令人腰痛，不可以咳，咳則筋縮急，刺肉里之脈，爲二痏，在太陽之外，少陽絶骨之後。王氏曰：肉里之脈，少陽所生，陽維脈氣所發，絶骨之後，陽維所過分肉穴也，在足外踝直上絶骨之端，如後二分筋骨間，可刺五分。

[*The Canon*] also states, "[A disease in] the vessel of the interior flesh will cause a person to have lumbar pain, who finds it intolerable while coughing; upon coughing, there will be tension and contraction of the sinews; pierce the vessel of the interior flesh, perform it twice; it is located outside of the tàiyáng [channel] and behind Jué Gǔ (GB-39) of the shàoyáng [channel]."[661]

Mister Wáng [Bīng] says, "The vessel of the interior flesh is engendered by the shàoyáng [channel], and it is effused by the yángwéi vessel qì; it is namely Fēn Ròu[662] (GB-38) located behind Jué Gǔ (GB-39),[663] where the yángwéi vessel traverses; it is located between the bone and sinew, 2 fēn behind the tip of the severed bone, which is directly above the outer ankle [bone]; one can pierce 5 fēn into it."[664]

---

660 *Sùwèn* Chapter 41 commentary by Wáng Bīng.
661 From *Sùwèn* Chapter 41.
662 I.e., an alternate name for GB-38.
663 I.e., an alternate name for GB-39.
664 *Sùwèn* Chapter 41 commentary by Wáng Bīng.

The Yīnqiāo Vessel

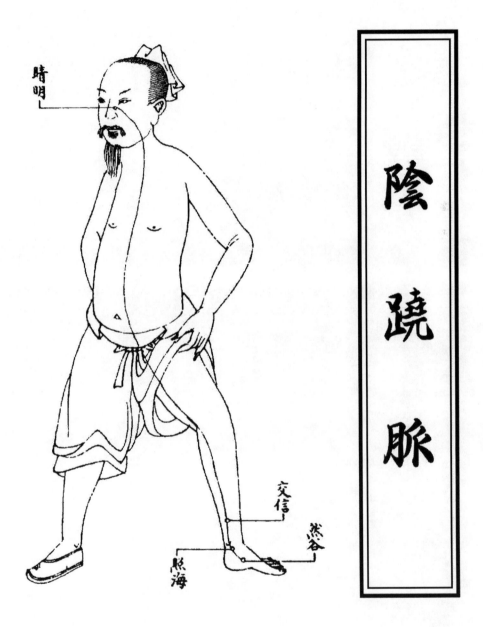

睛明

交信

然谷

照海

陰蹺脈

The Yīnqiāo Vessel

陰蹻脈

思蓮子曰：陰蹻者，足少陰之別脈，其脈起於跟中足少陰然谷穴之後，同足少陰循內踝下照海穴，在內踝下五分，上內踝上之二寸，在內踝骨上，少陰前，太陰後廉，筋骨間之交信穴，以此穴爲郄，

Master Sīlián says, the yīnqiāo is a branch vessel of the foot shàoyīn [channel]. This vessel commences from within the heel, behind Rán Gǔ (KI-2) of the foot shàoyīn [channel]; together with the foot shàoyīn [channel], it follows Zhào Hǎi (KI-6), which is 5 fēn below the inner ankle [bone]. It then ascends to 2 cùn above the inner ankle [bone] to Jiāo Xìn (KI-8), which is located in the space between the sinew and bone, above the inner ankle bone, in front of the shàoyīn [channel], and behind the ridge of the tàiyīn [channel]; this point also serves as the cleft point [of the yīnqiāo vessel].

遂直上循陰股入陰，上循胸裏出缺盆，上入人迎之前，至喉嚨交貫衝脈，入頄內廉，入鼻上行屬目內眥，與手太陽、足太陽、足陽明、陽蹻五脈，會於睛明穴而上行，女子以之爲經，男子以之爲絡。

Thereupon, it ascends in a straight line along the yīn of the thigh to enter the genitals, ascends following the interior of the chest to emerge at Quē Pén (ST-12), ascends to enter the front of Rén Yíng (ST-9), and arrives at the throat to intersect and pierce the chōng vessel. It enters the inner ridge of the cheekbone, enters the nose, and ascends to adjoin to the inner canthus; together with the hand tàiyáng, foot tàiyáng, foot yángmíng, and yángqiāo [vessels], these five vessels meet at Jīng Míng (BL-1); thereupon, it continues to ascend. In females, it is considered as a channel, whereas in males, it is considered as a network-vessel.[665]

陰蹻以交信爲郄，陰蹻爲病，陽緩而陰急，陽緩而陰急者，當從內踝以上急，外踝以上緩。

For the yīnqiāo [vessel], Jiāo Xìn (KI-8) serves as the cleft point.

---

[665] Regarding the yīnqiāo as a channel in females and as a network-vessel in males, see footnote 35.

When the yīnqiāo [vessel] is diseased, the yáng will be slack and the yīn will be tense.[666] Regarding "the yáng is slack and the yīn is tense," this refers precisely to the tension above the inner ankle [bone] and slackening above the outer ankle [bone].

寸口脈後部左右彈者，陰蹻也。此脈不動則陰蹻無病，如動則苦癲癇，寒熱，皮膚淫痹。又爲少腹痛，裏急，腰及髖髎下相連，陰中痛，男子陰疝，女子漏下不止。

When the pulse is flicking in the rear positions of cùnkǒu pulse on both left and right, this is the yīnqiāo [pulse].[667] When the pulses [at these positions] are not stirred, there is no disease in the yīnqiāo [vessel]. If they are stirred, one will suffer from epilepsy, chills and fevers, and spreading impediment in the skin. Also, there will be pain in the lower abdomen, internal urgency of the abdomen that radiates to the pelvis and coccyx, pain of the genitals, yīn mounting in males, and incessant spotting in females.

又曰：癲癇瘛瘲，不知所苦，兩蹻之上，男陽女陰。陰蹻在肌肉之下，陰脈所行，通貫五臟，主持諸裏，故名爲陰蹻之絡。

Another source states, "For withdrawal epilepsy with tugging and slackening, when there is an inability to identify where the pain is, [treat] the bottom[668] of the two qiāo [vessels], yáng [qiāo vessel] for males and yīn [qiāo vessel] for females."[669] "The yīnqiāo [vessel] is located underneath the flesh, which is where the yīn vessels travel, so that it communicates and interlinks with the five zàng-viscera, as well as takes charge of the interior; thus, it is named as the yīnqiāo network-vessel."[670]

陰蹻爲病，陰急則陰厥強直，五絡不通，表和裏病，陰病則熱，可灸照海、陽陵泉。陽陵泉乃足少陽之合也，筋病治此。照海乃陰蹻之本也。又曰：在裏者，當下。又曰：癲癇晝發，灸陽蹻，夜發，灸陰蹻。

When the yīnqiāo [vessel] is diseased, the yīn will be tense; as a result, there will be yīn reversal with stiffening and straightening,[671] failure of the five network-vessels to communicate, with harmony in the exterior but disease in

---

[666] From *Nànjīng* Difficulty 29.

[667] From *Màijīng* Vol. 10.

[668] "下 bottom" is originally "上 above" in the manuscript; however, it does not fit the context of the line here, and we have amended it in accordance with the *Língshū* and *Qíjīng Bāmài Kǎo* 奇經八脈考 (*An Investigation of the Eight Extraordinary Channels*, 1578 CE).

[669] From *Língshū* Chapter 73. Note: as this statement makes little sense if it were translated literally, we have adopted the interpretation by Mǎ Shì for elaboration.

[670] From the *Qíjīng Bāmài Kǎo* 奇經八脈考 (*An Investigation of the Eight Extraordinary Channels*, 1578 CE).

[671] From *Nànjīng* Difficulty 29.

the interior; as the yīn [aspect] is diseased, there will be fevers, one can moxa Zhào Hǎi (KI-6) and Yáng Líng Quán (GB-34).[672]

Yáng Líng Quán (GB-34) is the uniting point of the foot shàoyáng [channel]; for sinew diseases, treat this point. Zhào Hǎi (KI-6) is the root of the yīnqiāo [vessel].[673]

Another states, "As [the disease] is located in the interior, one ought to precipitate it." Another states, "For withdrawal epilepsy that occurs during the day, moxa the yángqiāo [vessel]; if it occurs at night, moxa the yīnqiāo [vessel]."

然陰蹻之脈亦能令人腰痛，痛引膺，目䀮䀮然，甚則反折，舌卷不能言，刺內筋爲三痏，在內踝上大筋前，太陰後上踝二寸所。

Nonetheless, [a disease in] the vessel of the yīnqiāo can also cause a person to have lumbar pain, pain that radiates to the breast, and dim vision; when it is severe, there will be [arched-back] rigidity and curled tongue with inability to speak; pierce the inner sinew 3 times,[674] which is located in front of the great sinew above the inner ankle [bone], at the place that is behind the tàiyīn [channel] and 2 cùn above the inner ankle [bone].[675]

王氏曰：陰起於然谷之下，上內踝之上，循陰股入陰，循腹入胸裏，出缺盆，上出人迎之前，入頄內廉，屬目內眥，會於太陽、陽蹻而上行，故其病如此，內筋即陰蹻之郄交信穴也。按昌陽之病狀，的是陰蹻脈所行部分之病，故宜取陰蹻之郄也。

Mister Wáng [Bīng] says, "The yīn [qiāo vessel] commences below Rán Gǔ (KI-2), ascends above the inner ankle [bone], follows the yīn thigh to enter the genitals, follows the abdomen to enter the interior of the chest, emerges at Quē Pén (ST-12), ascends to emerge at the front of Rén Yíng (ST-9), enters the inner ridge of the cheekbone, and adjoins to the inner canthus; it then meets with the tàiyáng and yángqiāo [vessels] and further ascends; therefore, it has such diseases. Furthermore, the 'inner sinew' is precisely Jiāo Xìn (KI-8), which is the cleft point of the yīnqiāo [vessel]." My observation is this, the disease signs of the glorious yáng are indeed diseases of the area where the

---

[672] From the Qíjīng Bāmài Kǎo 奇經八脈考 (An Investigation of the Eight Extraordinary Channels, 1578 CE).

[673] This passage also seems to be a paraphrase from the Qíjīng Bāmài Kǎo 奇經八脈考 (An Investigation of the Eight Extraordinary Channels, 1578 CE).

[674] For "3 times" here, it is actually "2 times" in the Sùwèn.

[675] From Sùwèn Chapter 41. Note: for "vessel of the yīnqiāo," while the original passage from the Sùwèn has "昌陽之脈 the vessel of glorious yáng," Wáng Bīng interprets this vessel as the yīnqiāo.

yīnqiāo vessel travels, thus it is appropriate to choose the cleft point of the yīnqiāo [vessel].

《靈樞》云：目中赤痛，從內眥始，取之陰蹻交信穴。又云：風痙反折，先取足太陽及委中及血絡出血。若中有寒邪，取陰蹻及三毛及血絡出血。

The Língshū states, "For redness and pain in the eyes that begins at the inner canthus, choose Jiāo Xìn (KI-8) of the yīnqiāo [vessel]."[676]

It also states, "For wind tetany with arched-back [rigidity], initially choose the foot tàiyáng [channel] and Wěi Zhōng (BL-40), and further let blood from the blood vessels. If there is a strike by cold evil, choose the yīnqiāo [vessel] and [the region of] the three hairs, and further let blood from the blood vessels."[677]

李氏曰：取太陽者，取足太陽之束骨也，在足外側小指本節後大骨下，赤白肉際陷中，可鍼三分，灸七壯。委中乃太陽經穴，陰蹻乃交信穴，三毛乃肝之大敦穴，血絡者，視其處有血絡盛滿者，當出其血也。

Mister Lǐ [Shízhēn] says, "Regarding 'choosing the tàiyáng [channel],' this means choosing Shù Gǔ (BL-65) of the foot tàiyáng [channel], which is located below the great bone behind the base joint of the little toe, on the outside of the foot, in the depression on the border of the red and white flesh; one can needle 3 fēn, and moxa 7 cones. 'Wěi Zhōng (BL-40)' is a [foot] tàiyáng bladder channel point; 'the yīnqiāo' refers to the point Jiāo Xìn (KI-8); '[the region of] the three hairs' refers to the liver [channel] point Dà Dūn (LR-1); regarding 'the blood vessels,' observe these places for the presence of blood vessels that are exuberant and full; [should these vessels be present], one ought to let blood."[678]

又經云：目閉者，責之陰蹻。

Moreover, *the [Jiǎyǐ] Jīng* states, "For closed eyes [which causes an inability to see], seek the yīnqiāo [vessel]."[679]

---

[676] From *Língshū* Chapter 23; however, the point mentioned, Jiāo Xìn (KI-8), appears to be a later addition.

[677] From *Língshū* Chapter 23.

[678] From *the Qíjīng Bāmài Kǎo* 奇經八脈考 (*An Investigation of the Eight Extraordinary Channels*, 1578 CE).

[679] This quote is a paraphrase from *the Qíjīng Bāmài Kǎo* 奇經八脈考 (*An Investigation of the Eight Extraordinary Channels*, 1578 CE); we have included the bracketed term from the original text to provide the full context.

The Yángqiāo Vessel

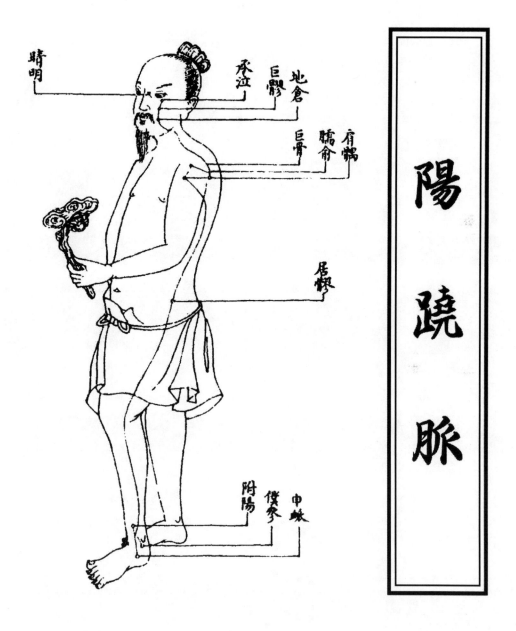

The Yángqiāo Vessel

陽蹻脈

思蓮子曰：陽蹻乃太陽之別，足太陽者，一身之巨陽，陽蹻者，主一身蹻動在陽分者。故脈之始起，發源於足太陽之脈。其脈起於足之後跟中，前出於足之外踝下五分赤白肉際陷中之申脈穴，又當踝後繞跟，以足太陽在跟骨下陷中，拱足而取之僕參爲本，遂上外踝上三寸，足太陽前，足少陽後，筋骨之間，太陽之附陽爲郄，

Master Sīlián says, the yángqiāo [vessel] is surely the divergence of the tàiyáng [channel]; as the foot tàiyáng is the great yáng of the entire body, the yángqiāo governs the Qiāo (Springing) movements in the yáng aspect of the entire body. Therefore, regarding where this vessel commences and begins, it emerges and originates from the vessel of the foot tàiyáng.

This vessel commences at the heel behind the foot, it moves forward to emerge at Shēn Mài (BL-62), which is located 5 fēn below the outer ankle [bone], in the depression at the border of the red and white flesh. Further, it encircles the heel behind the ankle and establishes Pú Cān (BL-61) of the foot tàiyáng [channel] as the root [of the yángqiāo vessel], which is located in the depression of the heel bone, to be found by arching the foot.

Thereupon, it ascends to Fù Yáng (BL-59) of the tàiyáng [channel], the cleft point [of the yángqiāo vessel], which is 3 cùn above the outer ankle [bone], in front of the foot tàiyáng, behind the foot shàoyáng, and between the sinew and the bone.

直上過膝，循股外廉，循後至胛上，會手太陽小腸經、奇經陽維於肩之後大骨下，胛之上廉陷中手陽明之巨骨穴，又會手陽明、手少陽之髆骨頭，肩端上，兩骨䯊陷宛宛中，舉臂取之有孔，手陽明之肩髃穴，遂過肩上頸，由足陽明胃經，挾結喉兩旁，動脈應手之人迎穴，

It ascends vertically to traverse the knee, follows the outer face of the thigh, follows towards the rear, and arrives at the top of the scapula to meet with the hand tàiyáng small intestine channel and extraordinary channel yángwéi vessel at Jù Gǔ (LI-16) of the hand yángmíng [channel], which is below the great bone behind the shoulder, in the depression on the upper ridge of the scapula.

It continues to the head of the humerus, where it meets with the hand yángmíng and hand shàoyáng [channels] at Jiān Yú (LI-15) of the hand yángmíng [channel], which is located at the edge of the shoulder, in the depression of the space where the two bones split, in the hollow that can be located by raising the arm.

Thereupon, it traverses the shoulder and ascends the neck by passing through Rén Yíng (ST-9) of the foot yángmíng stomach channel, which clasps the laryngeal prominence on both sides, where the pulsating vessel resonates with the hand.

過上至口吻旁，會手陽明、足陽明並任脈於足陽明胃經，口吻旁四分近下有微動之地倉穴，遂同足陽明而上行，挾鼻孔旁八分，直瞳子，平水溝，足陽明之巨髎穴，又後會任脈於目下七分，直瞳子，足陽明之承泣穴，遂上至目內眥，與足太陽、手太陽、足陽明、陰蹻五脈，會於足陽明之睛明穴，

It traverses upwards to reach the side of the mouth and meet with the hand yángmíng and foot yángmíng [channels], as well as the rèn [vessel] at Dì Cāng (ST-4) of the foot yángmíng stomach channel, which is located 4 fēn to the side of the mouth, where there is a faintly pulsating vessel underneath.

Thereupon, it ascends with the foot yángmíng to Jù Liáo (ST-3) of the foot yángmíng [channel], which is located 8 fēn to the side of nostril, in line with the pupil, and level with Shuǐ Gōu (DU-26).

Afterwards, it continues to meet with the rèn vessel at Chéng Qì (ST-1) of the foot yángmíng [channel], which is located 7 fēn below the eye and in line with the pupil.

Thereupon, it ascends to arrive at Jīng Míng (BL-1) of the foot tàiyáng[680] [channel] at the inner canthus; together with the foot tàiyáng, hand tàiyáng, foot yángmíng, and yīnqiāo [vessel], these five vessels meet here.

又循睛明上行入髮際，下耳後，入足少陽之風池穴而終。

It further ascends by following Jīng Míng (BL-1) into the hairline, then descends to and terminates at Fēng Chí (GB-20) of the foot shàoyáng [channel], which is located behind the ear.

陽蹻所過，皆手、足陽經，一始起於足太陽之申脈爲本，二會於足太陽僕參，三爲郄於足太陽之附陽，四會足少陽於足少陽之居髎，五會手太陽、陽維於手太陽之臑腧，

---

[680] "The foot tàiyáng" is originally "the foot yángmíng" in the manuscript, which is most likely a scribal error; therefore, we have amended it.

The entirety of where the yángqiāo [vessel] traverses is the hand and foot yáng channels; the first is the origin that commences at Shēn Mài (BL-62) of the foot tàiyáng [channel], which is the root of [the yángqiāo vessel];[681] the second meeting occurs at Pú Cān (BL-61) of the foot tàiyáng [channel]; the third is the cleft point at Fù Yáng (BL-59) of the foot tàiyáng [channel]; the fourth is the meeting with the foot shàoyáng [channel] at Jū Liáo (GB-29) of the foot shàoyáng [channel]; the fifth is the meeting with the hand tàiyáng [channel] and yángwéi [vessel] at Nào Shù (SI-10) of the hand tàiyáng [channel];

六會手陽明於手陽明之巨骨，七會手陽明、手少陽於手陽明之肩髃，八會手陽明、足陽明於足陽明之地倉，九同足陽明而上足陽明之巨髎，十會足陽明之承泣，其所過皆陽經舉動蹺捷之所，故曰陽蹺也。

The sixth is the meeting with the hand yángmíng [channel] at Jù Gǔ (LI-16) of the hand yángmíng [channel]; the seventh is the meeting with the hand yángmíng and hand shàoyáng [channels] at Jiān Yú (LI-15) of the yángmíng [channel]; the eighth is the meeting with the hand yángmíng and foot yángmíng [channels] at Dì Cāng (ST-4) of the foot yángmíng [channel];

At the nineth, it joins together with the foot yángmíng [channel] to ascend to Jù Liáo (ST-3) of the foot yángmíng [channel]; the tenth meeting occurs at Chéng Qì (ST-1) of the foot yángmíng [channel]. [The yángqiāo vessel] traverses entirely at these locations of the yáng channels, where one [can] make agile and Qiāo (Springing) movements, therefore, it is called the yángqiāo [vessel].

《難經》曰：陽蹺爲病，陰緩而陽急。《內經》云：陽蹺脈急，當從外踝以上急，內踝以上緩。

The Nànjīng states, "When the yángqiāo [vessel] is diseased, the yīn will be slack and the yáng will be tense."[682] The Nèijīng states, "When the yángqiāo vessel is tense, there ought to be tension above the outer ankle [bone] and slackening above the inner ankle [bone]."[683]

寸口脈前部左右彈者，陽蹺也。如脈不動則陽蹺無病，如動則苦腰背痛，又爲癲癎僵仆羊鳴，惡風偏枯瘴痺，身體強。又曰：陽蹺微澀爲風癎，並取陽蹺，在外踝直足絕骨端，乃足太陽之附陽穴也。

When the pulse is flicking in the front positions of the cùnkǒu pulse on both left and right, this is the yángqiāo [pulse]. When the pulses [at these positions]

---

[681] This may be a scribal error or that Yuè Hánzhēn may not have meant it literally, as Pú Cān (BL-61) is the root of yángqiāo vessel.

[682] From Nànjīng Difficulty 29.

[683] This is actually not from the Nèijīng as stated, but from Màijīng Vol. 2, Chapter 4.

are not stirred, there is no disease in the yángqiāo [vessel]. If they are stirred, one will suffer from lumbar and upper-back pain, also withdrawal epilepsy, sudden collapse, bleating like a sheep, aversion to wind, hemilateral withering with paralysis, impediment, stiffness and rigidity of the body.[684]

It also states, "When the yángqiāo [pulse] is slightly rough, there will be wind epilepsy; one should choose the yángqiāo [vessel], which is located at the tip of the severed bone and in line with the outer ankle [bone]."[685] This is referring to Fù Yáng (BL-59) of the foot tàiyáng [channel].

張氏曰：陽蹻在肌肉之上，陽脈所行，通貫六腑，主持諸表。陽蹻爲病，陽急則狂走目不眛，表病裏和。陽病則寒，可鍼膽經之風池，督脈之風府。又曰：在陽表者，當汗之。又曰：癲癇晝發，灸陽蹻。陽蹻之脈，亦能使人腰痛。

Master Zhāng [Yuánsù] says, "The yángqiāo [vessel] is located above the flesh, which is where the yáng vessels travel, so that it communicates with the six fǔ-bowels, as well as takes charge of the exterior. When the yángqiāo [vessel] is diseased, the yáng will be tense; as a result, there will be manic walking yet without blurred vision, with disease in the exterior but harmony in the interior. When the yáng [aspect] is diseased, there will be chills, one can needle Fēng Chí (GB-20) of the gallbladder channel and Fēng Fǔ (GB-16) of the dū vessel."

He also says, "As [the disease] is located in the yáng exterior, one ought to sweat it."

He also says, "For withdrawal epilepsy that occurs during the day, moxa the yángqiāo [vessel]." In addition, [a disease in] the vessel of yángqiāo can also cause a person to have lumbar pain.

《內經》云：腰痛不可舉者，申脈、僕參主之。皆太陽之穴，陽蹻之本也。經又云：會陰之脈，令人腰痛，痛上漯漯然汗出，汗乾令人欲飲，飲已欲走，刺直陽之脈上三痏，在蹻上郤下五寸橫居，視其盛者出血。

The Nèijīng states, "For lumbar pain with inability to hold [the body] upright, Shēn Mài (BL-62) and Pú Cān (BL-61) govern it."[686] These are both points of the tàiyáng [channel], as it is the root of the yángqiāo [vessel].

The Canon also states, "[A disease in] the vessel of meeting yīn[687] will cause a person to have lumbar pain, and pain that ascends with wet discharge of sweat; once the sweat dries up, that person will have a desire to drink fluid;

---

[684] From Màijīng Vol. 10.
[685] From Màijīng Vol. 10.
[686] This actually comes from Wáng Bīng's commentary of Sùwèn Chapter 41.
[687] This is identical with the name of Huì Yīn (REN-1).

once one finishes drinking the fluid, that person will have a desire to walk; pierce the vessel of straight yáng, perform it thrice. It is located above the qiāo with transverse [vessels] that lodge at 5 cùn below the cleft;[688] observe these places [for the presence of blood vessels] that are exuberant; [should these vessels be present], one ought to let blood."[689]

王氏曰：足太陽之脈，循腰下會於後陰，故曰會陰。直陽之脈，挾脊下行，貫臀至膕，過外踝之後，條直而行者，故曰直陽之脈。蹻爲陽蹻所生申脈穴也，蹻上郄下，乃承筋穴也，即腨中央如外陷者中也，太陽脈氣所發，禁鍼。但視其兩腨中央有血絡盛滿者，乃刺之出血也。

Mister Wáng [Bīng] says, "The vessel of the foot tàiyáng follows the lumbus to meet with the rear yīn[690] below, thus it is called 'meeting yīn.' The vessel of straight yáng clasps the spine as it descends, pierces the buttocks to arrive at the back of the knee, and traverses behind the outer ankle [bone]; as it travels on a perfectly straight [pathway], thus it is called the 'vessel of the straight yáng.' Regarding 'the qiāo,' it refers to the point Shēn Mài (BL-62), where the yángqiāo [vessel] is engendered. As for what is 'above the qiāo and below the cleft,' this refers to the point Chéng Jīn (BL-56), which is precisely the centre of the calf where [the flesh to] the sides appear to sink towards the centre, where the tàiyáng vessel qì emerges; needling is contraindicated. However, if one observes blood vessels that are exuberant and full in the centre of both of the calves, pierce them to let blood."[691]

經又云：邪客於陽蹻之脈，令人目痛，從內眥始，刺外踝之下半寸，即申脈穴也。左刺右，右刺左。陽蹻爲病，令人目不得瞑。

The Canon also states, "When the evil lodges in the vessel of yángqiāo, it will cause that person to have eye pain that begins at the inner canthus; pierce half a cùn below the outer ankle [bone]."[692] This refers precisely to the point Shēn Mài (BL-62); for the left [disease], pierce the right [point]; for the right [disease], pierce the left [point].

[Also], "When the yángqiāo [vessel] is diseased, it will cause that person to be unable to close their eyes."[693]

---

688 For "郄下五寸 5 cùn below the cleft," the primary manuscript originally has "膝下五寸 5 cùn below the knee." The editors of this manuscript, Zhāng and Zhà, amended it according to *Sùwèn* Chapter 41.
689 From *Sùwèn* Chapter 41.
690 I.e., the anus.
691 From Wáng Bīng's commentary of *Sùwèn* Chapter 41.
692 From *Sùwèn* Chapter 63.
693 From *the Jiǎyǐ Jīng*

The Chōng Vessel

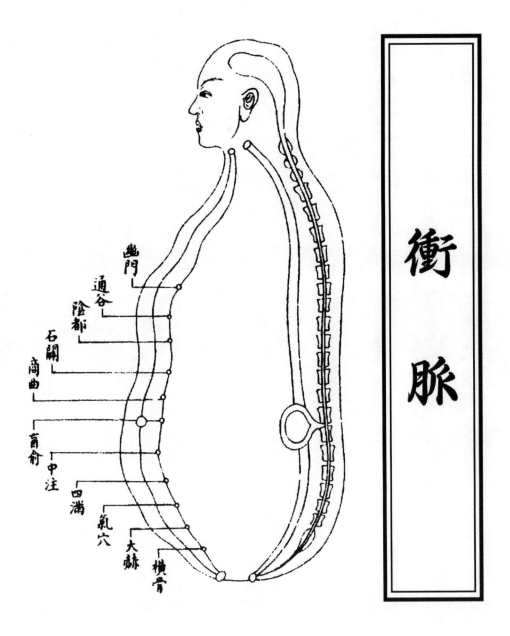

幽門

通谷

陰都

石關

商曲

肓俞

中注

四滿

氣穴

大赫

橫骨

衝

脈

The Chōng Vessel

衝脈

思蓮子曰：以其脈上衝於胸，下衝於足而得名也，其脈上下首尾不離乎足少陰之部分，又曰血海。

Master Sīlián says, [the Chōng] vessel receives its name because it Chōng (Surges) upwards into the chest and Chōng (Surges) downwards into the feet. From the above to the below, from the beginning to the end, this vessel does not depart from the vicinity of the foot shàoyīn [channel]; in addition, it is also said to be the sea of blood.

其脈與任脈同起於少腹之內胞中，其浮而外者，出於少腹毛中兩旁各二寸，橫骨兩端，動脈宛宛中，足陽明胃經之氣衝穴，

Both this vessel and the rèn vessel commence from within the womb[694] inside the lower abdomen. It moves superficially to the outside, emerging at Qì Chōng (ST-30) of the foot yángmíng stomach channel, which is located within the pubic hair [region], 2 cùn on each side [of the midline] on the lower abdomen, at the two tips of the pubic bone,[695] in the depression on the pulsating vessel.

足陽明胃經去腹中行各二寸，足少陰去腹中行五分，而衝脈所歷，在二經之間，循少腹橫而入於陰毛，骨形如偃月，去中行寸半，腎經之橫骨穴，歷腎經之橫骨上一寸，去腹中行寸半之大赫穴，又上歷大赫上一寸，去中行寸半之氣穴，

While the foot yángmíng stomach channel is 2 cùn on each side of the abdominal midline, the foot shàoyīn is 5 fēn on each side of the abdominal midline; and the chōng vessel travels between these two channels. Following the lower abdomen, it moves transversely to Héng Gǔ (KI-11) of the kidney channel, which is into the pubic hair [region], by the bone that resembles a crescent moon in shape, at 1 cùn and a half from the midline. It then passes through Dà Hè (KI-12), which is 1 cùn above Héng Gǔ (KI-11) of the kidney channel, 1 cùn and a half from the abdominal midline. It further passes

---

[694] Note: For men, this "womb" would likely refer to the elusive "精室 essence chamber/精宮 palace of essence," as discussed in *Nánjīng* Difficulty 36. Some commentators believe that such an anatomical structure is located between the bladder and small intestine.

[695] Whilst this is the same name as KI-11, it appears to be discussing the anatomy.

through Qì Xué (KI-13), which is 1 cùn above Dà Hè (KI-12), 1 cùn and a half from the midline.

遂上歷臍下兩旁腎經諸穴，中注下一寸之四滿，肓腧下一寸之中注，商曲下一寸之肓腧，此臍旁以下之穴也。

Thereupon, it ascends to pass through the various kidney channel points on the two sides below the umbilicus, which are namely, Sì Mǎn (KI-14) that is 1 cùn below Zhōng Zhù (KI-15), Zhōng Zhù (KI-15) that is 1 cùn below Huāng Shù (KI-16), and Huāng Shù (KI-16) that is 1 cùn below Shāng Qū (KI-17); these are the points that are located on the sides and below the umbilicus.

然臍下腎經五穴，諸書所載去中行多少分寸不同。《素》註載去中行各寸半，《銅人》載去中行各寸半，而有載各一寸者，仍以寸半爲是。

Nevertheless, for these five points of the kidney channel below the umbilicus, different distances from the midline have been recorded in various books. *The Sùzhù* records 1 cùn and a half on each side of the midline, *the Tóngrén* records 1 cùn and a half on each side of the midline [as well], yet there are others that record 1 cùn [on each side of the midline]; still, one should regard 1 cùn and a half as the proper [distance].

自肓腧挾臍旁而上行，歷腎經之商曲、石關、陰都、通谷、幽門，皆去中行各五分，上下相隔各一寸之穴，上至胸中，又上行通於咽喉，別而絡唇口。

From Huāng Shù (KI-16), it clasps the sides of the umbilicus and ascends, passing through Shāng Qū (KI-17), Shí Guān (KI-18), Yīn Dū (KI-19), Tōng Gǔ (KI-20), and Yōu Mén (KI-21) of the kidney channel; all of which are points that are 5 fēn on each side of the midline[696] and 1 cùn apart from each other vertically. It ascends to arrive within the chest, and further ascends to communicate with the pharynx and throat, where it diverges to network with the lips and mouth.[697]

經云：三陰之所交，結於脚也，踝上各一行行六者，此腎經之下行也，名曰太衝。王氏曰：腎脈與衝脈並下行，循足合而盛大，故曰太衝。

The Canon states "The intersection of the three yīn knots at the foot; for the one column that passes through the six [points] above each ankle [bone],[698]

---

[696] For "5 fēn on each side of the midline," the secondary manuscript has "1 cùn 5 fēn from the midline."

[697] This seems to be a paraphrase from *the Qíjīng Bāmài Kǎo* 奇經八脈考 (*An Investigation of the Eight Extraordinary Channels*, 1578 CE).

[698] For "踝上各一行行六者 for the one column that passes through the six [points] above each ankle [bone]," it is originally "踝上各一寸者 for what is 1 cùn above each ankle [bone]" in the primary manuscript. The editors of this manuscript, Zhāng and Zhà, amended it according to *Sùwèn* Chapter 61 and the secondary manuscript.

this is the descending pathway of the kidney channel, which is called the Tài Chōng (Great Surge)."[699]

Mister Wáng [Bīng] says, "The kidney vessel and the chōng vessel descend together, they follow the foot and join together; as such, there is an exuberant and large [vessel], thus it is called Tài Chōng (Great Surge)."[700]

《難經》曰：衝脈爲病，逆氣而裏急。

The Nànjīng states, "When the chōng vessel is diseased, there will be counterflow qì with internal urgency."[701]

《靈樞》曰：氣逆上，刺膺中陷下者與下胸動脈。腹痛刺臍左右動脈，按之立已，不已，刺氣街，按之立已。兩手脈浮之俱有陽，沉之俱有陰，陰陽皆盛，此衝、督之脈也。衝、督之脈，爲十二經之道路，衝、督用事，則十二經不復朝於寸口，其人怳惚狂癲。

The Língshū states "For counterflow qì ascent, pierce Yīng Zhōng[702] in the depression on the chest as well as the pulsating vessel that descends the chest. For abdominal pain, pierce the pulsating vessel on the left and right sides of the umbilicus and apply pressure [after needling], [the pain] will immediately cease; if it fails to cease, pierce Qì Jiē (ST-30) and apply pressure [after needling], [the pain] will immediately cease."[703]

When both wrist pulses are floating and possessing entirely yáng [qualities],[704] when [both wrist pulses] are deep and possessing entirely yīn [qualities],[705] and when both the yīn and yáng [positions][706] are exuberant, this is the pulse of the chōng and dū vessels. As the vessels of the chōng and dū are the pathways of the twelve channels, when the chōng and dū are in

---

[699] From *Sùwèn* Chapter 61. Note: although the "Tài Chōng 太衝 (Great Surge)" share the same characters as the point Tài Chōng (LR-3), most commentators, such as Wáng Bīng, Mǎ Shì, and Zhāng Jǐngyuè, seem to think that this is simply a name or a title for the kidney vessel, and that it has nothing to do with the point Tài Chōng (LR-3).

[700] From Wáng Bīng's commentary of *Sùwèn* Chapter 61.

[701] From *Nànjīng* Difficulty 29.

[702] I.e., an alternate name for LU-1.

[703] From *Língshū* Chapter 26

[704] I.e., floating, slippery, and long, as noted in *Màijīng* Vol. 1, Chapter 9.

[705] I.e., deep, rough, and short, as noted in *Màijīng* Vol. 1, Chapter 9.

[706] Note: according to *Màijīng* Vol. 1, Chapter 9, distal wrist pulse position is the yáng position, proximal wrist pulse position is the yīn position.

power,[707] the twelve channels will no longer assemble at the cùnkǒu [pulse]; the person will have abstraction,[708] mania and feeble-mindedness.[709]

又曰：脈來中央堅實，徑至關者，衝脈也，動苦少腹痛，上搶心，有瘕疝，遺溺，脇支滿煩，女子絕孕。又曰：尺寸俱牢，直上直下，此乃衝脈，胸中有寒痛也。

It also states, "For a pulse that is hard and replete in the centre that arrives directly on the guān [position], this is the chōng [vessel] pulse; when it is stirred, one will suffer from pain in the lower abdomen that ascends to prod the heart, presence of mounting-conglomeration with enuresis, propping fullness and vexation of the rib-sides, and infertility in women."[710]

It also states, "When the chǐ and cùn [positions] are both firm, [with the three] positions going up and down together, this is the chōng [vessel] pulse; there will be cold pain in the chest."[711]

李氏曰：凡臍之上下左右有氣，築築然牢而痛，正衝、任、足少陰、太陰四經病也。又曰：衝脈爲十二經之海，其輸上在於大杼，下出於巨虛之上下廉。又云：血海有餘，則常想其身大，不足則小。

Mister Lǐ [Shízhēn] says, "Whenever there is qì on the above, below, left, and right [sides] of the umbilicus, with discomfort that is firm and painful, this is precisely the disease of the four channels, which are namely the chōng, the rèn, the foot shàoyīn and tàiyīn.[712]

It is also stated, "Chōng vessel is the sea of the twelve channels; its transport above is at Dà Zhù (BL-11), and it emerges at the upper and lower great hollows[713] below."[714]

It is also said, "When the sea of blood has superabundance, one often feels oneself to have a large physical stature of the body; when it is insufficient, one [often feels oneself to] have a small physical stature [of the body]."[715]

---

[707] I.e., in power in order to engage with evil invasion in their respective domain.

[708] *The Practical Dictionary* "Inattention to present objects or surroundings, or low powers of mental concentration. It is a sign of heart disease."

[709] From *Màijīng* Vol. 2, Chapter 4.

[710] From *Màijīng* Vol. 2, Chapter 4.

[711] From *Màijīng* Vol. 2, Chapter 4.

[712] From *the Qíjīng Bāmài Kǎo* 奇經八脈考 (*An Investigation of the Eight Extraordinary Channels*, 1578 CE).

[713] I.e., ST-37 and ST-39.

[714] From *Língshū* Chapter 33.

[715] From *Língshū* Chapter 33.

The Dài Vessel

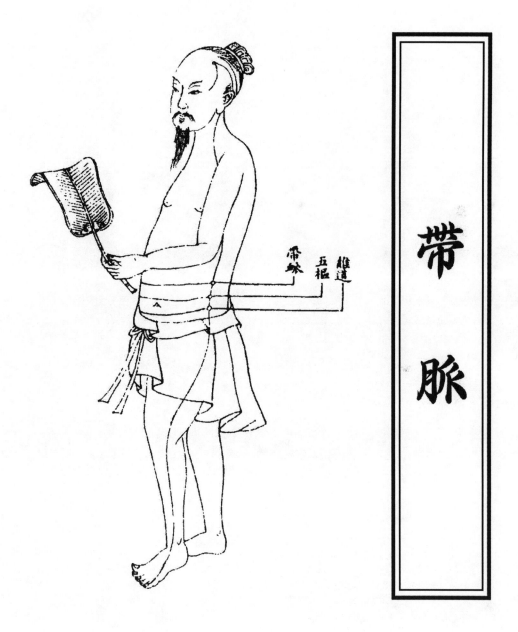

帶脈

The Dài Vessel
帶脈

思蓮子曰：帶脈者，周圍一身如束帶也。其脈起於季脇足厥陰之章門穴，此穴爲
足厥陰肝、足少陽膽經二脈之會，在季脇骨端，側臥肘尖盡處是穴，同足少陽循
帶脈穴，其穴在季脇下一寸八分陷中，又與足少陽會於五樞，在帶脈穴下三寸，
又與足少陽會於維道，在章門下五寸三分。

Master Sīlián says, the dài vessel encircles the body in a [horizontal] circuit, as though one is bound with a Dài (Sash). This vessel commences under the rib-side at the floating rib, at Zhāng Mén (LR-13) of the foot juéyīn; this point is the meeting of two vessels, the foot juéyīn liver and the foot shàoyáng gallbladder channels. This point is located at the tip of the floating rib under the rib-side, where the tip of the elbow touches while lying on one's side.

Along with the foot shàoyáng, [the dài vessel] passes through the point Dài Mài (GB-26), which is located in the depression 1 cùn 8 fēn below the floating rib under the rib-side.

It continues to meet with the foot shàoyáng at Wǔ Shū (GB-27), which is located 3 cùn below Dài Mài (GB-26). It further meets with the foot shàoyáng at Wéi Dào (GB-28), which is located 5 cùn 3 fēn below Zhāng Mén (LR-13).

《靈樞》又云：足少陰之正，至膕中，別走太陽而合，上至腎，當十四椎，出屬
帶脈。

The Língshū also states, "When the principal [pathway] of the foot shàoyīn arrives at the back of the knee, it diverges to unite with the tàiyáng, ascends to reach the kidneys, and emerges at the fourteenth vertebra to adjoin with the dài vessel."[716]

《難經》曰：帶脈爲病，腹滿，腰溶溶如坐水中。溶溶者，緩慢也。《明堂》
云：帶脈二穴，主腰腹縱，溶溶欲囊水之狀，婦人少腹痛，裹急後重，瘕癖，月
事不調，赤白帶下，可鍼六分，灸七壯。

---

[716] From *Língshū* Chapter 11.

The Nánjīng states, "When the dài vessel is diseased, there will be abdominal fullness, dissolution of the lumbus that appears as though one has been sitting in water."[717] Regarding this 'dissolution,' it refers to slackness and slowness.[718]

The Míngtáng states, "The two points of Dài Mài (GB-26) [on the two sides] govern slackness of the lumbus and abdomen with dissolution [of the lumbus] that resembles the appearance of a pouch of water, lower abdominal pain in women, internal urgency and heaviness in the rectum,[719] tugging and slackening, irregular menstruation, red and white vaginal discharge; one can needle 6 fēn and moxa 7 cones.

中部左右彈者，帶脈也。不動則無病，如動則苦少腹痛，引命門，女子月事不調，絕繼復下，令人無子，男子少腹拘急，或失精也。

When the pulse is flicking in the middle positions [of the cùnkǒu pulse] on the left and right, this is the dài [vessel] pulse.[720] When the pulses [at these positions] are not stirred, there is no disease. If they are stirred, one will suffer from pain in the lower abdomen that radiates to the mìngmén;[721] in females, there will be irregular menstruation with successions of amenorrhea and recurrence of menses, which leads to infertility; in males, there will be hypertonicity of the lower abdomen or seminal loss.[722]

---

[717] From *Nànjīng* Difficulty 29.

[718] From *the Qíjīng Bāmài Kǎo* 奇經八脈考 (*An Investigation of the Eight Extraordinary Channels*, 1578 CE).

[719] I.e., tenesmus.

[720] From *Màijīng* Vol. 10.

[721] This is likely the area of the lumbus, where Mìng Mén (DU-4) is located.

[722] From *Màijīng* Vol. 10.

Bibliography

Chace, Charles, and Miki Shima. An Exposition on the Eight Extraordinary Vessels: Acupuncture, Alchemy, and Herbal Medicine. Seattle: Eastland Press, 2010.

Dīng, Guāngdí. 諸病源候論校注 *[The Origin and Indicators of Disease, Revised and Annotated]*. 1989. Beijing: 人民卫生出版社 People's Medical Publishing House, 2013.

Dèng, Tiětāo. 子和醫集 *[Compilation Medical Works by Zhāng Zǐhé]*. 1992. Beijing: 人民卫生出版社 People's Medical Publishing House, 2014.

Dīng, Guāngdí, and Kuí Wén. 東垣醫集 *[Compilation of Medical Works by Lǐ Dōngyuán]*. 1992. Beijing: 人民卫生出版社 People's Medical Publishing House, 2014.

Ellis, Andrew, et al. *Grasping the Wind*. Taos: Paradigm Publications, 1989.

Gāo, Wǔ. 针灸聚英 *[Gathered Blooms of Acupuncture and Moxibustion]*. 1529, edited by Huáng Lóngxiáng. Beijing: 人民卫生出版社 People's Medical Publishing House, 2006.

Guō, Ǎichūn. 黄帝內經素問校注 *[The Yellow Emperor's Inner Canon: Sùwèn, Revised and Annotated]*. 1989. Beijing: 人民卫生出版社 People's Medical Publishing House, 2013.

Huá, Bórén. 古本十四經發揮 秘本十四經脈穴歌 合刊 *[Ancient Copy of Elaboration of the Fourteen Channels & Rare Copy of the Odes of the Vessel Points of the Fourteen Channel]*. 1341, edited by Chéng Dàn'ān, Taipei: 自由出版社 Freedom Book Press, 1976.

Huáng, Lóngxiáng. 中國針灸學術史大綱 *[The Historical Development of Acupuncture]*. 2001. Taipei: 知音出版社 Jyin Publishing Company, 2002.

Huáng, Lóngxiáng, and Yòumín Huáng. 针灸腧穴通考 *[Textual Criticism of Acupuncture Points]*. Beijing: 人民卫生出版社 People's Medical Publishing House, 2011.

Huángfǔ, Mì. 鍼灸甲乙經 *[The Systematized Canon of Acupuncture and Moxibustion]*. 259, edited by Huáng Lóngxiáng. Beijing: 人民卫生出版社 People's Medical Publishing House, 2017.

Lǐ, Jǐngróng, et al. 备急千金要方校释 *[A Thousand Gold Pieces Emergency Formulary, Revised and Elucidated]*. 1997. Beijing: 人民卫生出版社 People's Medical Publishing House, 2014.

Lǐ, Jǐngróng, et al.千金翼方校释 *[Wings of the Thousand Gold Pieces Formulary, Revised and Elucidated]*. 1996. Beijing: 人民卫生出版社 People's Medical Publishing House, 2014.

Lǐ, Shízhēn. "奇經八脈考 [Investigations on the Eight Extraordinary Vessels]." 本草綱目 *[Herbal Foundation Compendium]*. 1590. Taipei: 新文豐出版公司 Xīnwénfēng Publishing Company, 1987.

Líng, Yàoxīng. 難經校注 *[The Canon of Difficult Issues, Revised and Annotated]*. 1989. Beijing: 人民卫生出版社 People's Medical Publishing House, 2013.

Literature Research Center of the Zhejiang Traditional Chinese Medicine Academy. 丹溪医集 *[Compilation Medical Works by Zhū Dānxī]*. 1986. Beijing: 人民卫生出版社 People's Medical Publishing House, 2014.

Mǎ, Yuántái. 難經正義 *[Orthodox Concept of the Nànjīng]*, microfilm. C. 16th century. 寶命堂 Life-Treasuring Hall, c. 17th century.

Qián, Yǐ. 小兒藥證直訣 *[The Key to Diagnosis and Treatment of Children's Diseases]*. 1119, edited by Zhāng Shānléi, Taipei: 力行書局 Liehen Book Company, 1998.

Shěn, Yánnán. 脈經校注 *[The Pulse Canon, Revised and Annotated]*. 1989. Beijing: 人民卫生出版社 People's Medical Publishing House, 2013.

Sūn, Sīmiǎo. 備急千金要方 *[Thousand Gold Emergency Formulary]*. 652, edited by Xiāo Tiānshí, Taipei: 自由出版社 Freedom Book Press, 1976.

Sūn, Sīmiǎo. 千金翼方 *[Wings of the Thousand Gold Formulary]*. 682, edited by Xiāo Tiānshí, Taipei: 自由出版社 Freedom Book Press, 1976.

Tamba, Yasuyori. 醫心方 *[Heart of Medicine]*. 984. Taipei: 新文豐出版公司 Xīnwénfēng Publishing Company, 1976.

Unschuld, Paul S. *Huang Di Nei Jing Ling Shu: The Ancient Classic on Needle Therapy*. Oakland: University of California Press, 2016.

Unschuld, Paul S. *Huang Di Nei Jing Su Wen: An Annotated Translation of Huang Di's Inner Classic – Basic Questions*. Oakland: University of California Press, 2011.

Unschuld, Paul S. *Nan Jing: The Classic of Difficult Issues*. Berkeley: University of California Press, 2016.

Wáng, Déshēn, et al. 中國針灸穴位通鑒 [*Comprehensive Mirror of Chinese Acupuncture Point Locations*]. Qingdao: 青岛出版社 Qingdao Publishing Group, 1991.

Wáng, Huáiyǐn, et al. 太平聖惠方 [*The Great Peace Sagacious Benevolence Formulary*]. 992. Taipei: 新文豐出版公司 Xīnwénfēng Publishing Company, 1980.

Wáng, Táo. 重訂外臺秘要方 [*Essential Secrets from the External Official Library, Revised*]. 752. Taipei: 新文豐出版公司 Xīnwénfēng Publishing Company, 1987.

Wáng, Zhízhōng. 针灸资生经 [*The Classic of Supporting Life with Acupuncture and Moxibustion*]. 1220, edited by Huáng Lóngxiáng and Huáng Yòumín. Beijing: 人民卫生出版社 People's Medical Publishing House, 2007.

Wiseman, Nigel, and Ye, Feng. *A Practical Dictionary of Chinese Medicine*. 3rd ed., Taos: Paradigm Publications, 2014.

Wú, Qiān, et al. 醫宗金鑒：外科心法要訣 [*The Golden Mirror of Medical Ancestry: Core Methods and Key Essentials of External Medicine*]. 1742. Taipei: 新文豐出版公司 Xīnwénfēng Publishing Company, 1981.

Wú, Qiān, et al. 醫宗金鑒：刺灸心法要訣 [*The Golden Mirror of Medical Ancestry: Core Methods and Key Essentials of Needling and Moxibustion*]. 1742. Taipei: 新文豐出版公司 Xīnwénfēng Publishing Company, 1987.

Xǔ Shèn. 说文解字 [*Explaining Graphs and Analysing Characters*]. C. 2nd century CE. Beijing: 中華書局 Zhonghua Book Company, 1963.

Yáng, Jìzhōu. 针灸大成 [*The Great Compendium of Acupuncture and Moxibustion*]. 1601. Taipei: 大中國圖書公司 Greater China Book Company, 1994.

Yáng, Jìzhōu. 针灸大成 [*The Great Compendium of Acupuncture and Moxibustion*]. 1601, edited by Huáng Lóngxiáng. Beijing: 人民卫生出版社 People's Medical Publishing House, 2017.

Yang, Shouzhong, and Duan Wujin. *Extra Treatises Based on Investigation & Inquiry*. 3rd ed., Boulder: Blue Poppy Press, 1998.

Yang, Shouzhong, and Jianyong Li. *Treatise on the Spleen and Stomach: A Translation of the Pi Wei Lun*. Boulder: Blue Poppy Press, 1993.

Young, Wei-Chieh. 黃帝內經素問譯解 [*Deciphering and Explaining the Yellow Emperor's Inner Canon: Sùwèn*]. 2nd ed., 1990, Taipei: 志遠書局 Zhiyuan Book Company, 2011.

Young, Wei-Chieh. 黃帝內經靈樞譯解 [Deciphering and Explaining the Yellow Emperor's Inner Canon: Língshū]. 2nd ed., 1990, Taipei: 志遠書局 Zhiyuan Book Company, 2011.

Zēng, Fèng. 新雕孙真人千金方校注 [Newly Carved the Thousand Gold Formulary of Sūn the True Man, Revised and Annotated]. Beijing: 学苑出版社 Xueyuan Publishing, 2012.

Zhāng Jièbīn. 張氏類經圖翼 [The Illustrated Wings of the Classified Canon by Master Zhāng]. 1624. Taipei: 新文豐出版公司 Xīnwénfēng Publishing Company, 1976.

Zhāng, Yǐn'ān, and Mǎ Yuántái. 張馬合註素問靈樞 [Combined Annotations of Sùwèn & Língshū by Zhāng Yǐn'ān and Mǎ Yuántái]. 1910. Taipei: 廣文書局 Kwangwen Book Company, 1982.

Zhōu, Yìmóu, and Xiāo Zuǒtáo. 馬王堆醫書考注 [Investigation and Annotation of Medical Texts from Mǎwángduī]. Taichong: 樂羣書局 Lequn Book Company, 1989.

Index

Points Index

The Kidney Channel

KI-1	Yǒng Quán	Gushing Spring	湧泉	pg. 3, 7, 9-16, 20, 28, 72
KI-2	Rán Gǔ	Blazing Valley	然谷	pg. 3, 16-20, 29, 411, 413
KI-3	Tài Xī	Great Ravine	太谿	pg. 3, 19-23, 26, 269
KI-4	Dà Zhōng	Large Goblet	大鍾	pg. 3, 5, 23-27
KI-5	Shuǐ Quán	Water Spring	水泉	pg. 3, 26-28
KI-6	Zhào Hǎi	Shining Sea	照海	pg. 3, 28-33, 37, 411, 413
KI-7	Fù Liū	Recover Flow	復溜	pg. 3, 32-37
KI-8	Jiāo Xìn	Intersection Fidelity	交信	pg. 3, 29, 32-33, 36 – 39, 411, 413-414
KI-9	Zhú Bīn	Guest House	築賓	pg. 3, 39-43, 266, 397-398, 400
KI-10	Yīn Gǔ	Yīn Valley	陰谷	pg. 3, 43-44
KI-11	Héng Gǔ	Transverse Bone	橫骨	pg. 4-5, 45-50, 52-57-58, 62, 64, 66, 73, 236, 299, 425
KI-12	Dà Hè	Great Eminence	大赫	pg. 4, 45, 48-50, 425-426
KI-13	Qì Xué	Qì Point	氣穴	pg. 4, 48-49, 51-52, 426
KI-14	Sì Mǎn	Fourfold Fullness	四滿	pg. 4, 45, 48, 51-54, 426
KI-15	Zhōng Zhù	Central Pour	中注	pg. 4, 45, 48, 52, 54 – 55, 426
KI-16	Huāng Shù	Huāng Transport Point	肓腧	pg. 4, 45, 48, 54-57, 426
KI-17	Shāng Qū	Shāng Bend	商曲	pg. 4, 45, 48, 55, 57 – 58, 426
KI-18	Shí Guān	Stone Pass	石關	pg. 4, 45, 48, 57-60, 426
KI-19	Yīn Dū	Yīn Metropolis	陰都	pg. 4, 45, 48, 58, 61-62, 426

KI-20	Tōng Gǔ	Flowing Valley	通谷	pg. 4, 45, 48, 61-64, 426
KI-21	Yōu Mén	Dark Gate	幽門	pg. 4, 45, 48, 59, 62, 64-66, 426
KI-22	Bù Láng	Corridor Steps	步廊	pg. 4, 66-67
KI-23	Shén Fēng	Spirit Border	神封	pg. 4, 66-68
KI-24	Líng Xū	Divine Mound	靈墟	pg. 4, 67, 69
KI-25	Shén Cáng	Spirit Storehouse	神藏	pg. 4, 69
KI-26	Yù Zhōng	Lively Centre	彧中	pg. 4, 69, 70-71
KI-27	Shù Fǔ	Transport Mansion	腧府	pg. 4, 70-72

The Pericardium Channel

PC-1	Tiān Chí	Celestial Pool	天池	pg. 77, 79-82, 128-129, 146
PC-2	Tiān Quán	Celestial Spring	天泉	pg. 77, 79, 81-82
PC-3	Qū Zé	Marsh at the Bend	曲澤	pg. 77, 79, 83-85
PC-4	Xī Mén	Cleft Gate	郄門	pg. 77, 85-86, 89
PC-5	Jiān Shǐ	Intermediary Courier	間使	pg. 78, 86-89
PC-6	Nèi Guān	Inner Pass	內關	pg. 78, 89-90, 115-116
PC-7	Dà Líng	Great Mound	大陵	pg. 78, 91-93, 114, 234
PC-8	Láo Gōng	Palace of Toil	勞宮	pg. 78, 93-95
PC-9	Zhōng Chōng	Middle Surge	中衝	pg. 78-79, 82, 95-96, 110

The Sānjiāo Channel

SJ-1	Guān Chōng	Surging Pass	關衝	pg. 103, 109-111, 115, 121, 127
SJ-2	Yè Mén	Humour Gate	液門	pg. 103, 109, 111-113
SJ-3	Zhōng Zhǔ	Middle Pond	中渚	pg. 103, 109, 113-114
SJ-4	Yáng Chí	Yáng Pool	陽池	pg. 103, 104, 114-115

SJ-5	Wài Guān	Outer Pass	外關	pg. 89, 103, 109, 115 -116, 217
SJ-6	Zhī Gōu	Branch Ditch	支溝	pg. 103, 109, 116-119
SJ-7	Huì Zōng	Convergence and Gathering	會宗	pg. 103, 109, 118-119
SJ-8	Sān Yáng Luò	Three Yáng Network	三陽絡	pg. 103, 109, 118-120
SJ-9	Sì Dú	Four Rivers	四瀆	pg. 103, 109, 120
SJ-10	Tiān Jǐng	Celestial Well	天井	pg. 103, 109, 121-123
SJ-11	Qīng Lěng Yuān	Clear Cold Abyss	清冷淵	pg. 103, 123, 187
SJ-12	Xiāo Luò	Dispersing Riverbed	消濼	pg. 103, 123-124, 187
SJ-13	Nào Huì	Upper Arm Convergence	臑會	pg. 103, 109, 125-127, 187, 403, 405
SJ-14	Jiān Liáo	Shoulder Bone-Hole	肩髎	pg. 104, 109, 126, 187
SJ-15	Tiān Liáo	Celestial Bone-Hole	天髎	pg. 104, 109, 126-128, 187, 403, 405
SJ-16	Tiān Yǒu	Celestial Window	天牖	pg. 104, 109,127-130, 163, 177, 217, 364
SJ-17	Yì Fēng	Wind Screen	翳風	pg. 104-105, 128, 130-131, 128, 130-131, 134, 145, 156, 160, 163, 177
SJ-18	Chì Mài	Tugging Vessel	瘈脈	pg. 104, 131-132, 163, 177
SJ-19	Lú Xí	Skull Breathing	顱息	pg. 105, 132-133, 163, 177
SJ-20	Jiǎo Sūn	Angle Vertex	角孫	pg. 105, 109-110, 133-134, 163, 177
SJ-21	Sī Zhú Kōng	Silk Bamboo Hole	絲竹空	pg. 105, 110, 137, 156, 160
SJ-22	Hé Liáo	Harmony Bone-Hole	和髎	pg. 109-110, 136, 156, 160
SJ-23	Ěr Mén	Ear Gate	耳門	pg. 105, 109-110, 134-135, 163, 166

The Gallbladder Channel

GB-1	Tóng Zi Liáo	Pupil Bone-Hole	瞳子髎	pg. 105, 111, 134, 141-142, 144-146, 152, 155-156, 158, 160
GB-2	Tīng Huì	Hearing Convergence	聽會	pg. 141-142, 144, 157-158
GB-3	Kè Zhǔ Rén	Guest and Host-Person	客主人	pg. 141-142, 144, 152, 157, 159-161, 163, 177, 407
GB-4	Hàn Yàn	Submandibular Fullness	頷厭	pg. 105, 141-142, 144, 152, 162-165, 177
GB-5	Xuán Lú	Suspended Skull	懸顱	pg. 141-142, 144, 152, 164-166, 177
GB-6	Xuán Lí	Suspended Tuft	懸釐	pg. 105, 141-142, 144, 152, 163, 166-167, 177
GB-7	Qū Bìn	Temporal Hairline Curve	曲鬢	pg. 136, 141-142, 144, 152, 167-169
GB-8	Shuài Gǔ	Valley Lead	率谷	pg. 141-142, 144, 169-170, 377
GB-9	Tiān Chōng	Celestial Surge	天衝	pg. 141-142, 144, 152, 170-171
GB-10	Fú Bái	Floating White	浮白	pg. 141-142, 145, 152, 171-173, 377
GB-11	[Tóu] Qiào Yīn	[Head] Yīn Orifice	竅陰	pg. 141-142, 145, 152, 172-174, 179, 220, 377
GB-12	Wán Gǔ	Completion Bone	完骨	pg. 128-129, 141-143, 145, 152, 169, 172, 174-175
GB-13	Běn Shén	Root Spirit	本神	pg. 142-143, 145, 152, 163, 166, 175-176, 405-406
GB-14	Yáng Bái	Shàoyáng White	陽白	pg. 105, 142-143, 145, 152, 176-178, 231-232, 399, 405-406
GB-15	[Tóu] Lín Qì	[Head] Overlooking Tears	臨泣	pg. 142-143, 145, 152, 178-181, 216, 222, 232, 404-406
GB-16	Mù Chuāng	Eye Window	目窗	pg. 142-143, 145, 152, 180-181, 404, 406, 420

GB-17	Zhèng Yíng	Upright Construction	正營	pg. 142-143, 145, 152, 180-182, 404, 406
GB-18	Chéng Líng	Divine Support	承靈	pg. 142-143, 145, 166, 182-183, 404, 406
GB-19	Nǎo Kōng	Brain Hollow	腦空	pg. 134, 142-143, 145, 162, 166,-167, 183-185, 404, 406
GB-20	Fēng Chí	Wind Pool	風池	pg. 128, 130, 142-143, 145, 152, 176 -177, 179, 184-186 223, 404, 418, 420
GB-21	Jiān Jǐng	Shoulder Well	肩井	pg. 104, 127, 143, 146, 152, 186-188, 364, 404-406
GB-22	Yuān Yè	Armpit Abyss	淵液	pg. 80, 146, 188-189, 192, 231
GB-23	Zhé Jīn	Sinew Seat	輒筋	pg. 80, 146, 152, 189-192
GB-24	Rì Yuè	Sun and Moon	日月	pg. 40, 146-147, 152, 191-193, 231, 398
GB-25	Jīng Mén	Capital Gate	京門	pg. 147, 192-194
GB-26	Dài Mài	Dài Vessel [Point]	帶脈	pg. 147, 152, 194-197, 431-432
GB-27	Wǔ Shū	Pivot of the Five [Zàng-Viscera]	五樞	pg. 147, 152, 195-197, 431
GB-28	Wéi Dào	Yángwéi Path	維道	pg. 147, 152, 195, 198, 431
GB-29	Jū Liáo	Sitting Bone-Hole	居髎	pg. 147, 152, 192, 198-199, 403, 405, 419
GB-30	Huán Tiào	Ring Leaping	環跳	pg. 146-147, 153, 200-201, 403
GB-31	Fēng Shì	Wind Market	風市	pg. 148, 202-203, 224
GB-32	Zhōng Dú	Middle River	中瀆	pg. 148, 153, 203-204
GB-33	Yáng Guān	Yáng Pass	陽關	pg. 148, 204-205
GB-34	Yáng Líng Quán	Yáng Mound Spring	陽陵泉	pg. 148, 154, 204-205, 413
GB-35	Yáng Jiāo	Yáng Intersection	陽交	pg. 148, 153, 206-208, 403, 405

GB-36	Wài Qiū	Outer Hill	外丘	pg. 148, 153, 208-209, 211
GB-37	Guāng Míng	Bright Light	光明	pg. 106, 148, 153, 203, 209-210
GB-38	Yáng Fǔ	Yáng Assistance	陽輔	pg. 148, 153, 208, 210-211, 408
GB-39	Xuán Zhōng	Suspended Goblet	懸鍾	pg. 149-150, 153, 210, 212-214, 408
GB-40	Qiū Xū	Hill Village	丘墟	pg. 148-149, 153, 210, 215-216, 403
GB-41	[Zú] Lín Qì	[Foot] Overlooking Tears	臨泣	pg. 116, 149, 153, 215-217
GB-42	Dì Wǔ Huì	Earth Fivefold Meeting	地五會	pg. 149, 153, 218-219
GB-43	Xiá Xī	Clasped Ravine	俠谿	pg. 149, 153, 215-216, 218-220
GB-44	[Zú] Qiào Yīn	[Foot] Yīn Opening	竅陰	pg. 149, 153, 215, 220-221

The Liver Channel

LR-1	Dà Dūn	Great Mound	大敦	pg. 229, 233, 234-237, 258, 414
LR-2	Xíng Jiān	Moving Between	行間	pg. 229, 237-241
LR-3	Tài Chōng	Supreme Surge	太衝	pg. 218, 229, 240-246, 427
LR-4	Zhōng Fēng	Middle Boundary	中封	pg. 229, 233, 246-248, 251, 269
LR-5	Lí Gōu	Wormwood Canal	蠡溝	pg. 229, 247, 249-251
LR-6	Zhōng Dū	Middle Metropolis	中都	pg. 229, 247, 251-252
LR-7	Xī Guān	Knee Pass	膝關	pg. 229, 252-255
LR-8	Qū Quán	Spring at the Bend	曲泉	pg. 229, 233, 254-257
LR-9	Yīn Bāo	Enveloped Yīn	陰包	pg. 230, 233, 257-258
LR-10	Wǔ Lǐ	Five Lǐ	五里	pg. 230, 252, 258-259
LR-11	Yīn Lián	Yīn Corner	陰廉	pg. 230, 252, 259-262
LR-12	Jí Mài	Urgent Pulse	急脈	pg. 252, 259-262

LR-13	Zhāng Mén	Timber Gate	章門	pg. 146-147, 193, 195, 198-199, 231, 261-264, 306, 403, 431
LR-14	Qī Mén	Arranged Gate	期門	pg. 40, 42, 50, 146-147, 191-192, 231-232, 252, 261, 265-268, 366, 398

The Dū Channel

DU-1	Cháng Qiáng	Long and Strong	長強	pg. 4, 147, 256, 334, 336, 338, 342-346, 353, 391
DU-2	Yāo Shù	Lumbar Transport Point	腰腧	pg. 334, 343, 345-348
DU-3	Yáng Guān	Yáng Pass	陽關	pg. 334, 348-349
DU-4	Mìng Mén	Life Gate	命門	pg. 334, 343, 349-350, 432
DU-5	Xuán Shū	Suspended Pivot	懸樞	pg. 334, 343, 351-352
DU-6	Jǐ Zhōng	Middle of the Spine	脊中	pg. 334, 341, 343, 350-354
DU-7	Zhōng Shū	Central Pivot	中樞	pg. 334, 354, 392
DU-8	Jīn Suō	Sinew Contraction	筋縮	pg. 334, 343, 354-355, 361
DU-9	Zhì Yáng	Arrival at the Yáng	至陽	pg. 334, 343, 355-357
DU-10	Líng Tái	Divine Terrace	靈臺	pg. 334, 357-358
DU-11	Shén Dào	Spirit Path	神道	pg. 334, 343, 357-360
DU-12	Shēn Zhù	Pillar of the Body	身柱	pg. 334, 339, 343, 361-362
DU-13	Táo Dào	Kiln Path	陶道	pg. 334, 339, 343, 362-364
DU-14	Dà Zhuī	Great Vertebra	大椎	pg. 104, 127, 144, 163, 177, 334, 337, 339, 363-367
DU-15	Yǎ Mén	Mute's Gate	啞門	pg. 335, 343, 367-369
DU-16	Fēng Fǔ	Wind Mansion	風府	pg. 130, 184, 335, 340, 350, 360, 362-363, 369-372

DU-17	Nǎo Hù	Brain's Door	腦户	pg. 179, 335, 340-341, 372-373
DU-18	Qiáng Jiān	Unyielding Space	强間	pg. 335, 372-374
DU-19	Hòu Dǐng	Behind the Vertex	後頂	pg. 183, 335, 343, 373-375
DU-20	Bǎi Huì	Hundred Meetings	百會	pg. 181-182, 196, 232, 335, 340-341, 343, 374-379, 386, 392
DU-21	Qián Dǐng	Front of the Vertex	前頂	pg. 181, 335, 343, 376, 379, 383, 392
DU-22	Xìn Huì	Fontanel Meeting	顖會	pg. 181, 335, 344, 379-381, 383
DU-23	Shàng Xīng	Upper Star	上星	pg. 181, 335, 380-383
DU-24	Shén Tíng	Spirit Courtyard	神庭	pg. 142, 176-177, 335, 343, 377, 381-383, 392
DU-25	Sù Liáo	White Bone-Hole	素髎	pg. 335, 383-384
DU-26	Shuǐ Gōu	Water Trough	水溝	pg. 335, 343, 384-387, 418
DU-27	Duì Duān	Edge of the Opening	兌端	pg. 335, 387-388
DU-28	Yín Jiāo	Gum Intersection	齦交	pg. 283, 336, 365, 388-389

The Rèn Channel

REN-1	Huì Yīn	Meeting of the Yīn	會陰	pg. 276, 281, 285-288, 327, 334, 336, 345, 420
REN-2	Qū Gǔ	Curved Bone	曲骨	pg. 230, 252, 281, 285, 288-290, 338
REN-3	Zhōng Jí	Middle Pole	中極	pg. 4, 49, 230, 262, 281, 285, 288-291
REN-4	Guān Yuán	Origin Pass	關元	pg. 4, 51, 230, 252, 262, 281, 284-285, 289, 291-293, 305, 328
REN-5	Shí Mén	Stone Gate	石門	pg. 59, 282, 285, 293-295, 297-298
REN-6	Qì Hǎi	Sea of Qì	氣海	pg. 102, 282, 285, 295-297

REN-7	Yīn Jiāo	Yīn Intersection	陰交	pg. 52, 54, 77, 282, 285, 297-299, 302, 338
REN-8	Shén Què	Spirit Gate Towers	神闕	pg. 55, 282, 285-286 286, 299-301, 311, 327
REN-9	Shuǐ Fēn	Water Divide	水分	pg. 57, 282, 285, 301 -302
REN-10	Xià Wǎn	Lower Duct	下脘	pg. 58-59, 263, 282, 285, 301, 303 -304
REN-11	Jiàn Lǐ	Fortifying the Interior	建里	pg. 61, 282, 285, 303
REN-12	Zhōng Wǎn	Middle Duct	中脘	pg. 62-63, 77, 87, 232, 264, 282, 285, 304-308
REN-13	Shàng Wǎn	Upper Duct	上脘	pg. 282, 285, 305, 308-311
REN-14	Jù Quē	Great Gate Towers	巨闕	pg. 64, 264, 282,286, 308, 311-314, 398
REN-15	Jiū Wěi	Turtledove Tail	鳩尾	pg. 56, 282-283, 286, 288, 311, 314-315, 328, 337
REN-16	Zhōng Tíng	Centre Courtyard	中庭	pg. 66, 283, 286, 316
REN-17	Dàn Zhōng	Chest Centre	膻中	pg. 4, 77, 104, 111, 117-118, 163, 177, 283, 286, 316-317, 357, 364
REN-18	Yù Táng	Jade Hall	玉堂	pg. 283, 286, 317-318
REN-19	Zǐ Gōng	Purple Palace	紫宮	pg. 283, 286, 318-319
REN-20	Huá Gài	Florid Canopy	華蓋	pg. 283, 286, 318-320
REN-21	Xuán Jī	Jade Swivel	璇璣	pg. 71, 283, 286, 319 -321
REN-22	Tiān Tū	Celestial Chimney	天突	pg. 40, 42-43, 134, 283-284, 286, 316, 320-323, 392, 398
REN-23	Lián Quán	Ridge Spring	廉泉	pg. 25, 40, 42-43, 283, 286, 324-325, 398
REN-24	Chéng Jiāng	Sauce Receptacle	承漿	pg. 160, 163, 177, 283, 286, 290, 325 -326, 330

The Lung Channel

LU-1	Zhōng Fǔ	Central Administration	中府	pg. 370, 427
LU-2	Yún Mén	Cloud Gate	雲門	pg. 231
LU-5	Chǐ Zé	Cubit Marsh		pg. 154

The Large Intestine Channel

LI-5	Yáng Xī	Yáng Ravine	陽谿	pg. 97
LI-14	Bì Nào	Flesh of Upper Arm	臂臑	pg. 187, 403, 405
LI-15	Jiān Yú	Head of the Shoulder	五里	pg. 104, 403, 418-419
LI-16	Jù Gǔ	Great Bone	巨骨	pg. 364, 417, 419
LI-19	Hé Liáo	Grain Bone Hole	禾髎	pg. 156
LI-20	Yíng Xiāng	Welcome Fragrance	迎香	pg. 365

The Stomach Channel

ST-1	Chéng Qì	Tear Container	承泣	pg. 283, 418-419
ST-2	Sì Bái	Four Whites	四白	pg. 231
ST-3	Jù Liáo	Great Bone Hole	巨髎	pg. 230, 418-419
ST-4	Dì Cāng	Earth Granary	地倉	pg. 239, 418-419
ST-5	Dà Yíng	Great Reception	大迎	pg. 146, 158, 163, 177. 231
ST-6	Jiá Chē	Jaw Carriage	頰車	pg. 109, 146, 150, 158, 160, 162,-163, 166, 177, 239
ST-7	Xià Guān	Lower Gate	下關	pg. 159, 160, 163, 177
ST-8	Tóu Wéi	Head Corner	頭維	pg. 163, 166, 177
ST-9	Rén Yíng	Human's Reception	人迎	pg. 4, 29, 37, 160, 162, 231, 411, 413, 418
ST-10	Shuǐ Tú	Water Chimney	水突	pg. 187

ST-11	Qì Shè	Qì Abode	氣舍	pg. 187
ST-12	Quē Pén	Empty Basin	缺盆	pg. 29, 37, 104, 127 -129, 143-144, 146, 150, 154-156, 163, 177, 186-188, 190, 211, 284, 364, 370, 404, 411, 413
ST-19	Bù Róng	Not Contained		pg. 40, 231, 266
ST-28	Shuǐ Dào	Waterway	水道	pg. 147, 197
ST-29	Guī Lái	Returning	歸來	pg. 260
ST-30	Qì Chōn	Qì of Chōng Vessel	氣衝	pg. 8, 45-46, 146, 150, 195, 230, 242, 258-259, 262, 425, 427
ST-32	Fú Tù	Crouching Rabbit	伏兔	pg. 154, 190
ST-35	Dú Bí	Calf's Nose	犢鼻	pg. 204, 229, 253
ST-36	Sān Lǐ	Three Lǐ	三里	pg. 187, 264, 306
ST-37	Shàng Lián	Upper Ridge	上廉	pg. 5, 47, 428
ST-39	Xià Lián	Lower Ridge	下廉	pg. 5, 47, 428

The Spleen Channel

SP-1	Yǐn Bái	Hidden White	隱白	pg. 234
SP-4	Gōng Sūn	Grandfather and Grandson	公孫	pg. 90
SP-6	Sān Yīn Jiāo	Three Yīn Intersection	三陰交	pg. 3, 46, 229
SP-12	Chōng Mén	Gate of the Chōng Vessel	衝門	pg. 230
SP-13	Fǔ Shè	Bowel Abode	府舍	pg. 40, 42-43, 50, 230, 266, 397-398
SP-14	Fù Jié	Abdominal Bind	腹結	pg. 40, 230, 397
SP-15	Dà Héng	Great Horizontal Line	大橫	pg. 40, 50, 231, 261, 263, 397-398
SP-16	Fù Āi	Abdominal Loss	腹哀	pg. 40, 50, 192-193, 231, 263, 397 -398

SP-17	Shí Dòu	Food Hole	食竇	pg. 231-232
SP-18	Tiān Xī	Celestial Ravine	天谿	pg. 231
SP-21	Dà Bāo	Great Embracement	大包	pg. 231

The Heart Channel

HE-7	Shén Mén	Spirit Gate	神門	pg. 360

The Small Intestine Channel

SI-10	Nào Shù	Upper Arm Point	臑腧	pg. 404, 406, 419
SI-12	Bǐng Fēng	Grasping the Wind	秉風	pg. 104, 144
SI-14	Jiān Wài Shù	Outer Shoulder Point	肩外腧	pg. 364
SI-15	Jiān Zhōng Shù	Central Shoulder Point	肩中腧	pg. 364
SI-16	Tiān Chuāng	Celestial Window	天窗	pg. 134, 143, 156
SI-17	Tiān Róng	Celestial Countenance	天容	pg. 128-129, 134, 143, 156
SI-18	Quán Liáo	Cheek Bone-Hole	顴髎	pg. 105, 134, 146, 156, 158
SI-19	Tīng Gōng	Auditory Palace	聽宮	pg. 105, 134, 145, 156, 160

The Bladder Channel

BL-1	Jīng Míng	Bright Eyes	晴明	pg. 29, 31, 37, 105, 142, 179, 222, 336, 365, 377, 389, 411, 418
BL-2	Zǎn Zhú	Bamboo Gathering	攢竹	pg. 377
BL-4	Qū Chà	Deviating Turn	曲差	pg. 175-176, 377
BL-5	Wǔ Chǔ	Fifth Place	五處	pg. 181, 377
BL-6	Chéng Guāng	Receiving Light	承光	pg. 181, 377
BL-7	Tōng Tiān	Celestial Communication	通天	pg. 169, 181, 364, 377

BL-8	Luò Què	Declining Network	絡却	pg. 182, 364
BL-9	Yù Zhěn	Jade Pillow	玉枕	pg. 183, 364
BL-10	Tiān Zhù	Celestial Pillar	天柱	pg. 128-129, 143, 364
BL-11	Dà Zhù	Great Shuttle	大杼	pg. 5, 46, 144, 336-337, 370, 428
BL-13	Fèi Shù	Lung Transport	肺腧	pg. 267, 366
BL-15	Xīn Shù	Heart Transport	心腧	pg. 359
BL-16	Dū Shù	Dū Vessel Transport	督腧	pg. 47
BL-17	Gé Shù	Diaphragm Transport	膈腧	pg. 55-56, 355-356
BL-18	Gān Shù	Liver Transport	肝腧	pg. 267, 355, 366
BL-20	Pí Shù	Spleen Transport	脾腧	pg. 353
BL-23	Shèn Shù	Kidney Transport	腎腧	pg. 349
BL-31	Shàng Liáo	Upper Bone-Hole	上髎	pg. 147
BL-33	Zhōng Liáo	Central Bone-Hole	中髎	pg. 147
BL-35	Huì Yáng	Meeting of Yáng	會陽	pg. 334
BL-36	Chéng Fú	Receiving Support	承扶	pg. 107, 201
BL-39	Wěi Yáng	Winding Yáng	委陽	pg. 106-107
BL-40	Wěi Zhōng	Winding Centre	委中	pg. 5, 242, 399, 414
BL-45	Yī Xī	Yī Xī	譩譆	pg. 128-129
BL-54	Zhì Biān	Edge of the Sequence	秩邊	pg. 201
BL-56	Chéng Jīn	Receiving Sinews	承筋	pg. 421
BL-57	Chéng Shān	Receiving Mountain	承山	pg. 249, 408
BL-58	Fēi Yáng	Taking Flight	飛揚	pg. 41, 400
BL-59	Fù Yáng	Yáng Attachment	附陽	pg. 199, 202, 417, 419-420
BL-60	Kūn Lún	Kūnlún Mountains	崑崙	pg. 291
BL-61	Pú Cān	Attending Servant	僕參	pg. 399, 417, 419-420

BL-62	Shēn Mài	Shēn Vessel	申脈	pg. 32, 399, 403, 417, 419-421
BL-63	Jīn Mén	Metal Gate	金門	pg. 399, 403, 405
BL-65	Shù Gǔ	Bundled Bones	束骨	pg. 414

Alphabetical Index

fox-like 233, 313

fracture 115

fright 24, 83, 85, 87-88, 91-92, 112-113, 122, 132, 164, 169-170, 176, 179, 207, 239, 278, 309-310, 312, 315, 343-344, 350, 359, 361, 378-381, 383, 390-391, 393

  fright wind 169, 239, 379, 380, 393

fullness 12, 14, 18, 25, 41, 44, 47-48, 52-53, 56-57, 60-71, 78, 80-82, 90, 92, 95-96, 128, 162-163, 165, 170, 172, 189-190, 207, 209, 213-214, 216-217, 219, 223, 233, 239-240, 249, 255, 258, 261, 264-265, 267, 289, 294, 300, 309, 313-316, 318-320, 353, 357, 362-363, 366, 375, 378, 383, 399, 428, 432

  abdomen 25, 56-57, 64, 249, 255, 289, 353, 432

  chest 18, 63-64, 66-71, 778, 80-82, 92, 95, 128, 172, 189-190, 209, 216, 219, 223, 233, 265, 267, 313, 315-316, 319-320, 357

G

gallbladder 13, 18, 21, 40, 80, 104-106, 109, 111, 116, 127, 129, 139, 141-142, 144, 146, 149-152, 155, 160, 162, 164, 166-167, 169-176, 178-180, 182-186, 188-194, 196-200, 202-210, 212, 214-224, 231-233, 244, 247, 249, 262, 342-343, 364, 377, 398-399, 404-405, 407, 420, 431

Gān-erosion 326, 342, 344

  Gān diseases 344

  Gān of the teeth and gums 389

gasping 31-32

genital itchiness 30-31, 290

ghost evil 87

glomus 239, 267, 303, 313, 366

goitre(s) 125, 171-172, 184-186, 223, 323, 373

gǔ toxin 312

H

haemorrhoids 36, 214, 287, 310, 342-345, 353, 390

hardness 60, 216. 267, 298

headache 10-12, 80-81, 92, 110-114, 124, 133, 135, 150, 156, 164-165, 167, 170, 180-182, 185, 221-222, 267, 293, 315, 350, 359-360, 371, 374-375, 381

heart 69-70, 77-79, 82-87, 89-96, 101, 108, 111, 115, 118-119, 122, 173-175, 183, 211, 213, 217, 221, 230, 237, 240, 245, 256, 262, 264, 267-268, 270, 272, 282, 285, 287, 290, 292, 294, 296-297, 300, 302, 304-305, 307-312, 314-320, 322-323, 325, 328, 336357-360, 366, 368-369, 372, 374, 378, 388-389, 392-393, 397-399, 428

  heart pain 7, 13-14, 18, 22-23, 41, 65, 78, 82-83, 85, 87, 89-92, 96, 118, 217, 240, 245, 265, 296-297, 304, 308, 310, 312, 328, 354, 398-399 See also pain

  heart qì 66, 90, 92, 312, 359

  heartburn 323

heat 7-8, 10-13, 15, 17-18, 20-25, 30, 33-39, 47, 50, 54, 60, 62, 78, 81-84, 87, 90-92, 95-96, 114-115, 133, 150, 165, 167, 170, 173, 183, 191-192, 194-196, 210, 213, 216, 221, 234-325, 237, 241, 257-258, 263, 266-268, 270, 287, 290, 292, 297-298, 306-307, 309-310, 313, 324-326, 330, 344, 347-350, 353, 359-361, 365, 368-370, 372, 381, 387-389 See also damp heat

  generalized heat 165, 183, 309, 361

  in the mouth 7, 24-25

  in the palms 87, 90-92, 96

  on the bottom of the feet 10

  taxation heat 292

  vexation 7, 173, 221, 267, 313

heaviness 14, 30, 117, 126, 136, 183, 187, 196, 391, 399, 432

Hemiplegia 201, 206, 224, 326, 371, 378

humour ix, 19, 60, 84, 111-112, 188, 329

hunger 6, 122, 290-291

hypertonicity 78, 88, 90-91, 199-200, 206, 211, 213, 225, 247-248, 250-251, 270, 272, 285, 298, 348, 350, 366-367, 432

I

impediment 11, 19, 92, 95, 110-111, 121, 124, 156, 171-174, 201-204, 206-208, 211, 213, 217, 221, 224, 253, 298-299, 315, 319-320, 329, 347-348, 350, 399, 407, 412, 420

inability to raise 112, 115, 123, 125-126, 171, 187, 189, 221, 264

  to raise arm 112, 123, 125-126, 186-187, 264

  to raise elbow 110

456

457

257, 262, 265, 267-268, 312-313, 315-321, 323, 325, 353, 357-360, 366, 369, 397
lung connector 320-321
lustre 150, 218

M

malaria 21, 61-62, 80-81, 112-113, 115, 151, 185, 211, 216-217, 239-240, 248, 307, 347-348, 350, 359-360, 362-363, 365-366, 370, 378, 382
    intervallic malaria 80-81, 112, 185, 217, 239, 248, 350, 359, 363-363, 365-366, 378, 382
    See also cold malaria
madness 240
    See also mania
mania 10, 42, 87, 135, 207, 210, 214, 256, 270, 312, 330, 361, 391, 393, 428
    See also madness
menstruation 17, 27, 30-31, 37-38, 52-55, 88, 196, 217, 238, 243, 250, 258, 266, 284, 290, 296, 298, 432
    absence of 27, 37-38
    incessant 238, 298
    inhibited 217
    irregular 17, 30-31, 52-54, 88, 196, 250, 258, 290, 296, 432
mental depression 236, 250
metal 19, 33, 35, 57, 59, 86, 110, 149, 220, 229, 246, 248, 254
    metal point 248
ministerial fire 156, 170, 211, 214, 221, 236, 350
mother 12, 23, 26-27, 32, 34, 38, 42, 114, 220, 240, 254-256, 388
mother point 114, 254, 256
mounting 18, 21, 30, 38, 42, 47, 53, 56, 73, 197, 216, 232-233, 236, 239, 243, 247-250, 252, 255, 263-264, 268-269, 284, 289-290, 292, 294, 296-299, 313-314, 338, 350, 412, 428
    See also cold mounting
    downfall 42, 73, 268-269
    small intestine 243
    slumping 38, 232, 243, 255, 289
    sudden 243, 294
mouth sores 94, 325, 329

N

nape 9, 11-12, 40, 121, 124, 127, 129-130, 134, 143, 150, 163, 168, 171, 173-174, 176, 183, 185, 188, 208, 213, 267, 335-337, 340, 364-369, 371, 374-375, 388
nasal congestion 165, 179, 182, 380-381, 384, 388
near-sightedness 381-382
nightmares 221, 269
no desire to eat 6, 14-15, 110, 122, 167, 295, 313, 325
no pleasure in eating 23, 58, 65, 67-70, 198, 213, 248, 264-265, 270, 303-304, 353
nosebleed 12, 85, 94, 182, 186, 214, 257, 269, 298-299, 302, 369, 380, 384, 388
    See also incessant nosebleed
numbness 11, 224, 248, 270

O

oppression 12, 26, 115, 118, 187, 239, 250-251, 264, 268, 270, 315

P

pain 7-18, 21-25, 27, 29-31, 33, 37-38, 41-43, 44, 47-48, 50, 52-60, 62, 64-67, 69, 72-73, 78-83, 85, 87, 89-94, 96, 104, 108, 111-127, 130, 133, 136, 150-151, 154-156, 161-162, 164, 167-170, 172-174, 176-177, 179-181, 183, 185, 188, 193-194, 196-197, 199-204, 207-211, 213, 215-219, 221, 224, 232, 234-238, 240-241, 243-245, 247-249, 252-258, 260-261, 263-265, 267-268, 270, 272, 284, 287, 28--290, 292, 294, 296-299, 302-304, 306-310, 312-313, 315, 317-319, 323, 327-328, 337-338, 340, 342-343, 346-347, 349-351, 354-356, 361-362, 371, 373, 375, 379-381, 388-389, 391-392, 398-400, 407-408, 412-414, 420-421, 427-428, 432
    in the lumbar spine 24, 261, 263, 343, 355-356, 361-362
    lumbus pain 41, 122, 199, 224, 232, 247-248, 340, 347
    lumbar pain 14-15, 24, 41, 55, 194, 196, 201, 216, 238, 243, 261, 263, 296, 343, 346, 349-350, 355-356, 361-362, 391-392, 399-400, 407-408, 413, 420
    facial 373

T

X

Y

Z

2018

化性談

Discourse on Transforming Inner Nature

By Wang Feng Yi [王鳳儀]

Translated by Hausen and Akers

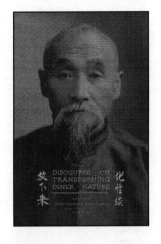

2019

經穴解

Explanations of Channels and Points VOl.1

By Yue Han Zhen [岳含珍]

Translated by Brown and Tsaur

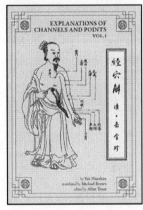

2020

太上感應篇

Tai Shang's Treatise on Action and Response:
A Commentary by Xing De [興德]

Translated by Hausen and Tsaur

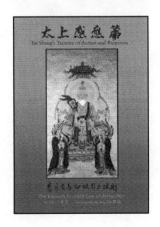

2020

Path of the Spiritual Warrior
Life and Teachings of
Muay Thai Fighter Pedro Solana

By Lindsey Wei

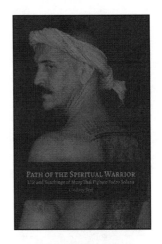

2020

景岳全書
Complete Compendium of Zhang Jingyue Vol 1.-3
By Zhang Jingyue

Translated by Tsaur and Brown

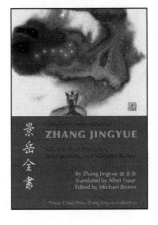

2020

修道四十九关
The 49 Barriers of Cultivating the Dao
By Xing De

Translated by Hausen and Tsaur

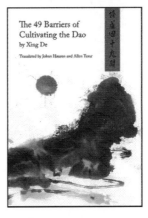

2021

太極拳行法釋要
The Heart Treasure of Taijiquan
By Ren Gang

Translated by Mattias Daly

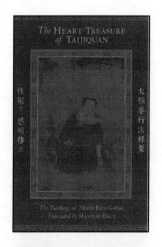

2021

道術
The Arts of Daoism
By Xing De

Translated by Hausen and Tsaur

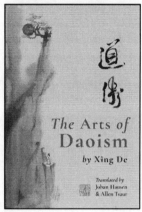

2021 (forthcoming)

蹺脈斠詮
An Archaeology of the Qiao Vessels

By Will Ceurvels

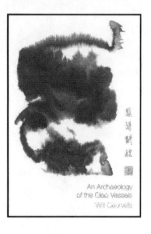

2021 (forthcoming)

周公解夢
The Duke of Zhou's Interpretation of Dreams

Translated by Nikita Bushin

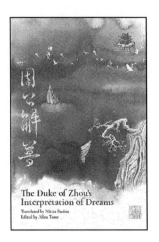

Made in the USA
Middletown, DE
28 April 2024

53579248R00281